Biomaterials

Biomaterials

A Systems Approach to Engineering Concepts

Brian Love

University of Michigan, Ann Arbor, MI, United States

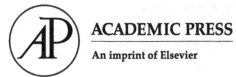

ACADEMIC PRESS

An imprint of Elsevier

Academic Press is an imprint of Elsevier
125 London Wall, London EC2Y 5AS, United Kingdom
525 B Street, Suite 1800, San Diego, CA 92101-4495, United States
50 Hampshire Street, 5th Floor, Cambridge, MA 02139, United States
The Boulevard, Langford Lane, Kidlington, Oxford OX5 1GB, United Kingdom

Notices
Knowledge and best practice in this field are constantly changing. As new research and experience broaden our understanding,
changes in research methods, professional practices, or medical treatment may become necessary.

Practitioners and researchers must always rely on their own experience and knowledge in evaluating and using any
information, methods, compounds, or experiments described herein. In using such information or methods they should be
mindful of their own safety and the safety of others, including parties for whom they have a professional responsibility.

To the fullest extent of the law, neither the Publisher nor the authors, contributors, or editors, assume any liability for any
injury and/or damage to persons or property as a matter of products liability, negligence or otherwise, or from any use or
operation of any methods, products, instructions, or ideas contained in the material herein.

British Library Cataloguing-in-Publication Data
A catalogue record for this book is available from the British Library

Library of Congress Cataloging-in-Publication Data
A catalog record for this book is available from the Library of Congress

ISBN: 978-0-12-809478-5

For Information on all Academic Press publications
visit our website at https://www.elsevier.com/books-and-journals

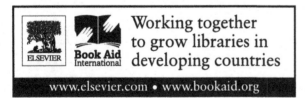

Working together
to grow libraries in
developing countries

www.elsevier.com • www.bookaid.org

Publisher: Matthew Deans
Acquisitions Editor: Laura Overend
Development Editor: Natasha Welford
Senior Project Manager: Priya Kumaraguruparan
Cover Designer: Miles Hitchen

Typeset by MPS Limited, Chennai, India

To Nancy, Francisco, and Benjamin

Contents

Author Bio

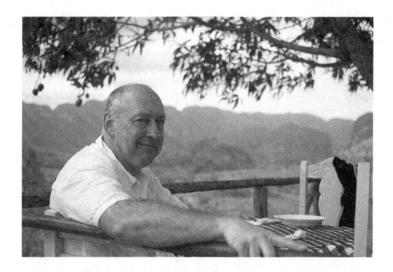

Dr. Brian J. Love is Professor of Materials Science and Engineering, Biomedical Engineering and Dental, and Biologic Materials at the University of Michigan, United States, where he heads a research group which is currently working on Biomaterials and Molecular and Cellular Biomechanics. He has held appointments at Virginia Tech, Wake Forest School for Biomedical Engineering, Georgetown School of Medicine and GIT, as well as working as an engineer for Texas Instruments. He is on the editorial board of two international journals and was on the Dean's list for Teaching Excellence (based on Student perceptions at Virginia Tech): 2004, 2002, 1998, and 1994. In addition, he was nominated for the WL Wine Award for Teaching Excellence in 2007.

Preface

Many believe that it is impossible to write a book relating to materials used in medicine. There are several reasons for this dilemma. Books that emphasize the materials' concepts are founded on volumetric replacement and biological response and less on a mechanical or other analysis of the design environment. The gap is even larger when considering organ function that will require materials integration. Other monographs that are focused on tissue engineering are also hard to gauge, because there is so much detail needed to define a scaffold structure, optimize the culturing environment, identify an implantation protocol, test in appropriate animal models, to establish when and how to assay, and to confirm a successful outcome. It is simply a grand challenge to settle on an optimum strategy to address a specific disease and that could be why tissue engineering has been so much the realm of vibrant research but not as many commercial products. Also depending on the cell source, one may need to consider long-term immune suppression to reduce the risk of host/ graft attack. It is simply hard to compare the promise of a tissue engineered solution with stopgap measures being implemented and optimized as current practice, even if an organic cellular solution is preferred. It is also harder to value new engineering approaches since the marketplace prevents one from disclosing a complete story, lest they give away a competitive corporate advantage. The clinical books are also focused more closely on the aspects of biocompatibility and the subtleties associated with materials, compositional variations, or/and end mechanical function are sometimes lacking. These comments are made not to criticize the discipline but more to establish the landscape. Many of them are excellent sources of information and I have cited them here.

There are many summaries of content in biomaterials that can satisfy the instructor and students of this discipline. For those who desire a textbook option, the choices coincide with what one is more comfortable supplementing. There are monographs and compendia in which often some of the most noted researchers are recruited to offer perspective on their area of expertise. These monographs are often quite deep, but for a senior/graduate class, foundation level materials to support what research reviews are about can be incomplete, and the links between one research topic and another require that all authors are aware of what the other authors are contributing. As a result there are often few examples or problems to consider more deeply.

There are several recent contributions to the discipline in biomaterials that do a more comprehensive job of satisfying the goal of establishing learning objectives in what look more like conventional textbooks. They all have their merits and it is encouraging to see the discipline taking such a wide variance on several conventional textbooks. I applaud the authors of new textbooks in the last several years, as I know that the original ideas go back a long time and it is not an easy process to complete anything like this. I remained committed to my own ideas that were likely formed during the same interval in which these other books have been produced. It is encouraging to see that, for example, there is more attention being placed on nanoparticles as part of enhanced diagnostics and phase contrast fluids; the commitment to include new and distinct areas of biomaterials offers both a distinct pivot in the engineering element of biomaterials and makes teaching biomaterials less of a history lesson.

The book is organized into 15 chapters and is structured as a cumulative presentation with three main themes, but with an understanding that the clinical relevance is distributed where it is sensible to do. The first section (Chapter 1: Cell Biology, Chapter 2: Cell Expression: Proteins and Their Characterization, Chapter 3: Bones and Mineralized Tissues, Chapter 4: Soft Tissues, Chapter 5: Property Assessments of Tissues, and Chapter 6: Environmental Effects on Natural Tissues) assumes that there is some basic understanding of biochemistry focusing not on the nuances of cell physiology, but more on the outcomes that arise in terms of cell expression, protein structure, and attributes to characterize both cells and proteins. These differences are used to justify the need to analyze normal and diseased tissues and fluid extractions focusing on diagnostics and gauging cell and tissue health adjacent to biomaterial installations. It is important to understand that structural proteins such as collagen keratin and silk have different sequences and forms (collagen has many different forms actually), and these are organizationally different than regulatory proteins (immunoglobulins), hormonal proteins (insulin and glucagon), and contractile proteins (actin and myosin) expressed in muscular tissues.

It is also worth noting that subsets of people can have different connective tissue structures, as noted in Chapter 3, Bones and Mineralized Tissues, and Chapter 4, Soft Tissues. It is known, for example, that people with Ehlers Danlos syndrome have hyperelastic skin (statistically different than the normal population) that makes them more flexible, but also at larger risk for aortic dissection and other cardiovascular abnormalities. Within bioengineering, we never explicitly discuss how subsets of people with a different collagen makeup have different clinical outcomes nor are we aware of its specific function for traces of other minute forms of collagen which might serve some crucial role in development. It is appropriate to at least sensitize engineers and scientists that a deeper understanding is needed considering proteins as tissue in the long run. There might be hundreds of similar examples each instructor could give to students and these are simply ice breakers to make students think whether it be for hard or soft tissues.

Chapter 6, Environmental Effects on Natural Tissues, is a perfect example of how a systems approach can be taken to understand disease progression in aging, chronic conditions, and diseases that remain frustratingly insoluble even now. By understanding the disease progression from a systems perspective, there is a chance to understand how to value organic, synthetic, and clinical efforts to manage disease. It can provide some insight why breast tissue self-examinations are a powerful first gauge in understanding the biophysical changes in tumorous tissues among others.

The second section (Chapter 7, Metallic Biomaterials, Chapter 8, Ceramic Biomaterials, Chapter 9, Polymeric Biomaterials, and Chapter 10, Nanomaterials and Phase Contrast Imaging Agents) presents the composition, structure, and performance characteristics of materials commonly accepted and used as biomaterials. Presented here is the engineering content to analyze the structure of these materials, how physical, electrical, and optical properties are measured, how these metals, ceramics, and polymers are produced, how phase determinations are performed, and pointing to opportunities to new materials development.

For example

- how are properties determined (mechanical behavior, yielding, etc.),
- how is it that structure is measured (X-ray diffraction and scattering, microscopy, etc.).

For that matter, dynamic issues such as how are changes in tissue structure (bone density, cataracts) arise in aging of natural tissues; how corrosion, amalgamation, and other chemical reactions that occur in vivo evolve; and how are these measured should be included. The scale of materials from nano to meso can be presented, showing examples where nanoscale matters (phase contrast fluids, drug delivery vehicles, diffusional barriers, etc.). Key science and mathematical content can support the quantitative elements of the course here (modulus and yield point determinations, Braggs Law, Snell's law, calorimetry, gravimetric determinations, etc.).

The final section (Chapters 11: Orthopedics, Chapter 12: Neural Interventions, Chapter 13: Cardiovascular Interventions: The Alliteration of P's Relating to Medicine. Proper Perfusion Prevents Pervasive Procedures Proffered to Improve Cardiovascular Health, Chapter 14: Artificial Organs, and Chapter 15: Special Topics: Assays Applied to Both Health and Sports) is a medical subdiscipline by subdiscipline area assessment that helps to define current issues being experienced by clinics now and for the immediate future. The main takeaway and the major crux of this book are focused on the fact that while tissue engineering might be the long-term future for medical engineering professionals and clinicians, graduating engineers and incoming medical professionals need to be much more aware of the current state of the art in a range of disciplines using materials as replacement tissues, organs, and repairs. Again, this book is more about the value of competitive technological interventions and clinical procedures that are used today and likely to be further optimized. This book is an empowering treatise that gives credit to how clinicians can design their own solutions based on their own problem solving skills. As an example, tissue engineering could be used to produce heart valves to fix compromised valves that are calcified but clinicians and medical engineers and scientists need to understand how clinicians fix defective valves today through their deployment of sutures, threads, annuloplasty rings, and scalpels. The theme is that graduating engineers who are taught a more objective view of the field of medical intervention need to have a stronger understanding of how medicine is practiced now in the clinic on their terms and using their language.

Five chapters in the final section is inadequate and I view only that the chapters are meant to expose students on how to view the subdisciplines. Clearly, more chapters tied to other clinical subdisciplines could be presented and it is possible to include supplemental content electronically if there is a desire. Other sub-disciplines could include ophthalmology and sensory augmentation, artificial skin and dermatological intervention, and drug delivery in comprehensive treatment, among others.

For more information about the book, please visit https://www.elsevier.com/books-and-journals/book-companion/9780128094785.

Acknowledgments

I would like to acknowledge the support and encouragement of colleagues and students at Virginia Polytechnic Institute and State University, Virginia Commonwealth University, Wake Forest University, and the University of Michigan, where I have been a faculty member in the academic enterprise. There are literally too many people to acknowledge along the way, but I would like to thank Tony Atala and Ed Damiano who provided example photographs that are included and useful insights linked with their own development activities. I would also like to acknowledge Kim Forsten-Williams who helped in scoping the original content with me. I would like to thank students who have taken my biomaterials and "skin as an engineering model system" classes as they have evolved. It was through teaching these, and interacting with the students that I learned along the way. Included among students who took an interest in the content were Mike Fischer, Graham Bilbey, and Quan Zhou and it was through our discussions that further refinements and calibrations were made. I'm indebted to Alexa Peltier who took cartoon drawings from me and made them respectable. Thanks everyone for your help and encouragement along the way.

I want to thank all of the students and post-docs who have worked in my research group over my academic career. My group has been smaller as a result of my attention to this book over the years while this has been written, and I am hoping that as I put the construction of this textbook to rest, I can commit more time to the research enterprise and new questions that remain unresolved and highlighted here. It would be fun to work on those in the future.

I want to thank my editorial team at Elsevier including Zara Preston, and most notably, Laura Overend who oversaw the original project concept evolve into a textbook proposal and Natasha Welford who has helped to focus on the final stages of the editorial development process which was both tedious and involved, especially for a nonmulti-tasker like me. I want to also acknowledge Priya Kumaraguruparan who guided me through the proof stage and Swapna Praveen who helped organize copyright approvals. I want to thank and formally acknowledge authors of other published materials who have been cited here and who have granted permission for me to use their figures and tables. The field is so large, the book is incomplete and unless I aimed for a 2000 page book, it will remain so.

Finally, I want to thank my friends and family who have kept me mostly sane through this whole process. The completion of this enterprise is a testimonial to the perseverance of setting a goal and trying to accomplish it. There have been late nights and early mornings dedicated to completing this and I am indebted to my wife Nancy who provided keen insights and a fresh perspective, and our sons Francisco and Ben who have helped in their own ways to allow me to finish this. I feel like a younger man being able to see the world through their eyes. I am pretty sure this monograph did not get done any faster as a result of our larger family, but it is sweeter to see that there is a brighter light at the end of this tunnel now. Finally thanks to the readers who have taken the time to go along for this ride as well.

CHAPTER 1

Cell Biology

Learning Objectives

By reading this chapter, the reader should be able to

1. Recognize the various naming conventions for cells including functions, tissues from which they are derived, morphological features, and what they ultimately produce as proteins.
2. Describe features and subunits of typical eukaryotic cells which include mitochondria, the nucleus, the cytosol, the lipid membrane, and other structural features that are tied to the cytoskeleton and to the glycocalyx.
3. Understand functions of cells, which include cell division, protein expression, extracellular sensing and communicating within the environment, assembly into larger tissue constructs, and cell death, whether by apoptosis, cell rupture, or some other mechanism.
4. Recognize cell types contained within blood, tissues, and organs.

1.1 Introduction

The genesis of living matter is regulated and organized by cellular production, encoded by different genetic sequences by cells in the presence of local tissues and fluids. There are a number of different classifications for cells in terms of their shape, function, location, and origin and these differences are noted in terms of their activities. The goal here is not necessarily to create a stand-alone cell biology textbook within this treatise. Other books are both more comprehensive and objectively, just better. There are some exemplary images and micrographs to represent detailed structural features of different cell types, organelles, and ensembles thereof. The goal here is to classify cells based on their attributes, functions, and influences sufficiently for bioengineers, and other interested scientists and engineers who have a working knowledge that is useful. A second goal is for readers to have sufficient background so that they can effectively communicate with collaborating life scientists using a more common language. Here the focus is also to identify both morphological features and chemical characteristics of normal eukaryotic cells, followed by a broader description of cellular physiology including the mechanics of cellular function.

Biomaterials. DOI: http://dx.doi.org/10.1016/B978-0-12-809478-5.00001-8

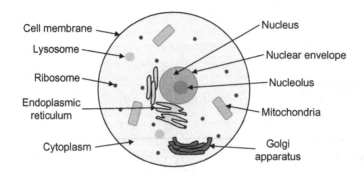

Figure 1.1
Schematic of the average eukaryotic cell showing mitochondria and other organelles contained within the cell membrane.

1.2 Cell Composition and Make-Up

Normal eukaryotic cells are highly organized and regulated structures and are shown schematically in Fig. 1.1. Eukaryotic (mammalian) cells are distinguished by a lipid bilayer that separates them from their environment. They contain a series of organelles (machinery) to drive cellular function. One such organelle is the nucleus that houses the genetic encoding (DNA, chromatin) and is contained by a separate lipid membrane isolating the DNA from the other organelles contained by the larger cell membrane. Examples of organelle machinery include the mitochondria that convert stored chemical energy channeled through adenosine triphosphate (ATP) into useable energy for cellular function, the endoplasmic reticulum (ER) that is involved in protein synthesis, and the Golgi apparatus that is involved in sorting and protein separations. Each distinct region is partitioned as a separate entity and identified as a different spatial location of the cell through microscopy. The cytosol makes up the fluid fractions of the cell outside of these functional domains with the proteins shuttled from one domain to the next as part of the production cycle. Also contained with the cell are filamentous proteins that compose the cytoskeleton. As a result, the cell has a mechanical structure with mechanical properties such as stiffness and recovery due to the equilibrium structure of the cytoskeleton. Pushing on a cell takes force to sustain the compression and cell retraction results upon unloading from the perturbed state. Contained both inside and outside of the cell and bound to the lipid bilayer are the so-called *receptor* molecules. Receptor proteins protrude either into the ECM or into the cell and are used to probe the external environment, communicate with neighboring cells, and respond through what is called receptor-binding links to trigger specific physiologic consequences.

1.2.1 The Nucleus

The nucleus of a cell is also bound by an internal lipid bilayer that separates the genetic encoding sequences (transcription) from the rest of the cytoplasm, as shown in Fig. 1.2.

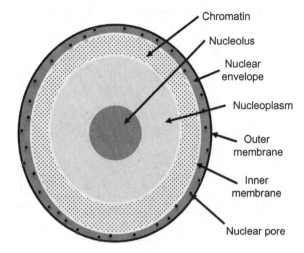

Figure 1.2

Structure of the nucleus in 2D. Note that the chromatin, uncoiled DNA occupies the space within the nuclear envelope. The nucleolus is found somewhere near the center of the nucleus. Pores are often found in the nuclear membrane that allow for trafficking of proteins between the nucleus and the cytoplasm.

The nucleus is often the largest and most easily identifiable organelle in a cell. Functions within the nucleus include controlling gene expression and mediating the replication of DNA during the cell cycle. Mutations in cellular DNA that lead to protein defects and the failure to control DNA replication usually trigger either apoptotic cell death during the normal cellular function or the formation of a cancer cell that grows in an uncontrolled fashion into a larger tumor mass.

1.2.2 The Endoplasmic Reticulum, ER

The ER houses a network of cisternae (sac-like structures) fixtured and shaped by the cytoskeleton, as shown in Fig. 1.3. A lipid bilayer isolates the cisternal space (or lumen) from the fluid region of the cell identified as the cytosol. The ER is involved in protein synthesis as the ribosomes are contained within a morphologically distinct region called the rough ER. The specific role of each ER is cell dependent, as not all cells produce proteins that are commonly transported (exocytosed) out of the cell. The ER ultimately sorts proteins that are conveyed out of the ER usually through a series of vesicles, lipid bilayers surrounding the secreted proteins. Ultimately, proteins are internally digested, internally sequestered, routed to the cell membrane, or exocytosed outside of the cell.

Protein folding occurs in the ER that is regulated by amino acid sequencing, the local charge, the presence of chaperone molecules to control local charge and ionic strength to

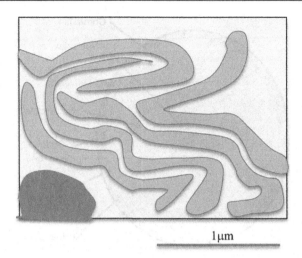

1μm

Figure 1.3
Schematic of endoplasmic reticulum (ER) in 2D: The rough ER possesses ribosomes
on its solid surfaces and newly formed proteins are conveyed in the interstices of the ER
to the Golgi apparatus. The gaps between solid surfaces of the ER are on the order
of 10s to 100s of nanometers.

drive the appropriate conformational shape. Defects linked with protein synthesis (primary amino acid structure) and folding (tertiary and quaternary structure) are often conveyed for digestion, while correct shapes are expressed appropriately. Inappropriately folded or amyloid protein structures that are expressed are the current focus of a range of age-related diseases called amyloid diseases including Alzheimer's disease, Parkinson's disease, Huntington's disease, and a host of tissue amyloidosis related diseases that are often encountered in the last hours of life [1].

1.2.3 Mitochondria

Mitochondria drive energy conversion in cells due to their production of ATP, used as a primary cellular source of chemical energy, as shown conceptually in Fig. 1.4. Individual cells can have multiple mitochondria which are also involved in a range of other cellular functions associated with the cell cycle, cell signaling, and apoptosis.

1.2.4 The Golgi Apparatus

The Golgi apparatus is an organelle downstream from the ER. Vesicles containing proteins are fused to the input region of the Golgi that causes the vesicle to break down and helps to convey the now liberated proteins into the entering lumen of the Golgi, as shown in Figs. 1.5 and 1.6. Once separated from the vesicles, many proteins are grafted with

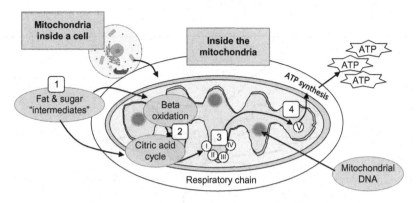

Figure 1.4

Conceptual picture of mitochondria and function. Carbohydrates and fatty acids are ultimately converted to adenosine triphosphate, ATP, through a process called oxidative phosphorylation. The source material is drawn from the cytosol (1) and undergoes a conversion first to acetyl coenzyme A (2) and then followed by a series of oxidative complexes (3) ultimately leading to ATP conversion in (4).

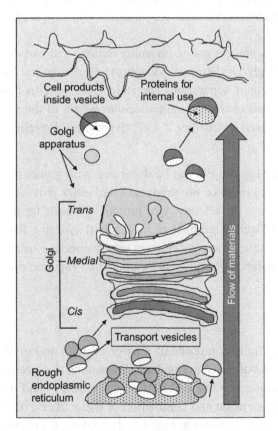

Figure 1.5

Proteins leaving the trans Golgi complex are either marked for internal use and consumption, recycled within the Golgi or conveyed in vesicles that facilitate transport into the cytosol destined for secretion as either growth factors, antibodies, cytokines, or some other expressed secretion.

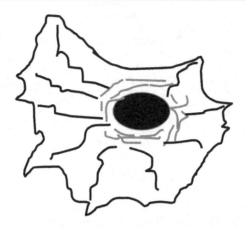

Figure 1.6
A schematic of the structural fiber make up within a moving cell. The microtubules shown in *blue* (grey in print version), actin and myosin filaments that interact to form intermediate filaments (shown in black), and other structural elements like lamellapodia that are stretched as the cell membrane also undergoes displacement or spreading.

hydrophilic phosphates (a process called phosphorylation) and carboxylic acids (glycosylation). Specific glycosylation or phosphorylation steps are kinds of labeling exercises that facilitate protein separations and to redirect proteins destined for different fates. There is often a small change in the molecular weight of the protein as a result of the grafting, which are discussed in Chapter 2, Cell Expression: Proteins and Their Characterization.

Other proteins synthesized in the ER can be decorated with glycosaminoglycans (GAGs) synthesized in the Golgi to produce proteoglycans and other polysaccharides. It is these labeling events that increase the selectivity of protein synthesis for a desired function. It is amazing to consider how well assemblies of these small systemic functions effectively work in concert to produce proteins that can organize into connective tissue, and how under homeostasis, there is a balance of inputs and outputs that regulate normal function.

1.2.5 Cell Structure

The cytoskeleton is essentially composed of a range of actin and myosin filaments, microtubules, and other tubules of intermediate dimensions that are expressed to reinforce the cell membrane structure, regulate cell movement (motility) and intracellular membrane protein transport by the extension and contraction of these fibers. An example schematic of the fibrous interior of a cell is shown in Fig. 1.6. The interaction between actin and myosin fibrils allows a cell to alter its shape including the formation of microvilli, lamellipodia, and filopodia; form contractile bundles; and enhance cell mitosis by restructuring the two cell surfaces from the one larger one. A great reference on cell structure is found in Chapter 11 of Ref. [2]. It is also the displacement of these fibers that enhances extracellular signaling and modulations in cell receptor interactions can also induce structural rearrangements of the cytoskeleton that can regulate cell gene activity and function as well.

1.2.6 The Membrane Structure: Phospholipids

The lipid membrane is composed of phospholipids, derived from glycerol. Two fatty acid substitutions are made on glycerol to form hydrophobic tails and to the center "ol" function is attached a hydrophilic phosphate group, as shown in Fig. 1.7. In solution, the tails and heads have sufficient mobility to reorganize (self-assemble) into lipid bilayers or vesicles in which the hydrophilic groups are pointed outward from the cell membrane, and the hydrophobic tails intermix among themselves, as shown in Fig. 1.8 to form the cytoskeleton [2]. The inner side is also hydrophilic by default. This resulting lipid bilayer structure is both stable and a relatively effective permeation barrier with a dimension on the order of 5−10 nm in thickness. The lipid membranes (nuclear and cellular) are organized such that the environments within the nucleus and within the cell are effectively isolated from the environments outside of the membrane. As a result, different chemistry can occur within the cell that would not be as well controlled as it is within each contained membrane region. While the membranes are effective barriers, they have their limits as stretching the membrane too far can cause the membrane to rupture, and proteins and ions contained in the cell can be released outside of the cell through various channels and pores. Also contained within the lipid bilayer are molecules that decorate the surface of the cell

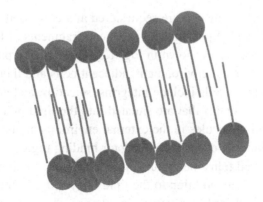

Figure 1.7
An example of a section of the phospholipid cell and nuclear membrane boundary. Lipid-rich legs extend from a hydrophilic phosphate function leading to an amphiphilic structure. Ensembles of these amphiphiles self-organize yielding a membrane barrier that can create hydrophilic environment both inside and outside of the cell.

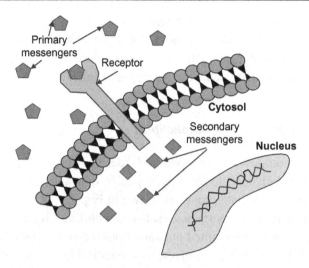

Figure 1.8

Pictures of model receptors: In this case, a transmembane protein extends from the lipid bilayer
presenting a tertiary/quaternary structure that surveys the local environment. Molecules
or proteins that interact with the protein can allow this cell to sense its external environment
without allowing transport across the membrane. Receptors can traverse the entire membrane
or not, depending on their molecular weight.

membrane either on the inside or outside of the cell which are used for communication.
The proteins that protrude through the lipid layer are called receptors.

1.2.7 Receptors

Some proteins synthesized by the cell are sequestered and expressed on its surface. These
bound molecules have phospholipid linkages that keep fragments of the proteins jutting out
into the cytoplasm. An example is shown in Fig. 1.8. These bound protein molecules are
available to sample the chemical environment, adjacent cells and their receptors, viruses,
etc. Examples of receptors on cells include integrins, selectins, and cadherins, which are
classes of transmembrane proteins that are situated into the lipid bilayer. Chemical reactions
that ensue between ligand molecules in the external environment and the bound proteins are
called receptor–ligand binding events, and receptor binding regulates cellular function,
particularly for the so-called trans-membrane proteins which contain extracellular and
intracellular protein linkages in addition to the lipid bilayer. Receptor binding is often
considered as kind of a "lock and key" effect; in other words, if the right ligands are
present in the environment and available to initiate receptor binding, this can set off a
cascade of conformational changes in the protein that can alter protein structure within the
cell, and can change cell function and protein production [3]. The specificity of receptor
binding is regulated often by the conformation of the extracellular membrane protein,

Table 1.1: Examples of receptors, ligands, and cells where these receptors are commonly found.

Receptor	Ligand	Cell Type(s)	Reference
Insulin receptor (IR)	Insulin	Adipocytes, myocytes	[4]
Fibronectin	Fibronectin	Fibroblasts	[5]
Fc_ε	Immunoglobulin E (IgE)	Basophiles	[6]
Interleukin 2	Interleukin 2	T lymphocyte cells	[7]
P2 type receptors	ATP	Epithelial cells, neural cells	[8]
Epidermal Growth Factor (EGF) receptor	EGF	Presented in overabundance in cancerous cells	[9]

and some receptors are more selective than others. Some examples of typical receptor/ligand linkages and the cell types to which they are found are included in Table 1.1.

As an example integrins are composed of two fragments, the so-called α and β fragments, that are coupled so that one integrin ($\alpha_6\beta_5$) targets one set of ligands. Other integrins composed of different combination of fragments are selective to some other series of ligands. It is possible to conserve one fragment (e.g., α_6) but still have a different ligand affinity due to the different β fragments. It is these decorations on the cell surfaces that regulate cellular communication and sensing with the extracellular environment. One can consider antibody–antigen interactions also as mediated by receptor binding.

The types of receptors include those like transmembrane receptors, channel-like receptors that create pores in the membrane, enzyme-based receptors activated by enzymes, G-coupled protein receptors where a signal activation outside the cell creates a signaling response within the cell, and intracellular receptors that upon direct interaction with a chemical cue, triggers a response. The action of the receptor binding to various chemistries is shown in Fig. 1.9.

Receptor binding is at the core of modern biotechnology as both drug discovery and tissue engineering are based on creating a more comprehensive understanding of cellular response ex vivo that can be translated into in vivo therapies without abusing surrounding cells not targeted for a response. Complications in regulating cell receptor binding relate to how fast therapies take hold and how permanent these induced changes remain. In other words, the answer to the question of how large of a dose is needed and for how long to induce cell apoptosis in a particular cancer cell requires an adequate understanding of the uptake rate and metabolism of a chemotherapeutic drug. Targeting receptors that interact with a fast kinetics of association might lead to therapies that require less persistence, thereby reducing the dose required to treat an oncology patient.

Receptor–ligand binding forms the basis of cell adhesion both between the same type receptor on different cells called homotypic binding and different receptors on different

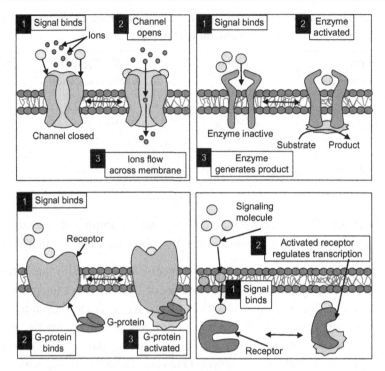

Figure 1.9

Receptor binding examples showing receptors activated through channel-like linkages (top left), through enzyme linkages, through G-protein coupling (bottom left), and through intracellular signaling (bottom right).

cells called heterotypic binding. Receptor binding can also be mediated by soluble catalysts that facilitate binding through an intermediate species. Calcium and zinc ions are potent intermediate facilitators of binding through receptors called cadherins. Ligand binding can also occur with receptors on surfaces of the extracellular matrix or other foreign bodies. A single cell expresses many different cell adhesion molecules, targeted for creating multiple binding efficiency.

Erythrocytes (red blood cells, RBCs) are decorated primarily with selectins and possess relatively weak interactions with other cell types. Erythrocytes exposed to shear often tumble where they bind and decouple to vascular wall surfaces with significant regularity. It suggests that a sufficient residence time with cells expressing selectins may be needed to form a stronger interaction. Clearly the presence of the selectins slows those interacting cells as they encounter the luminal wall of the cardiovascular network. Leukocytes (white blood cells) often express more integrins, and with a variety of α and β fragments, these cells can target a variety of foreign bodies that are presenting other ligands. Cadherins are transmembrane receptors that usually undergo heterotypic binding with another protein receptor called catenin, mediated by the presence of calcium ions.

How are these receptors manifested though and how fast are these extracellular connections made? There are models that describe the kinetics of binding and association, and they are likely influenced by temperature, pH, and ionic concentration [3]. Some receptors are only capable of linking with one type of ligand yielding significant selectivity while others have several possible ligands that can bind lowering selectivity. Ligand binding can trigger intracellular conformational rearrangements that can alter protein expression or cell function. Functionally, ligand binding and its impact on cytoskeletal reorganization as receptors toggle between a bound and unbound state is the mechanism by which a cell can react to external chemistry by altering its physiology and expression.

So the average eukaryotic cell possesses organelles, a membrane, a cytoskeleton, receptors, etc. Cells range on order of approximately 10 μm in diameter, with erythrocytes being slightly smaller and platelets much smaller than average. A lot more time is required for characterizing cellular response since there are clear differences in what specific cells are tasked to perform. Better ways are needed of distinguishing between different cells, which are collected from different locations, have different shapes and morphologies, and produce different proteins. The focus here is to classify cells extracted from different structures which should help to organize the terminology in terms of cellular production and morphology, key considerations that engineers and scientists might be more familiar with.

1.3 Cell Classifications

1.3.1 Stem Cells

There is much interest and focus on regenerative medicine applied to identifying, isolating, and ultimately characterizing the response of less-differentiated cells that maintain more regenerative capacity. Stem cells are identified both in terms of their renewal potential and their differentiation potential. A third discriminator for stem cells is the capacity to repopulate damaged, diseased, or replicated tissues as functional cells following some sort of transplantation procedure, whether by autografting (from the same person) or allografting (between different people).

Stem cells have been discovered in large numbers of different tissues and not all stem cells are the same. Within an adult population's bone marrow, both hematopoietic and mesenchymal stem cells can be isolated. These stem cells are separable by different labeling and isolation strategies, and they can transform into different terminal cell types. Hematopoietic stem cells, also known as universal blood stem cells, are essentially capable of producing all cell types resolved within blood. Other stem cells derived from marrow, called mesenchymal cells, can be directed into connective tissue, neurons, and myocytes, when coerced under the most appropriate culture conditions. It is also possible to extract stem cells from a growing embryo to form the so-called embryonic stem cells that have significant potential to be directed into a variety of terminal cell types.

Stem cells are graded in terms of the degree of differentiation potential available when isolated. As a result, stem cells are like trains on rails, as sufficiently differentiated cells are not capable of redirecting beyond one pathway might be considered as cells on a single track with one destination in mind or *unipotent*. These cells display an asymmetrical mitosis pathway, transforming to yield two daughter cells, a new stem cell and a second cell, committed to differentiate along one pathway yielding a cell with specific shape and functions.

Other, less-differentiated cells are like nodes with multiple pathways and destinations called cell lineages possible, depending on how the local chemistry (signaling molecules, pH, reactive oxygen species, etc.) and receptor binding affects cell differentiation. Depending on the possible pathways available, these cells might be defined as a specific number such as tri-potent (3), or an undetermined number such as pluripotent and multi-potent cells. Stem cells identified from blood remain the best-characterized at this stage, as hematopoietic stem cells isolated from red marrow express specific receptors such as CD34+ and are negative for other receptors such as CD10, CD14, CD15, CD16, CD19, and CD20. An example differentiation tree showing the evolution of a variety of cell types from the human universal stem cell is shown in Fig. 1.10. Other stem cells in different culturing conditions will lead to different terminal cell types.

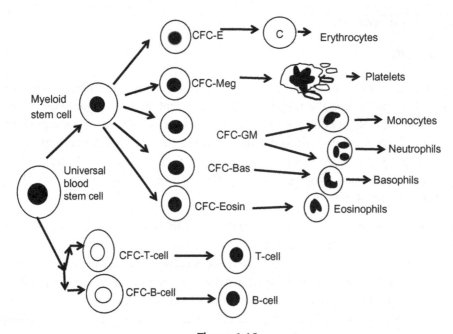

Figure 1.10
Decision tree of how a stem cell is differentiated from other more advanced cell types. *Redrawn from W.M. Saltzman, Tissue Engineering, Principles for the Design of Replacement Organs and Tissues, Oxford University Press, New York, 2004 [10].*

Stem cell isolation can be done by attaching biomarkers possessing antibodies for CD34. The receptor linkages will form a bound species that can be separated by electrophoresis, magnetic separation, centrifuge, etc. Cells that have antigens for these other markers such as CD10 are differentiated in ways that identify them as different from the cells that have the CD34+ receptors on them. There are many monographs focused on stem cell therapy and characterization and it is left to the reader to delve there for more comprehensive descriptions of the revolution in stem cell biology. It is important to note that there exists a wide distribution of localized stem cells within adult tissues and organs that can serve as near perennial sources of regenerative capacity. It is also important to note that finding an appropriate and robust cell type to address a specific disease is a challenge, and the development of the most successful ex vivo culturing conditions for that specific cell type remains a robust area of research support.

1.3.2 Differentiated Cells and Other Classifications

Stem cells that have been directed along a specific differentiation pathway usually proceed beyond a point of no return to form a terminal cell type which has a characteristic shape and structure, performs specific functions like protein synthesis, and lacks the potential to be redirected toward any other cell type. Those cells involved in constructing connective tissue are commonly synthesizing collagens with very subtle differences in primary amino acid sequence that can affect the composition and properties of the final tissues. Those cells forming more connective tissue are called fibroblasts, those involved in bone synthesis are called osteoblasts, and those forming cartilage are called chondrocytes. Osteoblasts are a subset of all bone-related cells classified as osteocytes. As it turns out in bone, bone is an evolving structural system, and those associated with synthesis are the osteoblasts, those involved in reducing less perfect bone stock are called osteoclasts. A key regulation between osteoblasts and osteoclasts yields someone who possesses no net change in bone density with age. One can consider osteoporosis as a regulation problem whereby the osteoclasts are more active than the osteoblasts for whatever reason yielding lower bone density with time.

1.4 Cells Associated With Specific Organs and Systems

Cells are also linked to specific organs from which they are identified. This tends to help in diagnosing and staging disease and identifying affected regions. Thus hepatitis is identified as an infection of hepatocytes in the liver, renal carcinoma as a cancer of epithelial cell lining in the kidney, astrosarcoma as a cancer of astrocytes found in the brain, and melanoma as a cancer of melanocytes, the pigment producing cells also found near the basement membrane in the epidermis. In the cardiovascular system, nonerythrocytes are defined as leukocytes, and a cancer arising from these cells is defined as leukemia. Sometimes designations of mutant cells are more nonspecific, in part since more than one cell type is involved in the larger tumor or disease. In mandibular jawbone cancers, the soft connective tissues associated with the palate are often the site for tumor initiation, but they invade the jaw with tumor growth making it also a bone cancer.

1.4.1 Cells Found in Blood

The universal blood stem cell is at the genesis of all cellular components found within blood. The pathway for the most common cell types found in blood associated with both perfusion and wound healing is regulated by the differentiation of the universal blood stem cells into first a myeloid stem cell, followed by more specific differentiation sequences defined by a colony forming cell (CFC) stage. The determination of differences at this stage leads to specific terminal pathways to form specific cell types found in blood. The most common classifications for blood cells include erythrocytes, platelets, monocytes, and polymorphonuclear (PMN) cells, also called neutrophils, eosinophils, and basophils. Distinctions between these cell types are based on size, morphology, and to some extent, function. Monocytes for example look relatively featureless as single cellular entities but polymorphonuclear cells have several distinct regions that represent partitioned functions in the cell. Since they are observably different, they can be isolated and compared in terms of their cellular activity, but both monocytes and neutrophils are involved in tissue digestion after wounding for example.

1.4.1.1 Platelets

Platelets are the only cell type substantially smaller in size (~ 1 μm) than other cells contained in blood. Nevertheless, platelets are large enough to avoid renal filtration that is based, in part, on pore size. Platelets regulate the coagulation cascade as it is the interaction between platelets and foreign bodies and turbulent flow that triggers their activation which transforms the receptors on their surfaces, and makes their membranes stickier and more likely to undergo a clotting formation, critical for controlling the bleeding response. Platelets normally are benign percolating through the vasculature by cardiac compression to create a pressure pulse to drive fluid flow.

1.4.1.2 Red Blood Cells (RBCs or Erythrocytes)

Erythrocytes are the perfusion workhorses in the cardiovascular system efficiently routing oxygen through hemoglobin binding. One misconception associated with Erythrocytes lack a easily identifiable nucleus like the other, more common eukaryotic cells. Nevertheless, this erythrocyte is a highly differentiated, terminal endpoint for the largest fraction of hematopoietic stem cells created in blood. Nature has optimized the RBC to have more hemoglobin as opposed to a nucleus that allows for more complete blood oxygen carrying capacity. There are known ways to stimulate the differentiation of a larger number of erythrocytes, including the use of drug therapy and steroids such as erythropoietin (EPO) to recruit more differentiation along this pathway. For cancer patients undergoing therapy who are easily fatigued, the presence of these stimulants can restore vitality by directing more stem cells to adopt the erythrocyte terminal pathway. Used in a healthy population, one can find oneself with a much larger fraction of RBCs than is physiologically normal. One could imagine the value of EPO among elite athletes who can harness these advantages into physiological differences and performance enhancements (see Chapter 15: Special Topics: Assays Applied to Both Health and Sports). Refinements in blood testing methods to determine what is a normal and a deviant cell count in both athletes and nonathletes would be useful in leveling the playing field.

1.4.1.3 White Blood Cells: Monocytes and Neutrophils

The demolition team associated with wound healing and recovery include the monocytes and PMN cells or neutrophils. These cells are identified earlier in the differentiation pathway and distinguished from those committed to forming erythrocytes. Monocytes and neutrophils compose the largest numbers of cells within the white blood cell or leukocyte system. These cells are also resident in blood and are recruited in larger numbers near a wound site requiring deconstruction. Neutrophils commonly are found first and rupture near these sites releasing their contents that include enzymes, amino acids, and reactive oxygen species. Neutrophils tend to lower pH as the released proteases yield more individual amino acids from the digested proteins. A schematic showing the co-mingled erythrocytes, monocytes, and platelets is shown in Fig. 1.11.

It is also these leukocytes that are expressed around implantation sites in an often-failed attempt to degrade these foreign bodies. Grafts made with hydrocarbons like polypropylene and polyethylene have no natural enzymatic interaction and are inert to the subsequent plume of metabolic agents released by monocytes and neutrophils.

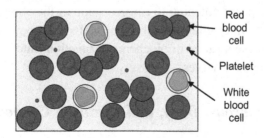

Figure 1.11
A conceptual representation of white and red blood cells colocated with smaller platelets found in the cell fraction found in blood. The RBCs are on the order of 6–8 μm in diameter, the leukocytes can be incrementally larger.

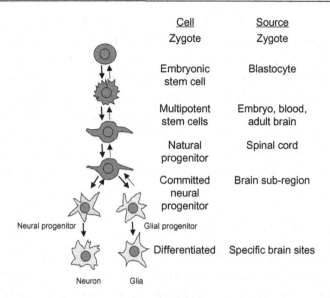

Cell	Source
Zygote	Zygote
Embryonic stem cell	Blastocyte
Multipotent stem cells	Embryo, blood, adult brain
Natural progenitor	Spinal cord
Committed neural progenitor	Brain sub-region
Differentiated	Specific brain sites

Figure 1.12

Map showing the classes of different cell types in the progression of the neurons formed in the system. *Redrawn from F.H. Gage, Mammalian neural stem cells, Science 287 (2000) 1433—1438 [14].*

1.5 Cells Found with the Nervous System

Neural stem cells have been identified from cerebrospinal fluid and from brain extracts from euthanized animals. These cells have shown the capacity to differentiate into both neuronal and glial cell types, as shown in Fig. 1.12. Since neuronal stem cells can be injected, they can adapt to the local microenvironment to be directed to their terminal pathway. As a result, there is hope that new neuronal stem cell development can displace lost function either by damage or by disease, which makes this an exciting time. It would be even more exciting if stem cells derived from one location had sufficient pluripotency that they could be reintroduced to replicate neuronal function. Repopulating functional neurons would have significant potential to reverse some of the complications of older age-accelerated dementia. Other glial cell sub-types include astrocytes due to their star shaped morphology and have a range of biochemical functions and Schwann cells that form the myelin sheath in peripheral nerves.

1.6 Cells Found in Fibrous, Bony, and Cartilage Connective Tissues

Thus, by bone marrow extraction, it is relatively easy to obtain a large number of potential bone marrow mesenchymal stem cells. By the proper selection of differentiation medium, these cells, once isolated, can be nudged to differentiate into fibroblastic, chondrocytic, adipocytic, or osteogenic pathways. These cells can be further subclassified among these broad classifications of connective tissue. Common differentiation medium formulations known to trigger more osteogenic response in cells include leptin which also tends to inhibit adipocyte response [11], while cartilaginous cells are commonly identified cocultured with transforming growth factor β [12]. Coculturing with insulin can coerce the stem cells to adopt the adipocytic pathway [13].

1.7 Reclassifying Cells Based on Organ Function and Physiology

1.7.1 Endothelial Vs Urothelial Cells

Certain specialized subsets of cells, rather than directed to generalized connective tissue such as bone or dermis, are directed toward organ development, with highly specialized functions associated with each organ types. For example, blood vessels contain several layers of cells organized as sheaths, as shown conceptually in Fig. 1.13. Blood interacts with the innermost cell lining called the intima that is linked with endothelial cells that are stretched and bound by tight junctions that strongly bind adjacent cells together. The inner region where blood flows is called the lumen. With inflammation, these tight junctions of the endothelial layer swell and break apart to some extent allowing migrating monocytes and PMN cells found in blood to both attach to these weakened areas and force their way out of the vascular network and into adjacent connective tissues, critical to part of the wound healing response. Adjacent to the endothelial cell layer are smooth muscle cells (myocytes) that allow for the pulsatile flow to create a resilient mechanical structure. And beyond the myocytes is fibrous tissue with connective tissue fibroblasts buried with the elastin and collagen matrix dispensed by these cells. Each cell type has its function, the endothelial cells to camouflage the tissue from a platelet activation response, the myocytes to create a rapid resilience in pulsatile flow and the fibrous tissue for broader mechanical strength and stiffness.

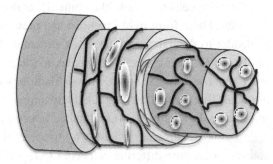

Figure 1.13

A representation of a blood vessel as a series of sheathes or tunics. The innermost layer (on the right) is the endothelial layer which form tight junctions between them. Intermediate sheathes consist of myocytes that give the blood its resilience. The outer region of a blood vessel consists of connective tissue and the fibroblasts cells that produce it on the outer layers of each vessel.

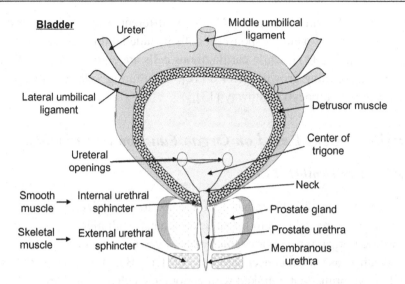

Figure 1.14
An example representation of the bladder and its relevant connections
from the kidneys to the urethra.

There are many other tissue-specific cells. For example along the excretory organs such as the ureter and the in the bladder, there are also endothelial cells which perform a similar function to line the wall of the ureter and bladder as the endothelial cells do in the bloodstream. These cells are alternatively considered as urothelial cells to distinguish the type of cell function (outermost layering of cells to contact the fluids) and their location. This example is shown in Fig. 1.14. There are many more examples.

In connective tissues, there are layers of cells that are often cogrown together, such as in skin, and other organs. The bladder is a simple example of an organ with a layered cellular morphology. In the bladder, there are cells that look like epithelial cells that line the inside of the bladder called urothelial cells. These form tight junctions and prevent the permeation of urine contained within the bladder to the interior of the tissue structure. The structural integrity of the bladder derives from the smooth muscle cells that make up the bulk of the bladder cross-section. One cannot construct a viable artificial organ without finding ways to incorporate both cell types as you need them both. But the bladder is a relatively simple organ as its designed function is to hold fluid and to signal to the brain when the bag is nearing capacity. The simplicity of the bladder's design is an attractive feature why tissue engineering has focused on its development and the ability to coculture differing cell types to replicate this tissue.

1.7.2 Metabolic Cells Found in the Pancreas

Digestive organs used in metabolism also contain functional cells that are tasked with specific functions such as expressing and releasing enzymes and proteins. In the pancreas, there is a functional release from relevant biomolecules, expressed from α and β cells described as islet cells or islets. Thus the pancreas secretes insulin after consuming sugars; the islet cells in the normally functioning pancreas can quickly respond by expressing insulin as needed. As the world population of diabetics rises, it will be necessary to harness how new islet cells can be regenerated or repopulated in these people who, for whatever reason, are incapable of producing insulin as part of the body's regulatory cycle. What a remarkable contribution this would be to medicine if pancreatic function could be restored effectively in a cellular therapy in a wider array of affected people.

1.7.3 Metabolic Cells Found in the Liver

Higher order organs active in metabolism secrete regulatory enzymes and proteins that are part of normal human physiology that lead to metabolic problems without proper cell function. The liver is an example of a highly perfused organ that is involved in breaking down foodstuffs. Hepatocytes, as islets within the liver, deliver a host of protein-byproducts and enzymes that are extremely useful for subsequent digestion. Components expressed by liver include bile that is critical for further food digestion; glycerol and other fatty acids are converted by liver output into glucose and ATP. Enzymes produced by hepatocytes reduce blood alcohol levels, and the other dietary proteins are reduced to their amino acid constituents by the presence of proteases also produced in the liver. When the liver is damaged by overexposure to toxins, or by bacterial colonization leading to inflammation broadly identified as hepatitis, the capacity for further regulatory management can be permanently compromised.

1.7.4 Sentry Cells

In Section 1.3, it was discussed that the T and B cells can be created by hematopoietic stem cells from universal blood stem cells. T and B cells are ultimately produced in the thymus and bone marrow, respectively, that are distributed within the lymphatic system and tissues as part of the acquired immune system and are often mentioned as lymphocytes. These cells are encoded with antibodies from prior bacterial and viral infections. When a patient is subsequently re-exposed, the infection is noted from the presence of an antibody—antigen interaction with T and B cells now encoded to look for a specific antigen. The immune system senses these insults faster in an attempt to ward off more comprehensive infection. We hear most about these cells when patients have low T or B cell counts either innately or through immunosuppressant therapies (e.g., transplant patients). As a result, these patients are at greater risk of infection due to their T-cell and B-cell deficiency and raise the chances of transmitting diseases to others.

Sentry T and B cells are often found within the lymph system also tracking within dermis. The presence of sensory cells found within dermal tissue is really at the origin of immunology and skin sensitivity tests as allergists make use of T- and B-cell response in skin to evaluate the size of a response to various antigens. In prior days, immunologists would expose a patient and observe responses within a series of days to evaluate the relative allergic sensitivity to typical antigens like pollen, nuts, and grains. Positive responses are really an indicator that the lymph system is overreacting to the antigens present during an immunological screening.

Skin has other types of cells and has its own regenerative capacity. The outer layer of skin contains the basement membrane that contains a layer of keratinocytes that regenerate and push away older cells away from the hydrolyzed membrane. New keratinocytes are formed through mitosis at the basement membrane, followed by an extrusion process as the cells age as there are no nerves of blood vessels external to the basement membrane. The proportion of solid intracellular protein, keratin, increases as these cells are separated from the membrane and they ultimately transform their cytoskeleton from oval-shaped cells containing a nucleus near the basement to a much flatter, pancake-like layer that is difficult to resolve the nucleus within aged cells called corneocytes. The removal of the corneocytes as they dehydrate and flake off is what we think of exfoliation. Thus keratinocytes can take a range of forms and shapes over the life of an individual cell. The mutation of cells at the basement membrane is the basis for diseases such as basal cell and squamous cell carcinoma that are distinguished based on cell shape. Closely associated with these superficial cancers are the much more serious malignant melanomas which are cancers of the adjacent melanocytes, which permeate much deeper and normally produce the pigment protein, melanin. Melanocytes are already closer to the bloodstream innately, and as such, metastasis is facilitated compared to carcinomas.

1.8 Observation of Cell Size and Morphology: Microscopy

Cells have structure and they undergo normal physiology expression as a result of appropriate cues. Proteins are produced that are harnessed by the cells in forming their cytoskeleton, and expressed in the production of larger tissues. From building block cells, cues are introduced that trigger alternative differentiation pathways that lead to different terminal cell types. It is useful to also consider how we observe structure and physiology in living cells.

There are many ways to analyze the structure and morphology of eukaryotic cells. Various microscopic tools commonly observe the phase structure of cells, in part to distinguish between different cell types, but also to observe differences in cytoskeletal structure. The most common microscopic tools are primarily based on optical microscopy, UV fluorescence microscopy, and confocal microscopy. More detailed probing of surface structure, surface interactions, and adsorption and contact mechanics are tied more closely to evaluations of mechanical interactions of cells and surfaces.

The elucidation of cell structure can be done simply, for example observing differences in nuclear structures between PMN cells (neutrophils) as opposed to monocytes can be resolved with optical microscopy at relatively low magnification with appropriate stains to identify the nuclear membranes. More detailed substructural detail using alternative stains and contrast agents can illuminate specific regions differently depending on the binding of the stains.

Cells can either be analyzed in an isolated condition for example in cell culture, or as part of a tissue biopsy extraction. Usually, tissue samples from biopsies are potted in wax or some other hardening encapsulant, from which specimens can be later sliced by a microtome into thin sections $\sim 10\ \mu m$ thick for later microscopy. Detailed pictures of the basement membrane of epidermis are readily resolvable. Eosin is a common nuclear stain to help identify both the nucleus and the nuclear transformation that arises due to exfoliation.

A limitation with fluorescence microscopy is that photobleaching can lead to lower fluorescence emission as continued imaging of the same specimen. This makes it more difficult to resolve protein architecture with subsequent reanalyses. Fluorescence imaging is still a very common tool in histology and the development of more robust staining procedures and imaging modalities remains at the forefront of newer diagnostic analysis.

1.9 Bacterial Cell Types

We are not made up just of eukaryotic cells. We are also continuously being exposed to bacteria some of which are probiotic like those found in the gut for example aid in digestion. Others are clearly pathogenic leading to the development of biofilms and a range of infections to which antibiotics are routinely prescribed. Bacteria constitute a separate class of living cells capable of invading mammals. Bacteria are distinguishable from eukaryotic cells in that there is no obvious membrane-bound organelle structure and no nucleus identifiable. There are whole books in microbiology focused on the functional anatomy and physiology of different species of bacteria, their interactions with host species, and under what conditions they are eradicated, etc. Some examples of significant bacterial diseases include cholera, leprosy, anthrax, and tuberculosis. There have been quantitative efforts in cellular biology to provide estimates of the number of eukaryotic and prokaryotic cells, the ratio of which has commonly been cited as large as 10/1 bacteria/eukaryotic [15]. Recent refinements and better estimates tend to suggest that there are approximately 40 trillion bacteria (4×10^{13}) dominated by those found in the colon [16]. Comparisons of human cells suggest that they are dominated by erythrocytes and when one considers that there is 5 L of blood, common estimates suggest that there are approximately 30 trillion human cells. Thus there are a comparable number of eukaryote cells and prokaryotic cells found in humans [16]. The awareness about increasing microbial resistance to antibiotic therapy has raised the interest in researching other biochemical pathways that can eradicate various infections. Nevertheless, it is important to note that not all bacteria are pathogenic requiring intervention.

In terms of pathogens, during flu season, there is an endless amount of throat culturing ongoing to determine the presence of infectious bacteria. The presence of bacteria usually triggers the proscription of antibiotic regimens to fight the infection. Patients with cystic fibrosis are particularly at risk for continued proliferation of bacterial biofilms expressed by pathogenic bacteria. Most common bacterial colonization arises with *Pseudomonas aeruginosa* that can eventually lead to sufficient scarring of the lungs requiring transplants if one cannot clear the infection. Significant bacterial colonization occurs on all mammalian surfaces though including enamel that is the genesis of dental caries. The primary pathogen of Streptococcus on enamel is *Streptococcus mutans* that consumes polysaccharides and expresses organic acids that can etch enamel if they continue to proliferate. Differences in the affinity for natural tissue to colonize bacteria could include differences in skin pH and hydration and differences in cleansing habits. While we think of bacteria as problematic, there are some probiotic bacteria that are enhancing our own viability.

1.10 Conclusions

Presented here is a description of cells defined based on function, location, expression, size and morphology, and distinguishing between eukaryotic and prokaryotic cell types. The content in this chapter presented solely so that there is a larger working knowledge sufficient to understand the rest of the book. There are substantially larger and more comprehensive treatments in the details on their descriptions. But functionally, engineers and scientists, not primarily educated in biochemistry or molecular biology, need an appreciation of the distinctions between various cell types, their exquisite interplay as functional synthesis and communication centers, and their transformations in both normal physiology and disease. While the cell plays a controlling interest and is clearly linked to viability, these functional centers are often embedded in the byproducts of cell expression. It is those polymerized amino acids transcribed and replicated in the cellular environment to express proteins that make the framework of the human skeleton, skin, organ boundaries, the vascular network, etc. With an understanding of at least basic distinctions between cell types, subsequent chapters will focus on proteins as material and tissue (see Chapter 2: Cell Expression: Proteins and Their Characterization), the structure of hard and soft tissues (see Chapter 3: Bones and Mineralized Tissues and Chapter 4: Connective and Soft Tissues), the means to evaluate tissues and structures (see Chapter 5: Property Assessments of Tissues) and aging-related effects on these structures (see Chapter 6: Environmental Effects on Natural Tissues).

1.11 Problems

1. Familiarize yourself with typical cellular dimensions for erythrocytes, fibroblasts, and monocytes. Explain why we often do not see scale bars on micrographs of cell structure.

2. Explain why RBCs and keratinocytes are described as eukaryotic cells, but often lack well-defined organelles such as the nucleus.

3. An overactive immune system is an indication of overly sensitive T and B cells that are responding to antigens presented within the bloodstream. Explain how pharmaceuticals regulate the cellular response in someone with intolerable allergies?

4. There are cord blood banks that have evolved to store umbilical cord blood from birth. Explain why might cord blood have value as a source of cells later in life?

5. Skin exfoliation is a critical step in regulating the balance between eukaryotic cells and prokaryotic cells. Explain how exfoliation affects bound airborne bacteria and aging keratinocytes?

References

[1] I. Cherny, E. Gazil, Amyloids: not only pathological agents but also ordered nanomaterials, Angew. Chem. Int. 47 (2008) 4062−4069.

[2] G.M. Cooper, The Cell, A Molecular Approach, ASM Press, Washington DC, 1997.

[3] D.A. Lauffenberger, J.J. Linderman, Receptors, Oxford University Press, New York, 1993.

[4] E.W. Lipkin, D.C. Teller, C. de Haen, Kinetics of insulin binding to rat white fat cells at 15°C, J. Biol. Chem. 261 (1986) 1702−1711.

[5] S.K. Akiyama, K.M. Yamada, The interaction between plasma fibrinogen with fibroblastic cells in suspension, J. Biol. Chem. 260 (1985) 4492−4500.

[6] J.J. Pruzansky, R. Patterson, Binding constants of IgE receptors on human blood basophiles for IgE, Immunology 58 (1986) 257−262.

[7] K.A. Smith, Interleukin 2: inception, impact, and implications, Science 240 (1988) 1169−1176.

[8] E.M. Schweibert, A. Zsembery, Extracellular ATP as a signaling molecule for epithelial cells, Biochim. Biophys. Acta—Biomembr. 1615 (2003) 7−32.

[9] A. Wells, EGF receptor, Int. J. Biochem. Cell Biol. 31 (1999) 637−643.

[10] W.M. Saltzman, Tissue Engineering, Principles for the Design of Replacement Organs and Tissues, Oxford University Press, New York, 2004.

[11] T. Thomas, F. Gori, S. Khosla, M.D. Jensen, B. Burguera, B.L. Riggs, Leptin acts on human marrow stromal cells to enhance differentiation to osteoblasts and to inhibit differentiation to adipocytes, Endocrinology 140 (1999) 1630−1638.

[12] C. Cicione, E. Muinos-Lopez, T. Hermida-Gomez, I. Fuentes-Boquete, S. Diaz-Prado, F.J. Blanco, Alternative protocols to induce chondrogenic differentiation: transforming growth factor-beta superfamily, Cell Tissue Bank. 16 (2015) 195−207.

[13] F.M. Gregoire, C.M. Smas, H.S. Sul, Understanding adipocyte differentiation, Physiol. Rev. 78 (1998) 783–809.

[14] F.H. Gage, Mammalian neural stem cells, Science 287 (2000) 1433–1438.

[15] T. Luckey, Introduction to intestinal microecology, Am. J. Clin. Nutr. 25 (1972) 1292–1294.

[16] R. Sender, S. Fuchs, R. Milo, Revised estimates for the number of human and bacteria cells in the body, PLoS Biol. 14 (2016) e1002533. Available from: http://dx.doi.org/10.1371/journal.pbio.1002533.

CHAPTER 2

Cell Expression: Proteins and Their Characterization

Learning Objectives

From this chapter, the following learning objectives should be achieved:

1. The conceptual difference between template synthesis of proteins as opposed to more conventional polymerization schemes as well as the link to polydispersity.
2. Simple determination of both number average and weight average molecular weight and interpretations of colligative properties.
3. The differences in amino acid make up in example proteins and the means by which proteins can be digested should be understood.
4. A functional understanding of electrophoresis as it relates to chain length, molecular size, and gel mobility.

2.1 Introduction

Proteins are polypeptides synthesized intracellularly within ribosomes and are commonly interpreted as the products of cellular expression including tissues that compose enzymes, growth factors, and connective tissues. Since each ribosome is influenced by conformational hindrance and electronic charge, those features regulate the selectivity to a specific amino acid or acids that can be added to a growing peptide chain. As a result, even in a realm where there are many different potential amino acids to choose from, high degrees of replication are commonly coupled with very narrow molecular weight distribution of the polyamide proteins that are produced. The templates used to synthesize these peptides are commonly replicated with such regularity that even with minor differences in sequences between chains of different protein structures yield very modest differences in protein length and molecular weight on the order or hundreds of Daltons with average molecular weights ranging from 3 to 300 kDa. The syntheses used to produce proteins are interesting from a conceptual comparison to chain growth that occurs through a condensation reaction at very modest conditions, and while the growth rates are likely slow, the sheer volume of cells that can have replicate function is so large that slower growth rates can be tolerated for growing replicated tissues. One can also compare protein synthesis to radical

Biomaterials. DOI: http://dx.doi.org/10.1016/B978-0-12-809478-5.00002-X

polymerization which when controlled usually has a small number of reaction sites and a much wider range of molecular weights distributed within the reaction mixture at the end of the synthesis. In this chapter, a deeper understanding of these distinctions coupled with how chain lengths within polymers and proteins are determined.

2.2 Protein Molecular Weight

If cells were monolithic in terms of their production and expression, the products of cellular expression would also be separate and distinct. But cells are often "lysed" in probing the results of a cell culture experiment. The normal components found in cell culture experiments would also include the eukaryotic cell membranes, receptors, other organelles, and the metabolites from the cell that are separated from what's actually produced. In other words, the proteins composing the cell factory are all part of a wider milieu of proteins colocated within a cell expressing a specific series of functional proteins. If the typical methods of polymer characterization were applied to resolve the molecular weight of a particular cell culture experiment, what one would identify are a series of narrow bands of proteins all with a generally specific molecular weights, and our common techniques to measure weight average and number average molecular weight could be applied. But perhaps other separation processes might yield more important and relevant information about individual proteins, their structure, and length. Protein separation is commonly performed using techniques like gel permeation chromatography (GPC) and electrophoresis in which separation is based on the ability of these protein molecules to percolate through beads or a porous gel structure. By capturing and separating elution fractions as a function of time, it is possible to isolate the individual proteins in different exudates.

Fundamentally, normal characterization applied to typical polymers produced by either conventional radical or condensation polymerization of even a single monomer yields a broad molecular weight distribution shown schematically in Fig. 2.1. The ability to distinguish between attributes like the weight and number average molecular weights is a key to understanding the breadth of the molecular weight distribution function, and the ratio of weight average molecular weight to number average molecular weight is linked with the breadth of the distribution function.

The average of a mixture of chains of varying length can be taken by either weighting it either based on the number of chains or the weight fraction of each chain length. The so-called number average molecular weight, M_n, is a quotient of sums following

$$M_n = \frac{\sum\limits_{i=1}^{\infty} n_i M_i}{\sum\limits_{i=1}^{\infty} n_i} \tag{2.1}$$

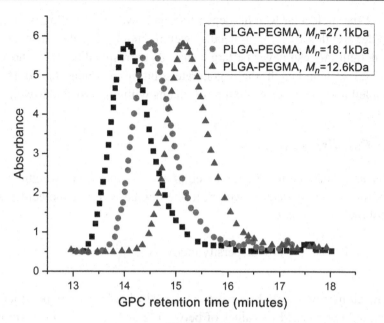

Figure 2.1
Example output of gel permeation chromatography on a Polylactic-glycolic acid/polyethylene glycol dimethacrylate copolymer solution as a function of the molecular weight [1]. The higher molecular weight polymers are too large to encounter the interstices of the gel and percolate through the gel faster.

where n corresponds to the number of chains of a characteristic molar mass, M. Thus we are simply generating a sum for the mass of the mixture of chains in the numerator and a sum of the number of molecules making up this mixture in the denominator.

We could also just as easily consider isolating the chains into groups of varying chain length, but rather than counting them we could assign mass fractions to each chain length. With that, we could assign an average identified as the weight average molecular weight which is a sum of product of the mass fractions and the molecular weight of each fraction divided by a sum of the mass fractions which is simply the mass of the total mixture of chains, highlighted in the following equation:

$$M_w = \frac{\sum\limits_{i=1}^{\infty} w_i M_i}{\sum\limits_{i=1}^{\infty} w_i} = \frac{\sum\limits_{i=1}^{\infty} n_i (M_i)^2}{\sum\limits_{i=1}^{\infty} n_i M_i} \tag{2.2}$$

Recognizing that the mass of the mixture is equal to the numerator of Eq. (2.1), on a weight basis, the weight average molecular weight, M_w, gives a higher weighting to the longer chain lengths in the mixture, and thus the same mixture of chains can yield two different interpretations of the molecular weight, depending on how the weighting is done. M_n is called a first-order weighting on the molecular weight and M_w is called a second-order weighting. By default, M_n can never be larger than its corresponding M_w. And when all chains have the same chain length, the degenerate solution in which M_n and M_w are equivalent is called a monodisperse mixture of chains with one molecular weight.

2.3 Protein Polydispersity

The relative disparity between number and weight average molecular weights is found as a ratio of the weight average molecular weight to the number average molecular weight, shown in the following equation:

$$\text{Polydispersity Index, PI} = \frac{M_w}{M_n} \qquad (2.3)$$

Proteins have much narrower polydispersities than radical polymerized polymers. Typical radical polymerized resins yield PI values of between 2 and 4, and specific anionic polymerization methods can yield polydispersities ranging as low as 1.05. Proteins, as a comparison, are templated from a fixed length of chain of messenger RNA, which regulates the protein chain length that strongly reduces the variability of the protein molecular weight. If postprocessing yields proteins that exist in solution in both a phosphorylated and an unphosphorylated form, the two different combinations will have slightly different molecular weights which are resolved as a more polydisperse mixture than if only one form existed. Picture two different fractions of a specific protein, one with a chain molecular weight of 65 kDa and a second, basically the same protein now phosphorylated on one end of the chain with a M_w of 65.1 kDa. The relative PI values are likely very close to 1, even more monodisperse than anionic polymerized resins. Functionally, these are two different proteins, one phosphorylated and one not and possess likely two different activities.

Conceptually, proteins and protein mixtures lysed from cells are better perceived as a formulated mixture of nearly monodisperse peptides rather than a broad distribution for normal polymers, with a molecular weight distribution function representative of what is seen in Fig. 2.2. After staining proteins and allowing for separation by electrophoresis, distinct lines are usually observed relating to the distance traveled under controlled voltage with smaller proteins moving more easily than larger ones. Around each monodisperse line is a small amount dispersion to account for the fact that in each spot of the template messenger RNA, it's possible that more than one amino acid can be attached to specific linkages in the protein chain.

As an example, separations data on cytoplasmic extracts of a murine embryonic fibroblast cell is presented in Fig. 2.3 [2]. The tool for separation is gel electrophoresis.

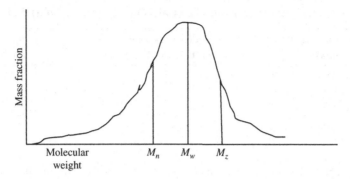

Figure 2.2
Molecular weight distribution for a heterogeneous polymer mixture.

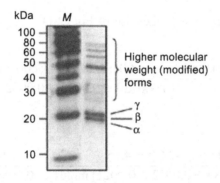

Figure 2.3
Electrophoresis gel separations data on the protein 4E-BP1, showing the separation of unphosphorylated from other grafted versions of 4E-BP1. *From A. Elia, C. Constantinou, M.J. Clemens, Effects of protein phosphorylation on ubiquitination and stability of the translational inhibitor protein 4E-BP1, Oncogene 27 (2008) 811−822.*

The relevant takeaway is that analyzing the cytoplasmic extract identifies three subtly different forms (α, β, and γ) of the translational inhibition protein, 4E-BP1. Molecular weight markers are run as a separate channel and indicate that all three forms of 4E-BP1 are found to have similar chain lengths, but that the α form is not phosphorylated and has a larger migration velocity than its other posttranslated forms, probably because it is smaller [3]. The α line is very faint; the β and γ lines are brighter. As a thought exercise, assume that the brightness of each line corresponds to the number of molecules tagged. For this example, the following data from this figure is available and summarized in Table 2.1.

- Based on a basis of 100 g of protein

Table 2.1: Data extracted from Elia et al., Oncogene 27 (2008) 811−822

Protein	Molecular Weight (kDa)	% of Fluorescent Tag Based on Line Brightness	# of 4E-BP1 Molecules* (Moles)
α 4E-BP1	19.0	15	7.89×10^{-4}
β 4E-BP1	19.6	42.5	2.2×10^{-3}
γ 4E-BP1	20.3	42.5	2.1×10^{-3}

Assuming a mass basis of 100 grams of protein that is ultimately analyzed.

Focusing on only the forms of 4E-BP1, if the goal is to resolve the number and weight average molecular weights of these mixtures, then assume a basis of 100 g of 4E-BP1. 15% of it is a, 42.5% of it is b, and the rest is c. To resolve the number of molecules in this basis, one needs to take the weight fractions of the fluorescent tags and divide that fraction by the assigned molecular weight of the fraction based on the molecular weight markers.

To solve for M_n of the mixture, one makes use of Eq. (2.1):

$$M_n = \frac{\sum_{i=1}^{\infty} n_i M_i}{\sum_{i=1}^{\infty} n_i} = \frac{0.000789*19,000 + 0.0022*19,600 + 0.0021*20,300}{(0.000789 + 0.0022 + 0.00021)\text{moles}}$$

$$M_n = \frac{\sum_{i=1}^{\infty} n_i M_i}{\sum_{i=1}^{\infty} n_i} = \frac{15\,\text{g} + 42.5\,\text{g} + 42.5\,\text{g}}{(0.000789 + 0.0022 + 0.0021)\,\text{moles}} = \frac{100\,\text{g}}{0.00508\,\text{moles}} = 19.68 \text{ kDa}$$

The determination of the weight average molecular weight, M_w, follows from Eq. (2.2):

$$M_w = \frac{\sum_{i=1}^{\infty} w_i M_i}{\sum_{i=1}^{\infty} w_i} = \frac{15\,\text{g}*19\,\text{kDa} + 42.5\,\text{g}*19.5\,\text{kDa} + 42.5\,\text{g}*20.3\,\text{kDa}}{15\,\text{g} + 42.5\,\text{g} + 42.5\,\text{g}}$$

$$M_w = \frac{285 + 833 + 862.75\,\text{g} - \text{kDa}}{15\,\text{g} + 42.5\,\text{g} + 42.5\,\text{g}} = \frac{1980.75\,\text{g} - \text{kDa}}{100\,\text{g}} = 19.8\,\text{kDa}$$

The ratio of M_w/M_n yields the PI, and for a mixture of three different variants of 4E-BP1, which is very narrow as a distribution. Note that there are higher molecular weight bands shown in Fig. 2.3 which are attributed to higher-order and crosslinked forms of 4E-BP1. This example shows how to use Eqs. (2.1)−(2.3), and when applied to proteins, the distribution function for soluble protein in solution looks more like a series of distinct polymers with fixed and narrow molecular weight distributions as opposed to one broad molecular weight distribution, as might be observed by Fig. 2.2. The very small difference in molecular weight between M_n and M_w suggests that these are very narrow molecular weight distributions, more common for proteins than for polymers.

It is possible that certain ribosome usually adds a proline peptide however it is only selective in excluding all but proline, glycine, or arginine. The difference in those individual amino acids is very small, but when hundreds of amino acids are linked together in a chain, some net number of substitutions yields a small level of dispersion in the molecular weight of the chain for peptides that have the correct amino acid chain length but variations in primary amino acid structure and composition. There might be an amino acid molecular weight difference of 10s to 100s of Daltons of variation if substitutions are possible. The ribosome is still attaching an amino acid, which could affect the secondary and higher-order structure of the protein, but the molecular weight would not be the ideal attribute to probe these changes.

Another influential factor affecting the molecular weight of a peptide is linked to the presence of other chemical moieties that are often enzymatically grafted onto the primary or side chain structure of the peptide. Example grafting procedures include phosphorylation, carboxylation, and amidazation which all can happen innately. The presence of a phosphorylated species also adds molecular weight to an otherwise native protein and can clearly affect its chemical potential, its tertiary and its quaternary structure in solution.

2.4 Biochemical Determination of Molecular Weight

Protein biochemists have separately developed the tools to effectively perform separations and resolved what proteins are contained within a specific cell culture through the combined use of electrophoresis and fluorescence marking of proteins. Electrophoresis is a separation tool similar to size exclusion chromatography with the driving force regulated by charge instead of pressure. The schematic associated with electrophoresis is included in Fig. 2.4. The gel used for the separations is actually composed of two resins of different molecular architecture. The actual separations are conducted using a "separating" gel, which has a relatively high molecular weight and is a fairly impermeable gel. Usually there is a lower molecular weight gel called a "stacking" gel used to allow easy percolation of the proteins to the boundary between the stacking and separating gels under low bias conditions. The number of individual experiments that can be conducted during each biasing of the electrophoresis unit is regulated by the number of fingers of the comb used to create gaps in the stacking gel as well as the quality of the gels that tend to deteriorate near the edges of each plate. Once each prong of the finger is removed, post-gelation, the small gap can be injected to initiate a subsequent electrophoresis experiment.

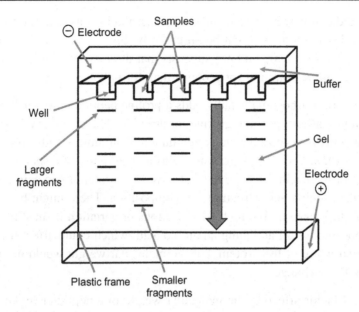

Figure 2.4
Schematic of electrophoresis unit [4]. Gel plates are made with cavities into which protein solutions can be added. Usually the gel is a two-stage gel with a stacking gel of weak separation potential, and a separating gel which is stiffer and more difficult to penetrate. When directly biased, negatively charged proteins are driven from the top fingers through the gel to the cathode, with smaller proteins having a higher drift velocity under the same bias conditions.

Electrophoresis is usually fractionated such that multiple experiments are conducted on one plate allowing a visual comparison of different cell culture experiments. Most separations are done with acrylamide gels of varying molecular weight and resin density. Biasing the reservoirs creates a positive charge at the bottom of the gel electrophoresis unit that attracts the negatively charged peptide solutions and drives proteins to percolate through the gel. Allowing for adequate time and power density to trigger separation, proteins separate by molecular weight, with the smallest proteins moving the farthest to the cathode during each electrophoresis experiment. If proteins are fluorescently tagged before electrophoresis, they will easily be identified as lines when imaged under a fluorescence reader linked with the movement of specific proteins with their own molecular weight and size.

Protein marker standards exist for calibration that contain ∼10 different proteins all fluorescently tagged with different colors. When electrophoretically separated, the gel is stained by 8−10 differently colored lines with each protein marker location being linked with a different molecular weight. Adequate separation is usually the gold standard. One can run the electrophoresis too short (not enough separation based on molecular weight) or too long (where the proteins all traverse the length of the channel again not yielding

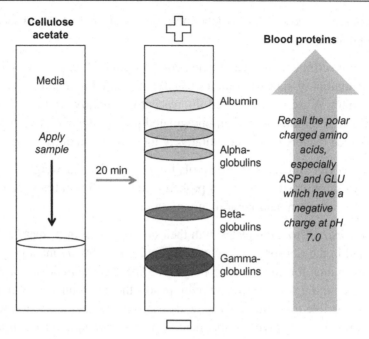

Separating serum proteins by electrophoresis

Figure 2.5
Albumin, being the lowest molecular weight protein commonly found in blood, has the highest drift velocity under bias conditions. Other soluble proteins includes α (thyroxine and retinol), β (*transferring*), and γ globulins. Other proteins are less inseparable with electrophoresis due to their insolubility and instability [5].

separation). A typical electrophoresis response is seen (Fig 2.5) on the serum (noncellular) component of blood.

The breadth of each line is linked with minor quality variations in the gel and differences in protein molecular weight. Subtle amounts of phosphorylation might yield the presence of a double line, one closely associated with the native protein and a second line nearby for the native protein with the phosphorylated graft. Interferences arise when multiple proteins have the same molecular weight, but for comparison studies, not every protein is marked making it easier to resolve subtle differences in cell culture conditions and their effect on cell expression.

When electrophoresis separates the contents of lysed cells, there are many different proteins usually included in the mix. Cellular engineering studies are often designed to show how the presence of minor modifications in culture conditions affects cell physiology, count, and subsequent expression as a function of culture time. If the culture conditions are such that there are differences between one cell culture reservoir and another based on cell expression, that is readily observable by labeling proteins of interest and observing them based on electrophoresis.

The most common electrophoresis experiments compare individual protein isolates in terms of up- or downregulation of specific proteins usually compared to a control protein that is perceived as invariant. A more pronounced fluorescent line relative to the control marker is qualitatively defined as an indicator of an upregulated protein. Quantitative tools based on digitized fluorescence readers do not quantitatively interpret the qualitative patterning.

More commonly, polymer characterization tools to probe molecular weight including light scattering and intrinsic viscosity have been probed using specific proteins including collagen, fibrinogen, albumin, and keratin, among others.

If proteins are synthesized from templates with their configuration of primary amino acid sequence controlled in the ribosome, it becomes difficult to simply define a polymeric repeat structure as is so common for homo- and copolymers. The sheer complexity of 20+ amino acids being organized through the ribosome often makes the determination of a replicated repeat structure impossible to identify. Thus, while chain length and molecular weight are common to both proteins and polymers, the identification of a simple repeat structure is not as clear but the tools to analyze these structures from primary amino acid sequencing are increasingly common. There are some sequences of local ordering commonly present. For example, certain common adhesion linkages are identified by a three amino sequence of arginine glycine and aspartic acid which together links as a trimer sequence denoted as a RGD sequence. It is also common that approximately every third amino acid is a glycine molecule. There are substitutions that are possible within these structures, yielding either functional or nonfunctional defects. The presence of genome maps helps to define templates for replication, but proteomic analysis is the ultimate characterization to determine the resulting protein structure and how variants are added to the subtly different proteins.

2.5 Protein Thermodynamics

With increased perfection in the scheme in which each protein molecule is produced, perhaps there is larger driving force for these molecules to interact or organize in solution. The driving force for a transformation is regulated by the structure of the protein, and the size and relevant protein−solvent interactions when dissolved in solution, which are regulated by the Second Virial Coefficient defined in solution thermodynamics when measuring colligative properties such as osmotic pressure for example which is used in the determination of number average molecular weight, shown in the following equation:

$$\frac{\pi}{RTc} = A_1 + A_2 c + \text{higher-order terms} \tag{2.4}$$

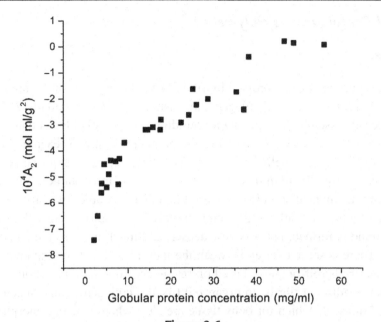

Figure 2.6

Measurement of the second virial coefficient, A_2, a measure of protein–solvent interactions as a function of globular protein concentration. *From V. Bhamidi, S. Varanasi, C.A. Schall, Langmuir 21 (2005) 9044–9050.*

where π is the osmotic pressure of the protein solution relative to the pure solvent, A_i are the virial coefficients, R is the gas constant, T is the absolute temperature, and c is the concentration of protein in solution. The first virial coefficient is the intercept of the line of osmotic pressure/concentration ratio with concentration in the limit of zero concentration and is equal to the inverse of the number average molecular weight of the protein added to the solution. The second virial coefficient corresponds to the slope of the osmotic pressure on this same curve and relates to the strength of polymer solvent interactions [6]. When the second virial coefficient is large and negative, there is a driving force for both protein aggregation and crystallization, both which reduce the surface area over which protein–solvent interactions occur in solution, as is shown in Fig. 2.6 [7,8]. Polypeptides, due to secondary bonding interactions, can be sufficiently attractive to remain in solution, but can also be induced into a crystal or gel state at sufficiently high concentration, or in the presence of triggers for the gel or crystal to form. Practically, concerns about the conditions that trigger protein gelation and crystal formation are of value both in resolving the solid-state phase structure (crystallography) and resolving the phase stability of supersaturated protein solutions relating to shelf life of proteins like insulin.

2.6 Typical Proteinaceous Polymers

2.6.1 Collagen

Connective tissue proteins are expressed by fibroblasts. Among the most important connective tissue proteins include collagen and elastin. Collagen is actually a hierarchically advanced tissue self-assembled from smaller building polypeptide blocks that organize into a series of triple helices. The building blocks are polypeptide strands each and the confirmation of a left-handed helix called α strands. Each strand is approximately 300 nm long and approximately 1.5 nm in diameter, and takes as its most stable form, a helical structure. When three helical strands are twisted together, the other two strands fit within the gaps formed by the first helix and a single molecule of approximately the same length as the single-strand is formed, but it is now denser, and much more stable and called tropocollagen. There is some overlap between the individual fibrils on the ends of tropocollagen as fibrils self-organize based on secondary bonding interactions that allow them to connect to adjacent fibrils. In organized fibrillar collagens, small spacings arise of dimension ∼67 nm wide which for bony tissue are sites where calcium phosphates precipitate to form mineral composites. Mineralization fills those void regions with mineral and helps explain why bony tissue is denser than demineralized proteins.

There are several variants associated with the α form of collagen strands and they are often noted as α1 and α2 or a1 and a2. There are more detailed distinctions that are beyond the scope of our discussion here, but in forming tropocollagen, collection of these varying strands yields subtle differences in terms of the resulting collagen structure. Small variations in the type of collagen are ultimately produced and as a result, there are more than 20 different collagen types that have been identified and natural tissue depending on tissue location and the cell type producing it. The most common forms of collagen are noted as type I, II, III, and IV. Type I collagen is commonly found within skin, tendon, the vasculature, other internal organs and is the main protein constituent in bone. Collagen I is also found within scar tissue. Collagen form I is made up of two α1 helices and one α2 helix as the main protein components that are wound together in forming tropocollagen I. Form II has three similar α1 fibers composing the tropocollagen molecule. Form III forms reticular fibers. Form IV is expressed at the basement membrane. A summary of details relating to collagen forms and structural details is included in Table 2.2

The production of tropocollagen is just one step in a much larger array of self-assembly steps required to compose natural tissue like skin or tendon. It is interesting to note the amino acid composition in different tissues, as a result of the different strands composing them, as noted in Table 2.3. Secondary bond interactions are required to link individual tropocollagen molecules together and there are separate self-assembly steps that are required to direct adjacent tropocollagen molecules into a larger array in the fibrillar

Table 2.2: Structural details and compositional make up of subunits making up collagen

Type	Chain Composition	Structural Details	Localization
I	$[\alpha 1(I)]_2[\alpha(I)]$	300 nm, 67 nm banded fibrils	Skin, tendon, bone, etc.
II	$[\alpha 1(II)]_3$	300 nm, small 67 nm fibrils	Cartilage, vitreous humor
III	$[\alpha 1(III)]_3$	300 nm, small 67 nm fibrils	Skin, muscle, frequently with type I
IV	$[\alpha 1(IV)]_2[\alpha 2(IV)]$	390 nm C-term. globular domain, nonfibrillar	All basal lamina
V	$[\alpha 1(V)][\alpha 2(V)]$ $[\alpha 3(V)]$	390 nm N-term. globular domain, small fibers	Most interstitial tissue, assoc. with type I
VI	$[\alpha 1(VI)][\alpha 2(VI)]$ $[\alpha 3(VI)]$	150 nm, N + C-term. glob domains, microfibrils, 100 nm banded fibrils	Most interstitial tissue, assoc. with type I
VII	$[\alpha 1(VII)]_3$	450 nm, dimer	Epithelia
VIII	$[\alpha 1(VIII)]_3$	?, ?	Some endothelial cells
IX	$[\alpha 1(IX)][\alpha 2(IX)]$ $[\alpha 3(IX)]$	200 nm, N-term. globular domain, bound proteoglycan	Cartilage, assoc. with type II
X	$[\alpha 1(X)]_3$	150 nm, C-term. globular domain	Hypertrophic and mineralizing cartilage
XI	$[\alpha 1(XI)][\alpha 2(XI)]$ $[\alpha 3(XI)]$	300 nm, small fibers	Cartilage
XII	$\alpha 1(XII)$	?, ?	Interacts with types I and III

From M.W. King, The Extracellular Matrix. Available from: <http://themedicalbiochemistrypage.org/extracellularmatrix.html>, 2010 [9].

proteins and ultimately tissues. The individual protein chains can be modified by enzymes including the hydroxylation of lysine and proline residues raising the amount of hydroxyproline in collagen.

Collagen can be reduced by reaction (digestion) with enzymes (called collagenases) to form protein fragments and more comprehensive digestion can reduce the tissue down to its amino acid constituents. These more detailed compositional analyses are commonly performed by liquid chromatography or mass spectrometry or through coupled techniques. Tendon and bone as adapted are shown in Table 2.3 from a couple of different sources [10,11]. For collagen, amino acid compositions have been determined for mammalian collagen in both bone and tendon.

2.6.2 Keratin

Keratins are a separate family of fibrous structural proteins that make up the main constituents of hair, nails, and hooves of other mammals. They are produced within cells identified as keratinocytes that are sequestered to the stratum corneum layer, that outermost, regenerative layer of the skin. Tight junctions form contacts between adjacent keratinocytes which serve to make the basement membrane rather difficult to permeate. Mitosis associated with keratinocytes occurs at the basement membrane and results in the

Table 2.3: Amino acid fractions/100 g of each tissue analyzed after 24 h of hydrolysis

AA Constituent in Collagen	AA Code	Bone (%(a))	Tendon (%(a))	Tendon (%(b))
Alanine	Ala	9.3	9	9
Glycine	Gly	26.2	26.4	35.1
Valine	Val	1.93	2.07	2.3
Leucine	Leu	2.09	2.12	1.3
Isoleucine	Ile	1.09	0.91	1.3
Proline	Pro	10.1	10.3	12.3
Phenylalanine	Phe	1.15	1.15	1.4
Tyrosine	Tyr	0.36	0.3	0.5
Serine	Ser	2.94	3	2.8
Threonine	Thr	1.5	1.51	1.9
Cysteine	Cys	~	~	~
Methionine	Met	0.43	0.47	0.6
Arginine	Arg	15.4	16	4.3
Histidine	His	1.41	1.31	0.3
Lysine	Lys	4.59	3.51	3.6
Aspartic Acid	Asp	3.84	3.94	4.7
Glutamic Acid	Glu	5.9	5.9	7.4
Amide		3.06	3.59	
Hydroxyproline	Hyp	8.2	7.5	9
Hydroxylysine	Hyl	0.58	1.45	N/A

Data from (a) J.E. Eastoe, The amino acid composition of mammalian collagen and gelatin, Biochem. J. 61 (1955) 589–600 and (b) C.H. Brown, Structural Materials in Animals, 1975, Pitman, London.

displacement of existing cells being pushed farther from it. Thus, the older the keratinocyte, the farther it is from the basement membrane and the more dehydrated it gets. Keratinocytes transform as part of this dehydration process as the mass fraction of insoluble keratin protein composing the cell continues to rise as a function of this aging process. The cells transform their shape, flatten and rupture looking nothing like the cells originally formed within the stratum corneum layer. The scrubbing action associated with using a loofah sponge in the shower or scratching the skin is a sufficient abrasive process to exfoliate these aged and transformed keratinocytes. The sloughing is removing both old cells, oils, and keratin protein in the process. While formed as a eukaryotic cell with a well-defined nucleus, as these keratinocytes age, the identification of a nucleus becomes more difficult. It is hard to call them eukaryocytes, but they clearly start out as such.

The size and molecular architecture of keratin are noted, as the size and type of the subunits are both species and site specific [12]. The identified range in molecular weight varies between 40 and 68 kDa, depending on the type of keratin subunit being expressed. In terms of structure, three basic types of keratins are produced, a so-called α form, a β form, and an irregular conformation. In terms of amino acid composition, keratins are noted for sizable amounts of cysteine that contain thiol functionality and are further capable of

Table 2.4: Amino acid composition of keratin found in hoof [13], hair [14], fingernail [15], and snake skin [14] The hoof is designated as high sulfur (high S) and low sulfur (low S). Only a limited direct determination of select amino acids was determined in [14]

AA Constituent in Keratin	AA Code	Hoof (Low S) (%) [13]	Hoof (High S) (%) [13]	Human Hair (%) [14]	Fingernail (%) [15]	Snake Skin (%) [14]
Alanine	Ala	3.2	7.2			
Glycine	Gly	7.2	6.3	4.3		13.1
Valine	Val	5.8	5.9			
Leucine	Leu	4.9	11.1			
Isoleucine	Ile	3.2	3.9			
Proline	Pro	13	2.4			
Phenylalanine	Phe	2.4	2.1	2.5	2.5	3.9
Tyrosine	Tyr	2.3	3.3	3	3	5.2
Serine	Ser	11.8	7.9			
Threonine	Thr	10.2	4.5			
Cystine	Cys	16.9	3.8	15.5	12	6.6
Methionine	Met	0	0.7			
Arginine	Arg	6	7.2	8	8.5	5.4
Histidine	His	0.9	0.8	0.6	0.5	0.4
Lysine	Lys	1	5	2.5	2.6	1.9
Aspartic Acid	Asp	4.3	10.1			
Glutamic Acid	Glu	6.9	17.7			

forming disulfide linkages. This is a good reason why the burning of hair tends to create such noxious fumes; it is the formation of hydrogen sulfide that is a gaseous reaction product of the combustion.

Prior work has resolved that keratin can be represented by two different structures being produced, with different molecular architectures and different amino acid compositions. The largest compositional difference is in the amount of cysteine found, and they are fractionated into high and low sulfur keratins and they are both found in the make-up of hair, hoof, and horn, all keratin-rich tissues. Mechanically, the high sulfur (high cysteine) proteins make up the matrix of these tissues that are reinforced by low sulfur α keratins that take a more fibrous structure. In hair, the α form is most commonly associated with a relaxed state, while the β form is induced when keratin is extended or stretched in the presence of higher humidity and temperature. Example determination of the low and high sulfur keratins found in the hoof are shown in Table 2.4.

2.6.3 Elastin

While keratin and collagen both form fibers and self-assemble into other structures and crystalline forms, there are other elastic proteins that cannot form more regular structures. Elastin is one such protein and is often found in many connective tissues such as skin,

Table 2.5: Amino acid composition of elastin found in the normal aorta, as determined by Kramsch, Franzblau and Hollander, [16]. The three amino acids denoted with * are lysine derivatives and are covalent bonding within the protein structure.

Elastin AA Constituent	AA Code	%
Cysteine (as cysteic acid)	CYS	0.1
Hydroxyproline	HYP	1.25
Aspartic Acid	ASP	0.6
Threonine	THR	1.2
Serine	SER	1
Glutamic Acid	GLU	2.1
Proline	PRO	12.7
Glycine	GLY	29.7
Alanine	ALA	21.1
Valine	VAL	13.1
Isoleucine	ILE	2.7
Leucine	LEU	6.5
Tyrosine	TYR	2.4
Phenylalanine	PHE	2.6
Isodesmosine	*	0.5
Desmosine	*	0.7
Lysinonorleucine	*	0.1
Lysine	LYS	0.7
Histidine	HIS	0.2
Arginine	ARG	0.8

commonly colocated with collagen. Thus, the make-up of these tissues is regulated by multiple cell types working harmoniously to synthesize a distributed matrix of different expressed proteins. The primary amino acid structure of elastin is more difficult to interpret due to the lack of structural regularity of elastin and the relative insolubility of the protein, but some measurements have been performed and summarized in Table 2.5. Nevertheless, there are ways to isolate elastin from elastin-rich ligaments.

Elastin has no long-range order and is not characterizable by techniques capable of resolving long and short range order such as X-ray diffraction which yields an amorphous halo. The mechanical behavior of connective tissues such as skin are commonly regulated by both the elastin and collagen components, and it is interesting to note that there is less elastin content reported in the composition of skin in Marfan's syndrome patients compared to normal populations who appear to have more resilient skin [17].

2.6.4 Albumin

Albumin is a ubiquitous protein expressed hepatically and found within blood and other tissues. Typical concentrations of albumin in blood range from 30 to 50 g/L [18]. Albumin is considered as a globular molecular transporter protein and is commonly used as a

Table 2.6: Composition of human serum albumin in terms of the amino acids found by digestion

Albumin AA constituent	Code	%
Alanine	Ala	4.6
Glycine	Gly	2.4
Valine	Val	5.3
Leucine	Leu	11.3
Isoleucine	Ile	2
Proline	Pro	3.2
Phenylalanine	Phe	7.5
Tyrosine	Tyr	4.8
Serine	Ser	3.2
Threonine	Thr	4.7
Cystine	Cys	5.6
Methionine	Met	1.3
Arginine	Arg	6.2
Histidine	His	4.8
Lysine	Lys	12.4
Aspartic Acid	Asp	10.2
Glutamic Acid	Glu	16.3

From C.W. Denko, D.B. Purser, R.M. Johnson, Amino acid composition in normal individuals and in patients with Rheumatoid Arthritis, Clin. Chem. 16 (1970) 54—57.

blocking protein to minimize other spurious binding events [19]. The globular structure is sufficient to shield the hydrophobic regions of the normal protein and allow albumin to remain soluble within blood. The molecular weight of human serum albumin is ~65 kDa [18,20], although albumin derived from other species such as the chicken egg suggests a lower molecular weight of between 34 and 40 kDa [21]. The amino acid make-up of human serum albumin extracted from blood [22] is listed in Table 2.6.

2.7 Conclusion

Proteins, as the expressed output from cells, are highly regulated, linear polypeptides, templated from DNA and postprocessed into phosphorylated or otherwise terminated structures that possess some unique attributes. One is that there is usually high specificity in the primary structural arrangement of amino acids that leads to intermediate to long chains that are nearly monodisperse. Proteins like other polymers have physically defined chain lengths, a chain molecular weight, and the chains can take many different conformations in solution that can affect their solubility, driving for larger agglomeration and protein—protein interactions. It is this size effect that can be leveraged through electrophoresis to discriminate between proteins of different chain length. By protease enzymatic digestion, one can resolve the composition of different proteins that are produced by fractionating them down to the amino acid or fragment level. The relatively low efficiency resulting from this high degree of perfection is accommodated by the presence of replicate cell structures performing parallel functions.

A second is that the protein produced is often a reasonable indicator of cellular health. Defects in the structure or chain length are likely indicators of mutations in the cell and under normal circumstances lead to programmed cell death or some other autophagy outcome. A third attribute of long chain architecture is that extended conformations can form larger structural assemblies leading to bones, skin, and tendons. If there are hydrophobic and hydrophilic regions along each chain, other structures can be formed based on the clustering of these regions along the chain that lead to receptor-type binding between molecules and localized arrangements of amino acids along chain segments for example. We might also consider that given that these are organic molecules, they have primary and secondary bonding characteristics as individual chains, a thermal conductivity, a conformational energy for their arrangement in solution, etc.

2.8 Problems

1. Explain in your own words how nature performs protein synthesis with more regularity and control than radical polymerization synthesis schemes.
2. The following gel electrophoresis analysis is completed for keratin extracted from Wool by Cardamone in lanes 1, 2, and 4 [23] and shown in Fig. 2.7. Keratin is identified in

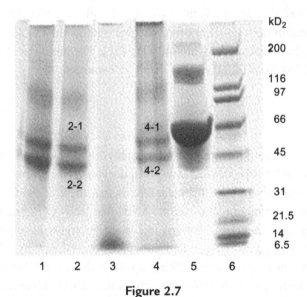

Figure 2.7

Gel electrophoresis of keratins resolved from wool. *From J.M. Cardamone, Investigating the microstructure of keratin extracted from wool: Peptide sequence (MALDI-TOF/TOF) and protein conformation (FTIR), J. Mol. Struct. 969(1−3) (2010) 97−105 [23].*

two different forms, one with approximately 45 kDa (designated 2), and a second larger form with a molecular weight of ∼65 kDa (designated 1). In lane 4, the brightness of the gel linked with the two keratin molecules is approximately the same, while in lane 2, the brightness of the lower molecular weight peak is nominally 30% more intense than the higher molecular weight one. If you can relate the brightness of each spot to the number of molecules making up each spot, explain how one could determine the number average and weight average molecular weights of keratin in lanes 2 and 4.

3. The osmotic pressure of a soluble 1 g of elastin protein solution 3.93×10^{-3} atm $- cm^3/g$ at 25°C. What is M_n? Assume low c regime, and the gas constant, $R = 0.08203$ L atm/mol K and start with equation 2.4.

4. If the same elastin solution was heated to 45°C, what would be the concentration dependence on the osmotic pressure assuming the structure was invariant to the heating.

5. Glutaraldehyde and Tannic acid are commonly used crosslinking agents for protein tissues [24]. The net result from treatment with tannic acid is an insoluble protein mass. Describe the mechanism of reaction between tannic acid or gluteraldehyde and proteins.

6. How might the higher-order structure of proteins alter their mobility during electrophoresis?

7. Compare the length of a normal protein molecule with that of the cell membrane. Can transmembrane proteins belong to both traverse the membrane and to extend into both the extracellular fluid and the cytosol or not? Explain your answer.

References

[1] A.O. Saeed, S. Dey, S.M. Howdle, K.J. Thurecht, C. Alexander, One-pot controlled synthesis of biodegradable and biocompatible co-polymer micelles, J. Mater. Chem. 19 (2009) 4529–4535.

[2] A. Elia, C. Constantinou, M.J. Clemens, Effects of protein phosphorylation on ubiquitination and stability of the translational inhibitor protein 4E-BP1, Oncogene 27 (2008) 811–822.

[3] C. Constantinou, M.J. Clemens, Regulation of the phosphorylation and integrity of protein synthesis initiation factor eIF4GI and the translational repressor 4E-BP1 by p53, Oncogene 24 (2005) 4839–4850.

[4] D.W. Ussery, Genetics 1998–2010. Available from: <http://www.cbs.dtu.dk/staff/dave/roanoke/genetics980211.html>.

[5] Kimball, Kimball's Biology Pages. Available from: <http://users.rcn.com/jkimball.ma.ultranet/BiologyPages/B/Blood.html>.

[6] F.W. Billmeyer, Textbook of Polymer Science, John Wiley, New York, 1971.

[7] V. Bhamidi, S. Varanasi, C.A. Schall, Langmuir 21 (2005) 9044–9050.

[8] I.W. Hamley, Introduction to Soft Matter, Wiley, Chichester, 2007.

[9] King, M.W. The Extracellular Matrix. 2010. Available from: <http://themedicalbiochemistrypage.org/extracellularmatrix.html>.

[10] J.E. Eastoe, The amino acid composition of mammalian collagen and gelatin, Biochem. J. 61 (1955) 589–600.

[11] C.H. Brown, Structural Materials in Animals, Pitman, London, 1975.

[12] H. Winter, J. Schweizer, Keratin synthesis in normal mouse epithelia and in squamous cell carcinomas: evidence in tumors for masked mRNA species coding for high molecular weight keratin polypeptides, Proc. Natl. Acad. Sci. U.S.A. 80 (21) (1983) 6480–6484.

[13] C. Marshall, J.M. Gillespie, The keratin proteins of wool, horn and hoof from sheep, Austr. J. Biol. Sci. 30 (1977) 389–400.

[14] R.J. Block, The composition of keratins—the amino acid composition of hair, wool, horn, and other eukeratins, J. Biol. Chem. 128 (1939) 181–186.

[15] H.O. Calvery, Some analyses of egg-shell keratin, J. Biol. Chem. 100 (1933) 183.

[16] D.M. Kramsch, C. Franzblau, W. Hollander, The protein and lipid composition of arterial elastin and its relationship to lipid accumulation and atherosclerosis, J. Clin. Investig. 50 (1971) 1666–1677.

[17] P.A. Abraham, A.J. Perejda, W.H. Carnes, J. Uitto, Marfan syndrome. Demonstration of abnormal elastin in aorta, J. Clin. Investig. 70 (1982) 1245–1252.

[18] MedlinePlus, Albumin-Serum. Available from: <http://www.nlm.nih.gov/medlineplus/ency/article/003480.htm>, 2010.

[19] K.D. McKeon, B.J. Love, The presence of adsorbed proteins on particles increases aggregated particle sedimentation, as measured by a light scattering technique, J. Adhes. 84 (2008) 664–674.

[20] B.D. Ratner, A.S. Hoffman, F.J. Schoen, J.E. Lemons, Biomaterials Science, an Introduction to Materials in Medicine, Academic Press, New York, 1996.

[21] F.W. Bernhart, Molecular weight of egg albumin, J. Biol. Chem. 132 (1940) 189–193.

[22] C.W. Denko, D.B. Purser, R.M. Johnson, Amino acid composition of serum albumin in normal individuals and in patients with Rheumatoid Arthritis, Clin. Chem. 16 (1970) 54–57.

[23] J.M. Cardamone, Investigating the microstructure of keratin extracted from wool: Peptide sequence (MALDI-TOF/TOF) and protein conformation (FTIR), J. Mol. Struct. 969 (1-3) (2010) 97–105.

[24] J.W. Payne, Polymerization of proteins with glutaraldehyde. Soluble molecular-weight markers, Biochem. J. 135 (1973) 867–873.

Further Reading

G.M. Cooper, The Cell, A Molecular Approach, ASM Press, Washington, D. C, 1997.

D.A. Lauffenberger, J.J. Linderman, Receptors, Models for Binding, Trafficking, an Signaling, Oxford University Press, New York, 1993.

B.D. Ratner, Biomaterials Science, An Introduction to Materials in Medicine, 3rd edition, Elsevier Academic Press, Amsterdam, 2013.

J.B. Park, R.S. Lakes, Biomaterials, An Introduction, 2nd edition, Plenum Press, New York, 1992.

J. Vincent, Structural Biomaterials, Princeton University Press, Princeton, NJ, 1990.

I.W. Hamley, Introduction to Soft Matter, Revised edition, Wiley, Chichester, 2007 Chapter 6.4.

P.T. Pugliese, Physiology of the Skin, Allured Publishing, Carol Stream, IL, 1996.

E.L. Smith, R.L. Hill, I.R. Lehman, R.J. Lefkowicz, P. Handler, A. White, Principles of Biochemistry, 7th edition, McGraw Hill, New York, 1983.

CHAPTER 3

Bones and Mineralized Tissues

Learning Objectives

In Chapter 1, Cell Biology Principles, distinguished characteristics between cell types are presented based on a range of identifying features. There are entire textbooks dedicated to cell physiology, ATP conversion and energy production, and synthesis, sorting, and recycling processes that occur within the cell. We also highlighted how cells communicate and how extracellular receptor interactions trigger intracellular structural and physiological changes. Also noted were features and function of a live cell, and that there are stages of cell life and death, the progression that can be tracked by observing dynamic cellular expression.

In Chapter 2, Cell Expression: Proteins and Their Characterization, the focus was on the output of cell expression, proteins conveyed from specific cell types. The length and types of amino acids consumed affect what is ultimately produced as a primary polypeptide structure and how it folds and rearranges to optimize its internal energy. Here, the focus is on cell activities that produce tissue enabled by enough ensembles of replicate cells to produce something larger. The initial goal is to discuss the production of bone and other specialized mineralized tissues like teeth. This chapter is organized around how different bone-forming cells produce different proteins and by these proteins have the capacity to self-organize, larger aggregates are coerced to form larger structures that can often mineralize. By reading this chapter, the learning objectives that the reader should achieve include:

1. An understanding that the most organized hard tissues (cortical bones) rely on a nourishment pathway and the replicating structure harnessed in a Haversian system.
2. Knowledge that the Haversian system extends about 200 μm in diameter with its own structure, and includes the mineral precipitates within these structures.
3. An awareness that variations in bone density relate to the ease with which local precipitation is possible within the nanopores of the proteins composing the organic fraction of bone.
4. A recognition that less organized, mineralized structures (cancellous or spongy bone) form near the growth plates of long bones and have completely different morphologies and properties.
5. And lastly, teeth also have their own growth pattern and structure, and development dictates cues for growth, eruption, and integration within the mandible and maxilla.

Biomaterials. DOI: http://dx.doi.org/10.1016/B978-0-12-809478-5.00003-1

There are whole books dedicated to bone and tooth structure and this is, at best, a fleeting synopsis for a developing engineer. Here the distinctions between subspecializations with dentistry have evolved where orthopedics seems to cover everything else.

3.1 Introduction

There are other more detailed descriptions about cartilage and cartilaginous structures that are normally found on the end of articulating bones and joints. Clearly joint degeneration is a factor and there are substantial efforts to characterize cartilage viability, chondrocyte activity, and persistence as a function of aging within orthopedics. Since joint replacement often resurfaces both articulating surfaces, the natural cartilage found on deteriorated joints is lost as part of normal joint replacement. In this chapter, the general attributes of bone and distinctions between different bone types are presented, but the reader is highly encouraged to look more deeply at more comprehensive descriptions for a complete view of both hard structures discussed here and soft tissues described in Chapter 4, Connective and Soft Tissues. A good reference book published recently is by Rodriguez-Gonzales which highlights clinical interactions of biomaterials used in hard tissue uses [1].

3.2 Cortical Bone

3.2.1 Cortical Bone Anatomy

The most organized sections of bone that correspond to the stiffest segments are called compact bone, or long bone, or cortical bone. Osteoblasts produce the collagen fibrils that are woven together through self-assembly to produce bone tissue. Resident osteoblasts also produce a range of other proteins in much lower concentrations including osteopontin and osteocalcin. The structural stiffness derives from the organization of three strands of collagen I that align in their interstices that allow for nanopores between the terminal segments of one grouping and the start of the next grouping, a schematic of which is shown in Fig. 3.1. Because of the regularity of the pores and the local tertiary structure that the side chains of the amino acids contained in each pore, these regions are where supersaturated calcium phosphate deposits ultimately precipitate. The two stiffening responses arise from the alignment of the organic polypeptides along the long direction and the presence of the inorganic nanoprecipitates that infiltrate the porous regions when collagen I is well organized.

The nanocrystals are so small as to create line broadening by X-ray diffraction, but are most often linked with then mineral calcium hydroxyapatite. An example of comparison of

(A)

(B)

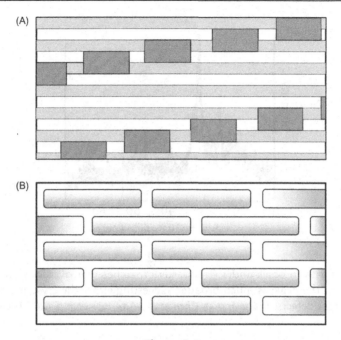

Figure 3.1

(A) 2-D representation of triads of tropocollagen fibrils self-assembled into large structures with identified gaps where bone mineral deposits precipitate. The gap dimensions are pores typically about 67 nm and the tropocollaten length dimension is approximately 300 nm. (B) Groups of mineralized tropocollagen fibrils also undergo a larger scale assembly forming collegen fibrils that are bound by extracellular matrix proteins.

a diffraction pattern from an elk antler and HAP is shown in Fig. 3.2. Clearly, the line broadening is observed for specific diffractions, and the results are noisy making it harder to discern smaller diffractions due to the signal/noise ratio from [2].

3.2.2 The 3.4.2: Haversian System

At larger scale, there is a separate self-assembly of living bone segments within long bone called an osteon or a Haversian system. Within each osteon, the center is called the Haversian Canal that contains the vascular network to nourish viable bone cells. Moving radially outward in the osteon, bone takes the form of a 2-D planar composite laminate that is wrapped into three dimensions in such a way that each layer is called a lamellar layer, as shown in Fig. 3.3.

An ensemble of osteons in a larger segment of tissue is shown in Fig. 3.4. There is a bonding interaction between layers identified as a cement layer. Individual living and dormant osteoblasts are housed in gaps identified in polarized light microscopy as dark circles called lacunae, with no more than one cell occupying each lacuna. The vascular

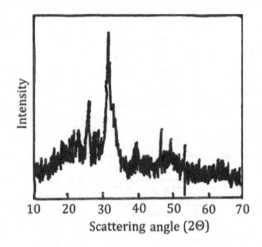

Figure 3.2
X-ray diffraction pattern of elk antler. The pattern matches that of calcium hydroxyapatite, but the breadth of the peaks is much broader suggesting either the crystals are very small or possess larger defects. *Redrawn from Chen et al., Acta Biomater. 5 (2009) 693−706.*

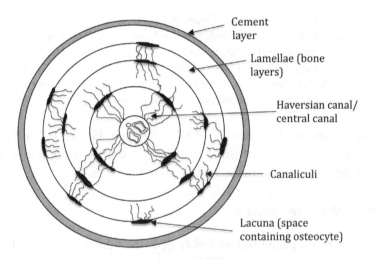

Figure 3.3
Schematic of the Haversian system, showing the interior canal, the lamellar layers of protein that are wrapped, the pore locations called lacunae, and the vascular connections that are linked radially, called canaliculi.

connections from the Haversian canal to the lacunae arise from very small capillaries known as canaliculi that nourish the lacunae. The canal of the osteon is typically <15 μm in diameter, and the outer reaches of each osteon are on the order of hundreds of microns (100−200 μm) in diameter [3] but these vary based on age, gender, mammalian type, etc.

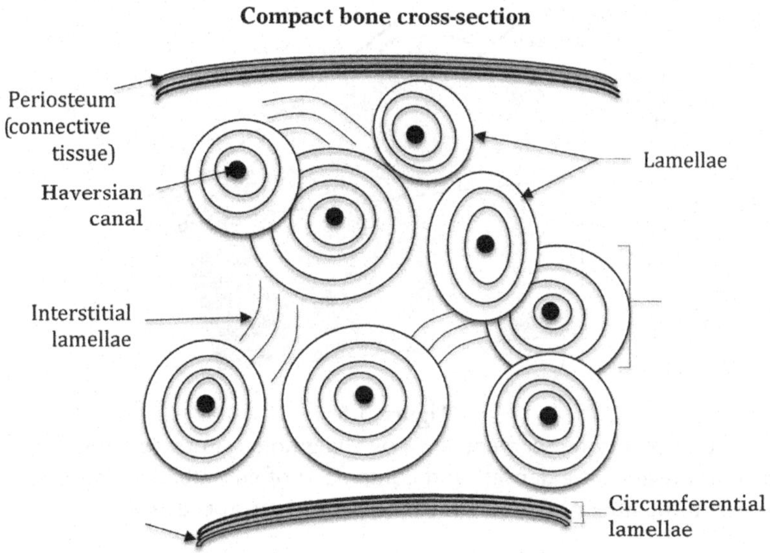

Compact bone cross-section

Periosteum (connective tissue)

Haversian canal

Interstitial lamellae

Lamellae

Circumferential lamellae

Figure 3.4
Groups of Haversian systems are commonly observed and linked as represented here.

During maturation, the annular osteon thickness is thin and tends to grow in dimension with age and the lamellae fill in from the outer regions of the osteon to the inner region. The threshold diameter is also linked with the perfusion requirements of the dormant and living cells with the tissue. For these to be stimulated through bone fracture or through an overstress condition, they need to remain viable. Thus, it is important to classify new bone growth primarily as lamellar thickening of existing osteons without the osteon growing radially, and recruitment of new osteons as bones long grow in a radial dimension.

This formation of organized bone occurs with axial alignment of the osteons in a kind of annular pipe arrangement with less organized trabecular bone found in the interior vascularity connections in the center of each osteon to allow individual osteons to be fed accordingly. A schematic of how the cortical bone alignment is arranged is shown in Fig. 3.5. Within any long bone, there are individual regions of bone stock that are more or less organized as a function of both the radius and the length, with differences in bone density as well.

To accommodate axial growth of long bones, the process of limb lengthening occurs at the ends of the bones called growth plates, junctions between well-developed cortical bone, and a less organized bone structure. Growth plates are usually defined as cartilaginous structures during pediatric development as limbs lengthen, the cortical bone extends maintaining the growth plate at the ends of these growing bones.

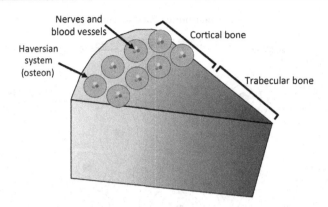

Figure 3.5

3-D wedge section of a bone segment showing the gradient in bone structure with radial dimension. The outer regions are densest and composted of ensembles of Haversian systems and closer to the hollow, marrow-filled center is the trabecular bone region.

Table 3.1: Long bone physical characteristics across a range of mammals

Species	Specific Gravity	H$_2$O Content (vol%)	Mineral Fraction (wt%)	Organic Fraction Converted From CO$_2$ (%)
Turtle	1.81	37	29.2	40.1
Frog	1.93	35.2	34.5	38.5
Polar bear	1.92	33	36.2	40.1
Human	1.94	15.5	39.9	41.8
Elephant	2.00	20	41.4	41.5
Monkey	2.09	23	42.6	41.1
Cat	2.05	23.6	42.2	40.5
Horse	2.02	25	41	40.5
Chicken	2.04	24.5	41.7	38.7
Dog	1.94	28	38.7	35.5
Cow	2.05	26.2	42.6	36.2
Guinea pig	2.1	25	43.5	37
Rabbit	2.12	24.5	45	37.2
Rat	2.14	20.2	49.9	38.3

Average values are reported +/−1 (SD). Reproduced from R.M. Blitz, E.D. Pellegrino, The chemical anatomy of bone, J. Bone Jt. Surg. Br. 51A (1969) 456−466.

Thus, long bones tend to be derived from the ossificiation of cartilaginous structures. Falls and overstress conditions in children often lead to fractures in and around the various growth plates, and with resetting and simple immobilization, often these resolve unremarkably.

3.2.3 Composition and Properties of Cortical Bone

In terms of mechanical behavior, bone response correlates with increased mineralization capacity and correspondingly, bone density as well. In Table 3.1,

Table 3.2: Example of how mechanical behavior is affected by human bone age

Ages (years)	No. of Femur Bones Tested	No. of Test Specimens Produced	Modulus of Elasticity (GPa)	Yield Stress (MPa)	Ultimate Stress (MPa)	Ultimate Strain
20–29	5	36	17.0 (2.24)	120 (6.2)	140 (10)	0.034 (0.0067)
30–39	2	11	17.6 (0.28)	120 (9.9)	136 (3.5)	0.032 (0.0092)
40–49	3	14	17.7 (4.45)	121 (8.4)	139 (10.7)	0.030 (0.004)
50–59	6	37	16.6 (1.74)	111 (11.9)	131 (12.6)	0.028 (0.0059)
60–69	8	42	17.1 (2.21)	112 (5.9)	129 (6.4)	0.025 (0.0055)
70–79	7	28	16.3 (1.78)	111 (6.3)	129 (5.5)	0.025 (0.006)
80–89	2	10	15.6 (0.71)	104 (5.0)	120 (7.1)	0.024 (0.0021)

Average values are reported +/−1 (SD). Reproduced from A.H. Burstein, D.T. Reilly, M. Martens, Aging of bone tissue: mechanical properties, J. Bone Jt. Surg. 58A (1976) 82–86.

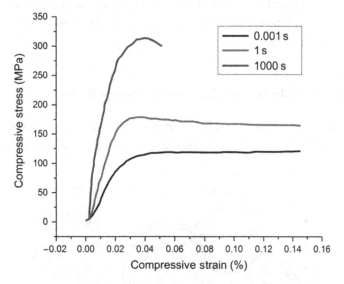

Figure 3.6

The compressive mechanical response of dry, deer antler cortical bone evaluated at three different strain rates. Note the rising E measured over the six orders of magnitude in strain rate. *Redrawn from M.A. Meyers, P.Y. Chen, Biological Materials Science, Cambridge University Press, Cambridge, UK, 2014.*

the density and composition of different long bones derived from different mammals are shown (From [4]).

There is a known loss of quasistatic mechanical stiffness and strength of long bone as a function of age, as indicated in Table 3.2. (From [5]).

And was discussed earlier, the viscoelasticity of the organic matrix affects the time-dependent mechanical behavior leading to a pronounced stiffening of the stress–strain response depending on a rising strain rate. An example is the representation on dry deer antler shown in Fig. 3.6 [6]. Static, elastic materials would behave independently of strain rate.

3.3 Cancellous (Spongy Bone)

3.3.1 Anatomy of Spongy Bone

Also found near the terminal ends and the interior of long bones is a different form of bone called spongy, trabecular, or cancellous bone, formed in the epiphyses of the femoral ball or the distal end of the femur, for example Ref. [7]. An example is shown in Fig. 3.7 near the proximal end of the femur where the terminus forms the femoral ball out of trabeculae [8].

In the trabecular regions, there is less protein organization yielding a lower mineral density in spongy bone than in cortical bone. Correspondingly, trabecular bone has a lower modulus of elasticity and a lower strength compared to that of compact bone. In terms of structure, in spongy bone, there is a disorganized array of mineralized bone struts called tribeculae (translation: small beam). These are distributed in three-dimensional space and when imaged, the phase contrast yields a complex, spongy appearance, hence its other name.

3.3.2 Composition and Mechanical Behavior of Spongy Bone

The mechanical behavior of cancellous bone specimens, both native (NCB) and treated with pereacetic acid/ethanol to demineralize fractions of the tissue, are shown below.

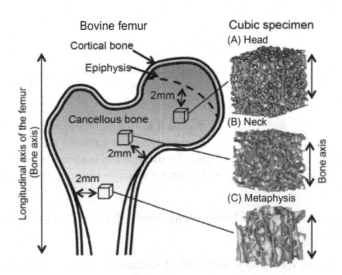

Figure 3.7
Gross morphological features of trabeculae or struts making up the femoral ball region as it progresses into the long bone region. Note the higher density of the cortical regions in the long bone and in the distal regions of the ball. *Reproduced with permission from K. Endo, S. Yamada, M. Todoh, N. Iwasaki, S. Tadano, Structural strength of cancellous specimens from bovine femur under cyclic compression, PeerJ (2016).*

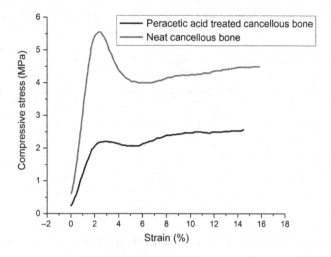

Figure 3.8

Compressive loading tests on cancellous bone specimens as received (NCB) and following acid exposure to extract the mineral constituents [9].

Removing some amount of the mineral reduces both stiffness and strength as noted here (from [9]) (Fig. 3.8).

With tissue aging, trabecular bone undergoes remodeling, as fractured and damaged trabaculae are dissolved and new matrix is deposited to create new trabeculae over time as part of the continued evolution of bone stock. There is more evolution in trabecular bone than in cortical bone that often is dormant until there is a fracture or significant bone hematoma or stress fracture. It has been reported that up to 6% of cancellous bone stock undergoes remodeling each year, and that exercise is a key to maintaining viable bone stock in trabecular bone since it is so much compliant than cortical bone. Peripheral cancellous bone turns over at roughly 2%/yr while more central cancellous bone can be as much as 8 times higher, leading to an average remodeling rate somewhere in between [10]. Remodeling translates into individual cracked trabecular components being redissolved and new structures being deposited to maintain the loading. Snapshot determinations of the composition and density of various cancellous bone segments have been determined long ago, with densities of ~ 1.9 g/cm^3 and comparisons of inorganic mineral ash content to organic matrix is roughly 2/1 [11] and are shown in Table 3.3.

Remodeling is accommodated by the presence of so-called osteoclasts that allow for drops in local pH sufficient to dissolve the mineral constituents within bone. A balance of osteoclasts relative to osteoblasts prevents any significant deviation in terms of overall bone density yielding something approaching steady state. Unsurprisingly, osteoporosis results in higher osteoclast activity and more bone mineral resorption relative to new deposition. As a

Table 3.3: Composition of inorganic and organic fractions from trabecular bone derived from several different animals.

Mammal	Trabecular Bone Fractions				Measured Density (g/cm^3)	Ratio of Ash/ Organic Mass Fraction
	Water	Organic	Volatile inorganic	Ash		
Steer	14.6% (1.0)	26.6% (0.05)	3.7% (0.1)	55.2%(1.7)	1.93	2.077
Dog	15.2% (0.8)	26.5% (0.1)	3.6% (0.0)	54.8% (1.4)	1.911	2.074
Human	14.0%(0.7)	25.8% (0.05)	3.7%(0.1)	55.9% (1.4)	1.924	2.177
Monkey	14.4(0.9)	27.3 (0.1)	3.6 (0.1)	53.8% (1.2)	1.878	1.97

From J.K. Gong, J.S. Arnold, S.H. Cohn, Compositon of trabecuilar and cortical bone. Anatom. Rec. 149 (1964) 319–324.

result, bone density, mineralization content, mechanical stiffness, and strength tend to decrease with age. This is one crucial reason why load-bearing exercise is so important for older patients as it stimulates further bone mineralization and helps to maintain sufficient bone density.

While there are single measurements to represent bone density, there may well be differences in terms of how much bone demineralization occurs in trabecular versus compact bone. Bone density measurements are essentially markers of more general health, and a more acute loss of bone density in a specific bone or region is more likely to generate bone fracture in that area or region.

3.4 Teeth

3.4.1 Tooth Anatomy and Evolution

Teeth and other cranial bones tend to form from the precipitation of minerals within mesenchymal tissues that occur during development including both the mandible and maxilla and the corresponding tooth structures. Teeth form from what are called germs that undergo a controlled precipitation that yields an inverted structure that presents itself as most living on the inside of each tooth, as shown in Fig. 3.9. In teeth, the dental root structure nourishes the cells found within internal cavity of the tooth structure. The root contains both blood vessels and nerves to nourish the tooth from the inside out. The root or pulp region is the softest section of the tooth as well. As one moves from the proximal center of each tooth distally, there is a bony deposit called dentin that includes a series of fluid pores called tubules. The mineral density found in dentin corresponds to a physical density of approximately 2.1 g/cm^3 [12] and an estimated modulus of elasticity of 18.6 GPa [13], on par with other long bone structures with similar mechanical behavior. The dentin tubules are radially arranged pointing outward from the pulpal region of the tooth to allow

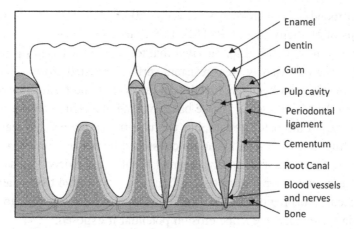

Figure 3.9
Schematic of a tooth structure showing the location of a molar within the lower jawbone, the mandible. The tooth is nourished from the inside.

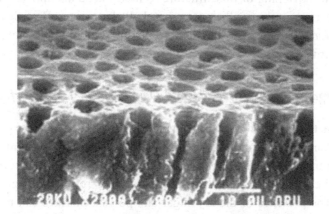

Figure 3.10
Surface structure of exposed dentin tubules observed by SEM. *From Marshall et al. G.W. Marshall, S.J. Marshall, J.H. Kinney, M. Balloch, The dentin substrate structure and properties relating to bonding, J. Dent. 25 (1997) 441–458.*

for fluid migration within the tooth, as shown in Fig. 3.10 [14]. It is thought that internal pressures exist in the tooth as tubules tend to leak when exposed from the outside during dental preparation for filling a tooth cavity. Maybe the tubules are linked with bone remineralization below the enamel as the tooth ages.

The most outward structure above the gum-line in the tooth superstructure is enamel, the hardest and least living substance found in man. Filled with as much as 98 wt% mineral constituents mostly in the form of hydroxyapatite and only a small fraction of protein, enamel tends to be highly impervious to bacterial colonization and very strong and stiff. The typical density of enamel found in humans ranges between 2800 and 3000 kg/m^3 [15] with an estimated modulus of elasticity of 83 GPa [13]. Before man ever made use of fire in cooking food for nourishment, it was critical for survival that teeth could tear and rip muscular protein tissue accordingly. These extremely wear-resistant surfaces resisted erosion. By ion exchange, one can replace fluoride for a hydroxyl function in the crystal and form fluoroapatite, an even harder substance in the MOH's scale. As we have evolved, our dental design requirements have reduced in terms of ultimate strength, but we have traded the need to tear and digest raw meat to now resisting excessive sugars that are consumed by bacteria on our enamel surfaces that produce fruit acids to etch and dissolve enamel. Challenges indeed. Subsurface adjacent to and below the gum-line, there is a section of bone-like connective tissue called cementum, that covers the apical (root) regions of the tooth that can also be susceptible to decay and erosion, if bacteria there create the same erosion potential if exposed.

These teeth are fixtured into the upper (maxilla) or lower (mandible) jaw by the presence of an oriented, collagenous layer identified as the periodontal membrane. The strong fiber alignment allows the stiffening of this structure to hold the cementum section of the tooth strongly in place. Strong impact collisions or baseballs bouncing off of faces can act to damage the membrane which causes the teeth to be much more compliant until this membrane has reformed.

3.4.2 Plaque, Organic Acids, Alter pH and Demineralize Tooth Surfaces

Understanding something of how teeth form and how their structures are compromised leads to an understanding of dental subspecialities. This time, lets go from the outside in. Dentists have been most commonly worried about general tooth decay, corresponding to a loss of enamel. A lack of brushing and flossing can lead to residual bacteria adhered to the enamel structure. The presence of dietary sugar and polysaccharides can metabolize into fruit acids by the biofilms on teeth that can lower oral pH and enhance the dissolution of mineral content in enamel. Your dentist, when probing your teeth, with a narrow, blunt edged instrument, is essentially doing a range of hardness tests. If, for whatever reason, your enamel (Knoop Hardness of 343 kg/mm^2 [13]) has decayed to a point of exposing dentin (Knoop Hardness of 68 kg/mm^2 [13]), the probe is more likely to stick in the softer dentin, versus caroming off the enamel. The softer exposed dentin regions are identified as dental caries, often rectified by removing the decayed enamel and the corresponding biofilm and addressing the gap in the tooth by a filling, which can be produced from any range of filling materials, as shown in Fig. 3.11. Composite restorative resins (Chapter 9: Polymeric Biomaterials) can be tinted to reflect remaining tooth structure allowing the filler to more accurately replicate the replaced tissue.

More involved caries typically require a larger resection of the tooth superstructure leading to the construction of dental crowns, bridges, and related bone implant strategies. These

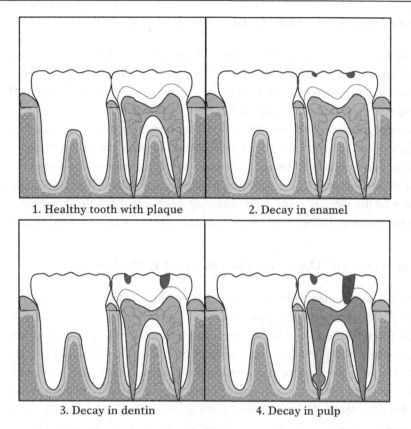

1. Healthy tooth with plaque
2. Decay in enamel
3. Decay in dentin
4. Decay in pulp

Figure 3.11
Schematic of caries ingression into an enamel surface.

dental reconstructions are for both function and aesthetic replacements. Functional crown restorations can be accomplished by gold and gold alloys (Chapter 7: Metallic Biomaterials) that are built following the use of impression compounds (Chapter 9: Polymeric Biomaterials) to define the existing tooth structure and bite surfaces prior to resection. Functional and more aesthetically representative tooth reconstructions are made from dental porcelains (Chapter 8: Ceramic Biomaterials), often cofired into precious metal bases that are then bonded to the residual tooth after the diseased tooth fraction has been removed and a base for the crown has been prepared.

If more than one tooth is involved, multiple crowns or assemblies of multiple superstructures can be constructed and installed as replacements. Even missing teeth in the mandible can be accommodated in a multiple-crown bridge arrangement where a single crown in the middle of three teeth is suspended and fixture by the adjacent crowned teeth. Biting on the suspended tooth is the equivalent of flexing the bridge, and as a result, much stronger and more highly alloyed compositions are required to produce a long-term functional outcome.

3.4.3 Dentin Exposure Through the Gum-line: Periodontal Disease

An alternative mode for exposing dentin comes from what is called gum recession. Bacterially laden gum tissues, again produced often from inadequate oral hygiene can lead to inflammation, redness, soreness, and if unresolved, gum disease which is often reflected as a loss of periodontal membrane coverage of the teeth, shown schematically in Fig. 3.12. If the gums recede enough, one can expose the periodontal bone structure much like dentin and the enamel in these areas are much thinner or nonexistent. In other words, tooth decay and bacterial infestation of bone can be also exposed requiring a similar caries response as would occur on the superstructure. People suffering from gingival recession are often referred to periodontists who are directly involved in restoring periodontal health, slowing the progression of gum-line recession and addressing other schemes to recover this exposed dentin.

3.4.4 Tooth Statics and Dynamics: The Origins of Orthodontia

And with increasing frequency, teeth erupt either encumbered by insufficient real estate in the oral cavity to be situated with appropriate spacing within the mandible and maxilla or otherwise misplaced. Often there is just not enough room for the last teeth in a mouth of 32 teeth including wisdom teeth to erupt without complicating where already erupted teeth are situated. The misplacement of teeth within the jawbone can be reorganized by the elective application of lateral forces that are commonly applied by archwires wound to brackets, adhered to teeth. There are other complications such as one tooth situated in front of another, impacted teeth that do not erupt sufficiently and remain more fully in the jaw, and other more refined bite problems such as an over/underbite, all of which can be planned for through a reorganization of the teeth that can occur over a period of years. But the outcomes are dramatic, as pointed out in Fig. 3.13.

Mechanically, the process of moving teeth requires a way to deliver small but controlled forces sufficient to dissolve the periodontal membrane in front of the tooth in the

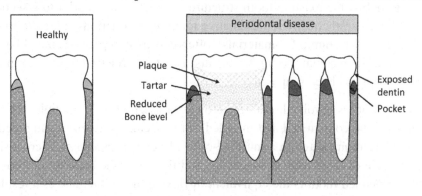

Figure 3.12
Schematic of tooth and gum structure undergoing periodontal disease.

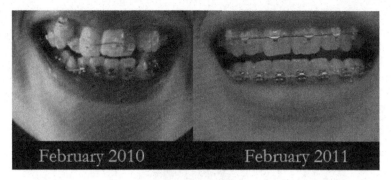

Figure 3.13
How 1 year of small lateral and vertical forces can rearrange tooth structures.

movement direction and reform the membrane on the trailing region of each tooth. Lateral forces are created by orthodontic archwires, commonly made from shape memory alloys like Nickel-Titanium, NiTi (discussed in Chapter 7: Metallic Biomaterials) that are soft when cooled and stiffen by a solid-state phase change as your mouth heats up the archwire. By bonding brackets to the teeth usually by mix and set acrylate chemistry (discussed in Chapter 9: Polymeric Biomaterials), the archwire can be fitted and attached to individual teeth and loaded to create the lateral force. Teeth can be moved up and down within the jawbones by the use of elastics that impart a retractive force upon jaw opening.

The subtlety associated with translating these teeth within the bone is achieved by applying sufficient force to cause millimeter level migrations between appointments. Typically treatment is finished within 2−3 years, followed by the installation of a removable retainer structure that can hold the translated teeth in place over a period of months while the periodontal membrane reforms to strengthen tooth attachments to the jawbones. It is clearly possible to apply more stress and yield larger translations and faster treatment periods, but that comes with the cost of a much more fragile tooth attachment to the bone while periodontal strengthening is occurring. A finite threshold unrelated to the mechanics of the applied force is that usually this tugging on the teeth creates some fairly significant pain responses and headaches.

Some of the same types of forces can be applied not through brackets but alternatively by the use of a series of dynamic retainers that are designed to apply the lateral forces but without a direct attachment. There is a system called Invisalign which is a customized mold making tool, linked with 3D renderings of a patient's tooth and jaw structure. This coupling allows a series (25−50) of customized plastic retainers, the first designed to apply the corresponding lateral forces simply by the patient installing the retainer, and each subsequent one designed to apply the forces but on a slightly altered tooth arrangement coerced by the prior retainer wearing, an example of which is shown in Fig. 3.14. The first

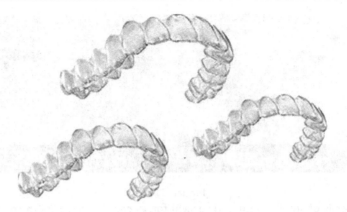

Figure 3.14
Three example retainers used with the Invisalign system.

retainer represents the initial state of where the teeth are positioned, and the last one best represents what how the teeth outcome should look after the treatment process is over.

With each retainer to be worn 20–22 hours/day, the same lateral forces can be applied without directly bonding brackets to teeth, and oral hygiene is better as the retainers can be removed for brushing and flossing. This is a great example showing two ways (physical attachment linked with archwires versus a progressive retainer system) to accomplish a similar outcome through completely different means, with different complexities. The presence of both systems as options offers orthodontists and general dentists a larger toolbox in personalizing how to accomplish tooth alignment.

3.4.5 Endodonics: Resolving the Dying Internal Structure of a Tooth

Within the tooth, there are instances when the tooth through some combination becomes infected, is damaged through blunt force, or the feeding blood vessels are blocked or severed, compromising the internal structure of a tooth or teeth. In instances when it is clear that the living section of the tooth is doomed, the non-living portions of the tooth can be retained through a process called a root canal procedure, often completed by another type of subspecialist, the endodontist. There is a finite window of time (often within a few days for a trauma case) in salvaging the nonviable elements of a dying tooth, as often with infection, the interior regions of the teeth darken as part of the decay and it is impossible to remove these discolorations.

During root canal procedures, access to the root and pulpal structure is created under anesthesia often from the top of the tooth or from behind the tooth. A more extensive and involved disinfection and cleansing of the interior regions of the tooth is commonly performed including the removal or cleansing of regions particularly in the feeding vessels if those are the origin of the infection, called a pulpotomy. Following disinfection, the tooth is packed with disinfectant-loaded elastomeric particles such as gutta percha or natural rubber to fill the cavity formed, followed by restoration of the pulp region to prevent an abscess and sealing of the residual tooth by installing a crown. After the root canal is finished, the tooth structure is essentially dead, but the tooth substructure remains and the region where the crown is located can be chewed on etc.

More refined schemes to perform root canal can be done by oral surgery while retaining the superstructure. So long as the hole made (usually in the back of the tooth) is large enough to lavage the region of infection and the root structure and feeding vasculature can be isolated and removed, a smaller incision can be made and more of the original tooth can be retained. The residual tooth can sometimes look a little different than surrounding teeth in part due to the translucency of the repaired tooth relative to the surrounding teeth, but the cementum and periodontal membrane often remain intact allowing the non-living tooth to remain years after the procedure.

3.4.6 Sealants as a Preventive Procedure to Fight Tooth Decay

It is also worth considering how the original formation of teeth makes us more or less susceptible to later dental erosion problems. An example is the construction of precipitating teeth structures required to form deciduous and permanent teeth. The process of forming teeth is essentially a nucleation and growth process, and often times, to form larger teeth like molars, one needs more than one nucleating structure called a germ to form the precipitated composite. Teeth form months and years in advance of their eventual eruption within the subgingival region and if one does diagnostic imaging preeruption, one will often identify early precipitates as tooth precursors. Molars can be seen to evolve from 3 to 7 grains and each peak in the molar is linked with the edge of an individual germ. Thus, a molar is the confluence of several germs, and somehow, during development, these germs need to undergo coalescence in order to form a unified tooth structure. What this means is that there are germ or grain boundaries forming at the interfaces between where distinct grains coalesce. This can be seen as a top view looking down on a molar structure, where multiple grains coalesce. If the surface energy of the germ surfaces is high, there is a larger driving force for these surfaces to form single integrated surface minimizing the surface area in the process. If the surface energy of each germ surface is low, one might find a longer grain boundary between grains, and an easier, shorter pathway for fruit acids to infiltrate the surrounding enamel and into dentin. On the surface of a molar, one might identify these long, craggy and deep junctions where the grains should coalesce but if they do not coalesce, it is easier for bacteria to get lodged in the interstices of the molar grain boundaries. These features are called pits and fissures and can be early indicators for the formation of dental caries in younger patients since these features are more susceptible to decay, and example of the tooth morphology and the pits that require sealing are shown in Fig. 3.15 [16].

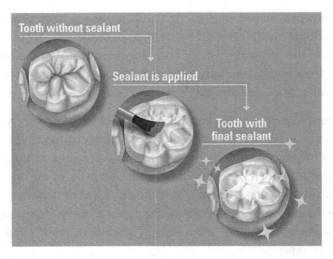

Figure 3.15

Top view of pits and fissures in a natural tooth formed from several grains. The cleaning and subsequent sealing of the gap regions has a large effect on reducing caries in these pit locations. *Reproduced with permission from Dental Sealant FAQ: What are Dental Sealants? (2016). Available from: https://www.cdc.gov/oralhealth/dental_sealant_program/sealants.htm.*

It is commonly too hard to discriminate between some with a few pits and fissures and another patient in which pits and fissures are pervasive to all teeth. As a result, general dentists tend to think of all patients with pits and fissures and schemes are deployed to fill all patients in all these potential pit and fissure regions with occluding resins (Chapter 9: Polymeric Biomaterials) that prevent further sugar metabolism deep within these fissures after a thorough cleaning in the dentist's chair.

3.4.7 Oral Surgery, Bone Implants, and Fracture Fixation

And finally in terms of subdental disciplines, there are more typical surgeons involved in resections called oral surgeons. These doctors are solicited in rebuilding and stabilizing bone structure in trauma cases, resecting tumorous bone and soft tissue in oral cancer cases, placing bone implants tied to permanent prosthetic plates and implants, etc. The bone implants used for oral rehabilitation are typically titanium and the plates used for fracture fixation are typically produced from stainless steel, treated much like other fracture fixation plates discussed in Chapter 11, Orthopedic Biomaterials and Strategies. Combinations of wires, plates, and screws are often required to stabilize traumatic fractures of the mandible and other dental structures. Examples of the types of interventions and repairs involved to deal with dental fractures are shown in Fig. 3.16 [17].

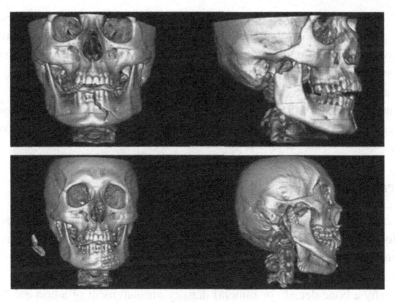

Figure 3.16
Pre-op and follow up CT renderings of two different fractures observed as a bulk submandibular fracture and a right condylar fracture, both resolved by four hole fracture fixation plates.
Reproduced with permission from J.N. Shi, H. Yuan, B. ZXu, Treatment of mandibular condyle fractures using a modified transparotid approach via the parotid mini-incision: experience with 31 cases, PLoS 1 (2013).

3.5 Conclusions

It is understood that the directed self-assembly of well-organized proteins, produced from osteoblasts, is directly linked with the capacity to trigger subsequent mineralization in bone. It is also understood that there is a trade-off between the maximum potential for mineralization and the capacity to retain a viable structure. The precipitates take a nanostructured form within nanopores directed to mineralize with a form most closely linked with calcium hydroxyapatite. The mechanical behavior of mineralized tissues correlates with both the amount of total mineral content and with the degree of organization of the proteins leading to mineral precipitation. One reading this chapter should come away with a sense of how even one bone or tooth structure can retain multiple forms of bone structures within it. For more organized tissues, the concept of a larger vascular building block has been forwarded, with the Haversian system being limited to a few hundred microns in diameter. A larger bone structure will have more Haversian systems as opposed to fewer larger ones.

Comparisons have been made between trabecular bone and cortical bone, and the structure and evolution of the two forms are quite different. While both have what are determined as quasistatic mechanical behavior, it is still worth noting that bone structures still have a viscoelastic feature.

We have also discussed both tooth structures and specialized mineralized tissues. Comparisons are made between bone and tooth structure in terms of how each remain viable, and given the location and the requirements to retain adequate oral hygiene, it is not a surprise to see that dental practice is both more specialized with more subspecialities given it easy accessibility, the challenges of being immersed in an environment of oral microflora, and more history of use regarding potential dental materials. It is worth noting that challenges in either oral health or skeletal health are not necessarily conserved between them.

3.6 Problems

1. If most crystals have very sharp diffraction patterns, explain what attributes (size, shape, form) of bone mineralization leads to the formation of broader, more diffuse diffraction patterns when evaluating bone?
2. Explain the components making up the anatomy of an osteon.
3. Explain why a bone density or mineral density measurement of a cortical bone might be misleading if a bulk measurement of the bone was used vs a higher resolution technique?
4. Compare osteoblast activity in a child with an active growth plate vs an adult who has a stress fracture resulting from an overuse injury (e.g., too much running too quick). What is different between them and what kinds of biochemical or physical cues trigger new bone synthesis in each.
5. Evaluate the modulus of elasticity of deer antler and the corresponding yield strength tested as a function of three strain rates in Fig. 3.6. Note that the faster the antler is tested, the more brittle it becomes, a hallmark of viscoelasticity.
6. Consider the vascular network of cancellous bone. Explain why you would consider the vascular organization more or less organized than in an osteon?
7. Consider orthodontia as a mechanical test. Where on the mechanical stress—strain diagram is the loading pattern to initiate tooth movement?
8. Explain whether you would expect a tooth that has undergone a root canal procedure to be more brittle, less brittle or about the same, as a result of the procedure?
9. Identify pathways and locations for caries formation.
10. Explain why dental sealants function to block caries formations as a preventative procedure?

References

[1] F.A. Rodriguez-Gonzalez, Biomaterials in Orthopaedic Surgery, ASM Publishing, Materials Park, OH, 2009.
[2] P.Y. Chen, A.G. Stokes, J. McKittrick, Comparison of the structure and mechanical propeties of bovine femur bone and antler of the North American Elk, ACTA Biomater. 5 (2009) 693—706.

[3] M. Viceconti, Multiscale Modeling of the Skeletal System, Cambridge University Press, Cambridge, UK, 2012.

[4] R.M. Blitz, E.D. Pellegrino, The chemical anatomy of bone, J. Bone Jt. Surg. Br. 51A (1969) 456–466.

[5] A.H. Burstein, D.T. Reilly, M. Martens, Aging of bone tissue: mechanical properties, J. Bone Jt. Surg. 58A (1976) 82–86.

[6] M.A. Meyers, P.Y. Chen, Biological Materials Science, Cambridge University Press, Cambridge, UK, 2014.

[7] S. Bhat, Biomaterials, Alpha Science International, LTD, Harrow, UK, 2005.

[8] K. Endo, S. Yamada, M. Todoh, N. Iwasaki, S. Tadano, Structural strength of cancellous specimens from bovine femur under cyclic compression, PeerJ (2016).

[9] J. Rauh, F. Despang, J. Baas, C. Liebers, A. Pruss, M. Gelinsky, et al., Comparative biomechanical and microstructural analysis of native versus peracetic acid–ethanol treated cancellous bone graft, Biomed. Res. Int. 2014 (2014).

[10] A.M. Parfitt, What is the normal rate of bone remodeling, Bone 35 (2004) 1–3.

[11] J.K. Gong, J.S. Arnold, S.H. Cohn, Compositon of trabecuilar and cortical bone, Anatom. Rec. 149 (1964) 319–324.

[12] K. Chatterjee, Chapter 6: Dentin, in: Essentials of Oral Histology, Jaypee Brothers, 2006

[13] R.G. Craig, J.M. Powers, J.C. Wataha, Dental materials, seventh ed., Mosby, St Louis, 2000.

[14] G.W. Marshall, S.J. Marshall, J.H. Kinney, M. Balloch, The dentin substrate structure and properties relating to bonding, J. Dent. 25 (1997) 441–458.

[15] S.M. Weidmann, J.A. Weatherell, S.M. Hamm, Variations of enamel density in sections of human teeth, Arch. Oral Biol. 12 (1967) 85–97.

[16] Dental Sealant FAQ: What are Dental Sealants? (2016). Available from: <https://www.cdc.gov/oralhealth/dental_sealant_program/sealants.htm > .

[17] J.N. Shi, H. Yuan, B. ZXu, Treatment of mandibular condyle fractures using a modified transparotid approach via the parotid mini-incision: experience with 31 cases, PLoS 1 (2013).

CHAPTER 4

Connective and Soft Tissues

Learning Objectives

After reading this chapter, the reader will be able to:

1. Understand the composition of tissues making up the circulatory system, connective tissues linked with skin and organs, and other structures that do not mineralize.
2. Recognize the alchemy that goes into integrating ensembles of different proteins that compose larger biological structures and organs.
3. Correlate the distinctions between composition, structure, and resulting mechanical behavior in soft tissues.
4. Recognize the pivotal role water has in softening many soft tissue structures, which complicates structural analysis of tissues from explants, as tissue aging and dehydration affect properties profoundly. The issue of water in tissue is at the origin of how large a cosmetics industry exists today.
5. And finally, the ties between how disease states are manifested in soft tissues both in terms of structure and properties will be referenced.

4.1 Introduction

In Chapter 3, Bones and Mineralized Tissues, the links between organized collagenous protein expression, directed assembly, and the ability of those organized proteins to mineralize were presented. It is certainly conceivable that there can be enough defects in the collagen I primary amino acid structure and higher order structures to prevent mineral formation. Hence proteins, even formed from collagen I, are only capable of mineralization if the protein structure is well organized.

In delving deeper in this chapter, it will become clear that many proteins devoid of mineral content are involved in composing human tissues. These bioviscoelastic solids are substantially more compliant, flexible, and capable of much larger displacements than mineralized tissues and compose a larger volume of human tissues and organs. Collagen, keratin, elastin, actin and myosin fibers, proteoglycans, and other proteins are commonly comingled and undergo their own forms of self-assembly to produce larger structures such as blood vessels and other segments of the vasculature, epidermal, and dermal tissues found in skin, hair, leaflets in cardiac valves, etc. Many of these soft tissues include cells that

Biomaterials. DOI: http://dx.doi.org/10.1016/B978-0-12-809478-5.00004-3

require oxygenation to keep the tissue viable in the long run. The heart is noted as a cellular organ that is extensively perfused. Without a vibrant and continuous blood supply to oxygenate its muscle cells, ischemic heart attack without a rapid intervention destroys the muscle cells and renders some fractions of the morbid heart muscle incapable of the same level of contraction before the event.

In this chapter, some very unique structures are discussed in detail. We also have books that discuss in great detail [1–4], subsections of this chapter. The hope here is to simply offer a few ideas about how to think about soft tissues, their composition and make-up, and some unique features of both internally- and externally-interconnected structures that are composed of soft tissues. It is also worth noting that with many different forms of soft tissue, there is some regenerative capacity noted with skin, hair, and nails to create new connective tissues continuously or semicontinuously or "on demand."

4.2 Protein Structure and Composition in the Circulatory System

The average blood vessel is one such soft tissue; a bioviscoelastic solid whose response is critical to sustain blood perfusion. We, humans, are composed of reams of vascular connections all distributed throughout the body. Laying our blood vessels end to end in an average person results in estimates of a combined length well into the thousands of kilometers [5]. The largest blood vessel is the aorta, which is approximately 1 inch in diameter in the average adult, while capillaries are more in the order of $5-10 \, \mu m$ in diameter.

Each vessel wall consists of three concentric layers, each with a different composition. The innermost layer is called the intima, the middle layer is called the media, and the outer layer is called the adventitia. Each layer is optimized by nature to yield a functioning structure that is viable for the long term. The innermost, intimal layer contains endothelial cells that form tight junctions to decrease the permeability of blood components out of fluid flowing through it. The presentation of endothelial cells on the inner surface tends to suppress platelet activation and maintains the viscosity of the fluid within the vessel. The intima also commonly contains a thin layer (80 nm thick) called the basal lamina, and in larger vessels, there are layers that contain an array of elastic fibrils, collagen fibrils, and some smooth muscle cells (SMCs). Whatever is contained in the intima has to transition to the medial layer; thus there is likely some sort of transition between the types of cells and proteins found as one moves from the intima to the medial layer.

The intermediate layer in the composite vessel sheath is called the medial layer and is made up primarily of SMCs. Encased with the SMCs are bundles of collagen, layers of elastin and these components are all found within a larger network of elastic fibrils. It is the perturbation of these elastic fibrils both within and external to the SMCs that results in a mechanical resilience or retraction force in the blood vessels to pulsatile pressures from cardiac output pushing blood into the aorta. As a result with each pressure pulse, the medial layer expands radially and recovers back to a baseline dimension or lumen dimension with each successive recovery. Depending on where one looks, the pressure pulse is rather large near the aorta, and as one moves to more peripheral vessels, the size of each pressure pulse diminishes. So the intermediate medial layer's crucial function is to provide the functional retraction response.

The adventitial sheath in the average blood vessel is composed of fibroblasts, collagen, proteoglycans, and some nerve connections. The adventitia layer is designed to support the medial layer, and to prevent any larger distortion of the tissue, for example, there should be a stress concentration due to a local variation in the thickness of the medial layer. The fibroblasts can supplement the amount of connective tissue found within each adventitial layer, and the mean pressure creates a smaller overall displacement of the vessel, with a larger adventitial thickness.

It is exquisite how nature can direct the culturing of endothelial cells, SMCs, and fibroblasts harmoniously to produce this composite sheath in such a wide variety of compositions and to direct them accordingly to where they are needed for higher strength, higher resilience, etc.

Nature recognizes that pulsatile flow near the heart requires one type of resilience and more peripheral vasculature does not have the same overpressures and mechanical design requirements. As a result, average vessel composition and properties change as a function of how much farther down the distribution network an artery is from the heart. Table 4.1 shows the relative amounts of elastin found in the medial layer of arterial tissue within

Table 4.1: Elastin content measured in arterial tissue taken from various arteries depending on location from the heart

Artery	Medial Elastin Fraction (%)	1 SD	Medial Elastin Fraction (%)	1 SD
	From Dinardo et al.		From Fung	
Femoral	14.3	1.29%		
Renal	8.8	1		
Abdominal aorta	12.2	2.71		
Carotid	17.3	1.71		
Mammary	42.7	2.43		
Thoracic aorta	55.2	2.43	36%	~10%
Coronary	4.3	3.85		
Pulmonary			16.7%	~5%
Plantar			3.3%	~2%

Source: Data is taken from C.L. Dinardo, G. Venturini, E.H. Zhou, L.S. Watanabe, L.C.G. Campos, R. Dariolli, et al., Variation of mechanical properties and quantitative proteomics of VSMC along the arterial tree. Am. J. Physiol.-Heart Circ. Physiol. (306) (2014) H505–H516; Y.C. Fung, Biomechanics: Mechanical Properties of Living Tissues, Springer, New York, 1993.

different arterial regions [6,7]. One would expect that the arteries containing much larger elastic fiber content are much more likely to recover or retract to each pressure pulse from the heart. Those arteries much farther away sense less pulsatile flow and do not have the same resilience requirements as the more peripheral pressure pulses are damped or dissipated along the vasculature.

The variation in protein composition manifests itself in terms of differences in mechanical behavior when arterial segments from different artery locations are mechanically loaded in static tension. Fig. 4.1 shows the mechanical response for relaxed bovine aorta, carotid artery, and vena cavae when cut into longitudinal segments and tested along the vessel direction, i.e., longitudinally or sectioned and stretched transverse to the vessel direction using a uniaxial loading frame [8]. Each shows a characteristic high compliance at low strain followed by a steeper, strain-hardening region. The network of elastin fibers acts as a crosslinked network and retards further stretching as the linkages between network segments become more taut. This behavior is analogous to other lightly crosslinked rubbery polymers.

Even under normal physiologic pressures, the elastic fibers are more taut but the structural fibers are still rather wavy and unaligned. In more hypertensive vessels, a larger fraction of the structural collagen fibers found in the adventitia is load bearing, with a much more pronounced effect on reducing compliance, a key feature in hypertension [9].

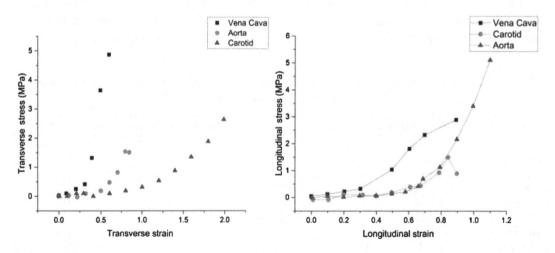

Figure 4.1
Mean incremental tensile stress—strain curves for the aorta, vena cava, and carotid artery evaluated in the transverse (L) and longitudinal directions (R). *Reproduced with permission from F.H., Silver, P.B. Snowhill, D.J. Foran, Mechanical behavior of vessel wall: a comparative study of aorta, vena cava, and carotid artery, Ann. Biomed. Eng. 31 (2003) 793—803. [8].*

Venous tissue is structurally different, that is more compliant than arterial tissue, and can expand under much more mild pressurization conditions. It is likely due to subtle variations in the organization of the adventitial layers and perhaps a looser medial network that allows for this larger response to pressure. The difference between venous and arterial tissue also suggests why there is a distinction in the biomechanics of the anastomosis between the arterial segments and the graft segments extracted from the saphenous vein during autografting for coronary bypass (Fig. 4.2).

Clearly, nature has designed a larger degree of elastic resilience into tissues more likely to sense peak pressures in arterial vasculature linked with the coordination of valve openings and closings in the heart. People with coronary artery blockages would benefit from bypass procedures that used vascular substitutes with a similar degree of elastin content included to replicate the behavior of the blocked artery when it was viable. Often, for bypass, it is more of a function of what is available and its viability. There are other types of cardiovascular

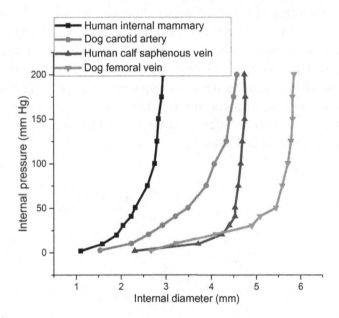

Figure 4.2

Data comparing arterial and venous radial displacement with internal pressurization. *Reproduced from P.B. Dobrin, Mechanical behavior of vascular smooth muscle in cylindrical segments of arteries in vitro, Ann. Biomed. Eng. (12) (1984) 497–510; F.N. Littooy, J. Golan, B. Blakeman, J. Fareed, P.B. Dobrin, Intimal hyperplasia and medial thickening in autogenous vein bypass grafts: influence of anastomoses and platelet-inhibiting drugs, Assoc. Acad. Surg., Abstracts Sci. Papers (1981); P.B. Dobrin, T. Canfield, J. Moran, H. Sullivan, R. Pifarre, Coronary artery bypass: the physiological basis for differences in flow with internal mammary artery and saphenous vein grafts, J. Thorac. Cardiovasc. Surg. (74) (1977) 445–454; P.B. Dobrin, A.A. Rovick, Influence of vascular smooth muscle on contractile mechanics and elasticity of arteries, Am. J. Physiol. (217) (1969) 1644–1652 [10–13].*

complications that can arise within arterial tissue that possesses a specific biomechanical response and it is not always exactly replicated.

With an aging cardiovascular system, cholesterol-based plaques deposited within the medial and adventitial layers can often result in arteriosclerosis, a perceived hardening of the arteries that also leads to more retarded behavior during pulsatile flow. Hardening can occur not only within the coronary arteries but also more systemically. Arteriosclerotic arteries extend less under pressure and recover slowly with longer time constants when unpressurized. The lack of a volumetric capacity increase due to the vessel expansion under pulsatile pressure can raise the arterial pressure required to provide sufficient perfusion. Under these instances, the composition of the arteriosclerotic vessels is clearly different than a normal adult vessel.

There are other pathologies that are known to result in connective tissue disorders that affect cardiovascular performance. An example is Marfan's syndrome in which there is a clear issue with the resilience of the blood vessels from one loading to the next. The Marfan's aorta is composed of substantially less elastin (57 vs ~30%) on a dry weight basis of total protein, while more collagen was also found in the Marfan tissue, relative to controls [14]. That subtly is borne out when doing mechanical assessments of Marfan vessel tissue. Fig. 4.3 shows data comparing the aorta response, from a loading and a reloading event, of a normal person with a patient suffering from the connective tissue disorder Marfan's syndrome [15]. Clearly the elastic quality of the Marfan aorta is less responsive than the control group during a 2nd loading.

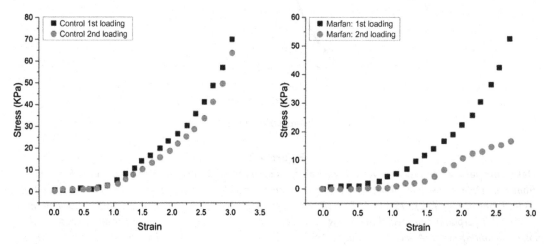

Figure 4.3
Comparison of the stress–strain diagrams of aorta tested twice in succession between a control group and one suffering from Marfan's syndrome [15]. Consider the wide distinction between the second loading response after an initial unloading.

There are other broader connective tissue disorders such as Ehlers Danlos syndrome, commonly related to Marfan's syndrome that affects the quality of the vasculature structure. While Ehlers Danlos is more commonly linked with hyper-elastic skin, the presence of more extensive bruising is also found suggesting that the vasculature can be more easily ruptured in Ehlers Danlos patients relative to control populations [16]. One complication is that Ehlers Danlos tends to be graded based on skin extensibility, which has made it more complicated in fully characterizing the distinction.

4.3 Protein Structure of Valvular Tissue and Leaflets

Valves found in the heart are complex organizations of connective tissue generally organized to direct one-way flow of blood when these function correctly. There are four valves found within the heart—the aortic valve, the mitral valve, the pulmonary valve, and the tricuspid valve. The walls of each valve are like other vascular tissue in that endothelial cells line the intima region of each valve. They are designed to be structurally inert while the leaflets are more compliant and under chamber pressures to open and close in coordinated ways by a common overlapping leaflet strategy. The valves have a specialized tissue called a hinge that directs leaflet growth toward the center of the valve where blood flows through it. The leaflets are very flexible, soft tissues coated with endothelial cells on their blood contacting surfaces, like other segments of vascular tissue.

Between the chamber regions, each leaflet has a series of layers called lamina. As many as five distinct layers can be found making up the lamina. The layers consist of collagen, elastic fibers, and within the interstices of the connective tissue, smooth muscle and fibroblastic cells are also found, not unlike that making up the vessel wall. The thickness of the aortic leaflets is $\sim 1.7\,\mu m$ which is thin enough to be almost transparent. The leaflets thicken near the hinge region where it interfaces with the wall of the valve [17]. These very thin leaflets jut out into the flow region are very compliant and successfully overlap to seal the gap between chambers or between a heart chamber and the corresponding artery to which it is linked. An example is the aortic valve, shown in Fig. 4.4, demonstrates the leaflet alignment during the systole cycle (open valve condition) and the diastole cycle (closed valve condition). A separate image of a pulmonary valve, identifying the left anterior leaflet (L.A.L.), the right anterior leaflet (R.A.L.), and the posterior leaflet is shown in Fig. 4.5.

4.3.1 Valve and Leaflet Defects

Later in Chapter 13, Cardiovascular Interventions, there is a larger discussion about clinical interventions relating to conditions that lead to cardiac regurgitation. Generally, any structural or aging phenomenon that retards the ability of leaflets to overlap and seal

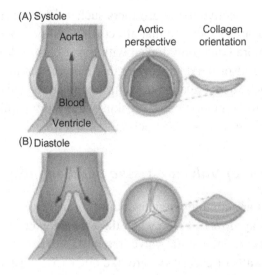

Figure 4.4

Schematic of the aortic valve in both systole (open) and diastolic (closed) conditions. *Reproduced with permission from J.D. Hutcheson, E. Alkwas, W.D. Merryman, Potential drug targets for calcific aortic calve disease, Nat. Rev. Cardiol (11) (2014) 218–231 [18].*

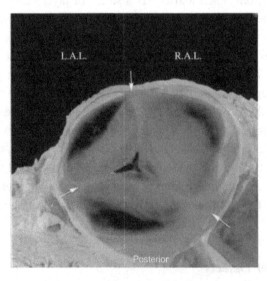

Figure 4.5

The pulmonary valve identifying the three distinct leaflets composing it. *Republished with permission from M. Misfeld, H.-H. Sievers, Heart valve macro- and microstructure, Philos. Trans. R. Soc. Lond., B: Biol. Sci. (362) (2007) 1421–1438 [17].*

adequately resulting in some amount of back flow or regurgitation. This back flow has a profound effect on cardiac efficiency and is clearly noticeable for a patient under load. Stress tests are easy indicators for someone with a cardiac insufficiency and once that insufficiency is diagnosed, the larger question is what is the root cause. Insufficiency could result from a lack of heart muscle coordination requiring a new pacing strategy or from seal problems. One common problem that affects the sealing efficiency and results in regurgitation is the precipitation of inorganic calcium salts onto the leaflet surfaces. As these precipitates nucleate and grow on these very flexible leaflets, the responsiveness of the leaflets to flow become much more sluggish. The leaflets harden and thicken, and often one leaflet does not mesh with the other leaflets as seamlessly. If leaflets are required to have facile movement to rapidly seal with each cycle of cardiac coordination, often the inability to seal in a timely manner results in regurgitation. Some of these regurgitation events require new valve assemblies to replace normal valvular function.

The hardening of arteries linked with arteriosclerosis can also harden the leaflets. These leaflets are designed to be very responsive and if that response is affected either by calcium deposits on the surface or fatty deposits within the lamina, the same general endpoint is achieved. Again, there are more details provided in Chapters 6 and 13, Environmental Effects on Natural Tissues; and Cardiovascular Interventions.

4.3.2 Aneurysms and Fistulae

Arteries are designed to withstand relatively high-cardiac output pressures and veins tend to be more expansive operating at lower pressure but accommodating any dynamic volume flow characteristics since they are a more complaint tissues. There are statistical fluctuations in the thickness and composition of vessel wall, and at any sustained load imparted by the dynamic blood pressure, some areas are inherently at higher stress. So as long as wall stresses are fully relieved with each cardiac cycle, the vessels are stable. But if the internal pressure is sufficiently high because the patient is hypertensive, or segments of the walls are weak enough, the weakened sections can bulge under load and those bulges can grow and ultimately rupture. These localized bulges are called aneurysms, discussed in Chapter 13, Cardiovascular Interventions. Fundamentally, the largest interest in addressing aneurysm is related to better diagnostics (see Chapter 10: Nanomaterials and Phase Contrast Imaging Agents) and understanding the link between other connective tissue attributes and the risk factors for aneurysm. With so many aneurysm conditions remaining undiagnosed, more sophisticated screening tools will have a big impact.

The formation of a fistula is the result of any abnormal anastomosis between blood vessels. The ones that are a larger concern are when arterials at high pressure and veins commonly at lower pressure form junctions, as the large pressure drop forcing blood through capillary flow regions results in a much lower pressure normally acting on veins. Without the capillaries in the resistive network, the natural arterial pressure on a vein causes a large expansion in its vessel diameter. Fistulae can occur under a variety of conditions including congenital formations, but perhaps more often, that arise from infection or from inflammation and the junctions randomly form.

With fistulae, the issue is whether the downstream vasculature is viable with the increased pressure. The resulting connective tissue composition and architecture are important regulating factors. Any abnormalities in either the composition or the properties of the expanded vessels puts those with an fistula at risk for a bleed.

4.3.3 Aortic Dissection

If the internal vascular pressure is sufficient to rupture a blood vessel wall, whether it is from an anastomosis, an aneurysm, or some other vascular anomaly, the outcome will result in a bleed, which could be clearly observable by diagnostics. It is possible to tear at layers of the sheath composing a blood vessel if the cohesive linkages between the layers are not strong without causing a complete rupture. This type of anomaly is called a dissection, which usually results in tearing between the endothelial and the medial layers of the vessel. Dissection as a significant vascular event has been diagnosed more directly in the aorta, probably due to the life threatening complications if sufficient amount of blood seeps into the forming cavity space within the vessel to create an insufficiency through the normal aorta.

Aortic dissection is life threatening, and commonly requires vascular grafts to replace the failed vessel. Aortic dissection is unsurprisingly linked with hypertension as higher pressures will tend to stress weaker tissues more, and approximately 20% of the cases are linked with connective tissue disorders including Marfan Syndrome, Ehlers Danlos syndrome, and other conditions where the cohesiveness of the connective tissue is in question. Those patients afflicted with other connective tissue disorders tend to present at ages between 30 and 40, much earlier than those suffering from hypertension. There are also some grades to an Ehlers Danlos diagnosis, so perhaps there are subpopulations within these designations at more risk for these vascular tearing events. Synthetic grafts are the common fix for those who are diagnosed early enough to designate them for surgery. Because of the rapid decline in patients during dissection if it is occurring away from a clinic, minutes matter. Again, more details are found in Chapter 13.

4.4 Dermal Tissues, Including Hair and Nerves

4.4.1 The Skin

The skin (also called the integument) is one of the largest organs in humans on a volume basis. There are distinct layers of connective tissue as one traverses from the outermost layers of skin to sublayers with both different compositions and functions. Skin is exceedingly well designed to address a number of different functional design requirements. There are several different barrier features that skin performs including the sustenance of internal pressure in vivo and containing vital organs contained within, there also is a mechanical protection attribute for mechanical contusions and impacts imparted on skin are dissipated as the impact is transmitted through and while bruising and hematomas result, often internal organs are spared. Furthermore, the skin acts as a reasonable chemical barrier with its combination of lipophilic and hydrophilic elements. It is also resistant to parasitic attack and the capacity to exfoliate the outer layers allows skin to have a reasonable bacterial resistance as well.

In addition to the role as a mechanical insulator, skin also acts as a reasonable mediator of both hypothermic and hyperthermic excursions, maintains internal temperatures under steady state that allow active metabolism, and allows sweat release during an overheated condition that allows the skin surfaces to be cooled through passive free convection of the sweat off of the skin surfaces.

Skin also contains hair bulbs and shafts, sweat pores, and functional heat and pressure sensors coupled with a nervous system network to convey signals and to detect tissue responses accordingly. Also contained within skin are connective tissue proteins such as collagen, elastin, keratin, and proteoglycans from which much of skin's mechanical behavior can be derived. Also contained in skin are blood vessels, fibroblastic cells and other cell types, and sentry cells such as T and B cells linked with the acquired immune response.

4.4.2 The Subcutaneous or Adipose Tissues

The innermost layers of the subcutaneous or sub-Q-dermis, are filled with adipocytes (fat cells) from which skin's thermal insulating capacity is enhanced. The adipocytes tend to form fat globules and there is a vasculature that can feed the cells found within the subcutaneous fat layer. The thickness of human adipose tissue or subdermis depends on anatomical location, sex, and relative obesity. Fat layer thicknesses between 20 and 50 mm are common [19], and with increasing human obesity, even thicker fat layers can be found. The human adipose layer is much thinner than that of the arctic animals; for example, fat layer thicknesses measured on Antarctic mink whales also depends on sex and anatomical location, but the layer thicknesses on the dorsal side of the mature males range on average from 40 to 170 mm in thickness; and for pregnant females from 44 to 180 mm in thickness [20]. The thicker fat layer in mink whales is one good reason why cold-water mammals are viable by insulating their vasculature more effectively than humans who are susceptible to hypothermia.

The notion of liposuction is linked with extracting liquid and gel-like fat tissue from the subdermis in an attempt to reduce body mass. It happens naturally with aging, where there is a common redistribution of subcutaneous fat that no longer keeps the outer layers of skin so taut from internal pressure. Hence, the origin of crow's feet and frowning brows, not from any deep change in the dermal or epidermal structure, but more from the fact that these tissues are not as stretched and relax. More on the relaxation of dermal tissues is included in Chapter 6, Environmental Effects on Natural Tissues, relating to environmental aging of tissues.

4.4.3 The Dermis

Moving outward from the subcutaneous dermis, the dermis layer is encountered, which is also a strong function of anatomical location. Around the head, dermal thickness is on the order of 1 mm thick and ranges in general from 0.3 mm to ~1.3 mm [21]. More generally across the body, the dermal thickness ranges between 0.3 and 4 mm in thickness and consists of two distinct layers. There is a thinner papillary layer near the epidermal junction that includes ridges and asperities to conform to the epidermal feature dimensions and is mostly composed of collagenous and elastic fibers, capillaries to nourish the epidermal layers and nerves [22]. Below the papillary region is the reticular dermis which is thicker than papillary dermis and consists of an interwoven series of collagen fibers contained within an elastic fiber network [23]. Also contained with the dermis is a substantial amount of hydrophilic proteoglycans that tend to swell dermal tissue and to make it appears softer. Dry connective tissue in skin has roughly 70% collagen, the bulk of the remaining tissue is elastic fibers, and as little as 0.2%–0.5% proteoglycans [24]. But these hydrophilic gels swell substantially (as much as 1000 times their own weight) and ultimately make up a relatively large fraction of the tissue mass once fully hydrated. The bulk of the hair cells, nerve fibers, and other structural features of the sensory system are also found in the reticular dermis layer. Within mature skin, some number of dormant fibroblasts exist that can be activated to form new connective tissue after wounding.

It is the interconnectedness of the elastic network and the collagen I fibers from which the skin derives most of its mechanical response and properties. It is also known that during wound healing, the new skin tissue deposited is less organized and contains more collagen III than the virgin tissue. There are also other unknowns about traces of other collagens and their role in regulated tissue behavior. There are also known genetic defects that affect the network density of the elastic network and can result in substantially more stretchable skin than again what is commonly found. Skin is clearly viscoelastic meaning that the tissue response depends on the scheme for loading (see more in Chapter 5: Property Assessments of Tissues), and is also Non-Hookean in that a nonlinear strain-hardening response occurs as the network is stretched. If simple, quasistatic mechanical loadings are imparted on skin and if it is assumed that most of the strain is accommodated in the dermis region, a reasonable assumption provides its relatively thickness, estimates for the Young's modulus of elasticity, a measure of resistance to deformation of the skin ranges from 0.42 MPa for normal younger skin to 0.85 MPa for more mature skin [25]. Distinctions in mechanical behavior depend on the level of displacement. A higher modulus tissue might be more linked with strain hardening in the tissue, and perhaps not a direct measurement of a linear stress−strain diagram. It could be that with age, more network crosslinks form through and that could be the distinction between younger and older skin on the outside. Clearly variations in the amount of hydration in the tissue could also be a significant effect on the volume fraction of polysaccharide in any tissue specimen and that is a concern with any measurement that uses extracted tissue that is not properly conditioned.

It is worth noting that the dermis is also a regenerative organ and is a cellular tissue as well. There are several subtypes of dermal fibroblasts found in dermis are capable of producing connective tissue [26]. There are probably other subfunctions that target the specificity of the different subtypes in many ways. These distinctions remain an interest from a research perspective. There are also muscle cells found within tissue that are exceedingly important to allow for contractile responses during wound healing. There are also hemipoetic stem cells present [26] that may in fact be directed to form specific fibroblasts or muscle cells when appropriately activated. There are open questions about how active aging dermal fibroblasts constituted in skin are in older, more mature patients [27]. There are also questions about how much turnover is there within dermal tissues, particularly as dermal fibroblasts age with their owner.

Dermal tissue is also laid down in a subtly oriented fashion, which is more pronounced if one creates a circular hole in tissue, that hole shape is altered by the relative alignment of the fibers making up the dermal network. The general alignment of soft tissue fiber networks has been established and anatomical maps of these alignments are available and noted as Langer's lines [28].

4.4.4 The Stratum Corneum and Epidermis

Perhaps the most interesting and unique architecture in skin is linked with the epidermal layer, an avascular and regenerative tissue that is nourished by osmosis and permeation through nearby vascular regions. A cartoon schematic of the epidermis including the dermis junction is shown in Fig. 4.6. The epidermis varies in thickness from 0.05 mm on the eyelids to about 1 mm in other areas of the body. Generally if the dermis is thin, so is the corresponding epidermal layer to which it is attached.

The business end of the epidermis is the proximal region of this tissue, which is called the basement membrane. This membrane is identified by a single layer of keratinocytes, cells that produce keratin as they age, that are all organized and aligned with tight junctions between them which tend to distort their shape into more box-like structures. The layer of cells follows that asperities in the epidermal structure, for example, the basement membrane keratinocytes are also aligned into the pore where a hair protrudes through it. These cells are clearly identified as eukaryotic cells as the nucleus is clearly identifiable. There are no blood vessels in the epidermal layer, so hydration and growth factors required for cell activities have to be derived by permeation across the membrane.

Cells found at this boundary undergo mitosis, that is creating new cells at the same junction between the dermis and epidermis and the process of continuously forming new cells acts to distend the existing cells from the basement membrane where they are less nourished. Keratinocytes are programmed to produce keratin as they age, and as a result, older cells possess more solid protein than newly formed cells. Aging of keratinocytes, as they are conveyed away from the membrane, raises the relative ratio of solid/liquid fraction in them, and ultimately triggers other types of structural changes that alter the shape, composition, and cohesive strength between one cell and its nearest neighbors.

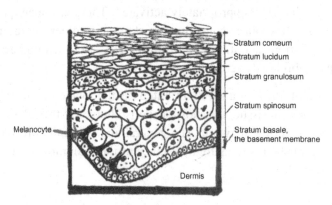

Figure 4.6

The identification of layers present in the epidermis. The most hydrated keratinocytes are found at the basement membrane, and are dislodged by continued expression of new cells. Structural changes in the shape, size, and solid phase fraction of each cell arise with cell age and the progression is linked with the layers here. Hardened corneocytes, the outermost cells that have flattened and released their lipiphilic residues are flaked off by exfoliation shown at the top.

Pigmentation in skin arises from specialized cells called melanocytes. These cells tend to be slightly larger (~ 7 to 8 μm in diameter) than keratinocytes and are also found at the basement membrane. Nominally, there are ~ 1000 melanocytes found/mm^2 of membrane, $\sim 5\%$ to 10% of the basement membrane constitutes melanocytes [29]. The melanocytes produce pigment-containing melanosomes that are uptaken and precipitated in adjacent keratinocytes. Depending on the amount of melanin produced, there are fundamental differences in the level of pigmentation. It is not necessarily more melanocytes but the same melanocytes are more efficient at expressing melanosomes in darker skinned individuals [29].

Sectioning of a typical epidermal tissue sample resolves several distinct layers that essentially represent the entire cycle of aging of keratinocytes as they form at membrane and are exfoliated on the outer surfaces, presented schematically in Fig. 4.6. As skin cells are displaced from the basement membrane, they progress through several different states or layers, identified as the stratum basale, the stratum spinosum, the stratum granulosum, and the stratum corneum. Keratinocytes progress through these stages as they are progressively displaced from the stratum basale and transform. For example, the tight junctions between cells tend to disappear as cell are displaced, they still retain an identifiable nucleus in the stratum spinosum, but they become more rounded, constituting a layer of ~ 8 cells thick or ~ 40 μm. Keratinocytes found in the stratum granulosum tend to flatten as more keratin is found in the cytosol, they lose their identified nucleus and initiate apoptosis, with the layer being ~ 4 cells thick. The stratum corneum is the outermost layer and consists of 20–30 layers of pancake-like cells that have flattened extensively, ruptured, and released their lipid-rich fractions in the interstices between pancakes. The relative cohesive strength of the stratum corneum is regulated by both the lipids holding the individual pancake layers together and the overall level of hydration. If the tissue is more dehydrated, there is less cohesive energy holding dead keratinocytes or corneocytes together. The process of scratching or abrading skin on its surface is called exfoliation, usually resulting in the sloughing of a whitish residue of dead corneocytes. To summarize, there are gradients in the level of hydration, the level of precipitated protein, and intracellular cohesive strength as one traverses from the stratum basale to the stratum corneum.

Any effort to leverage skin as a medium for molecular transport leads to the revelation that any functional molecule requires facile permeation through both lipophilic corneocytes and hydrophilic keratinocytes closer to the basement membrane. There is a rationale why only small molecules with a relatively low molecular mass and amphiphilic characteristics have the best chance to permeate skin. It also explains why skin is such an effective barrier. Nonetheless, some molecules percolate through, and can often lead to a dermatitis problem if these molecules are adding to the T-cell and B-cell sensitivity subsurface to the basement membrane.

It is also worth noting that any wound that occurs within the epidermis will leave no scar, as the outer tissue is completely regenerated with each successive turnover of the cells at the basement membrane. Wounds that pierce the basement membrane will bleed if they ultimately rupture components of the vasculature that are only found below the membrane. Deeper wounds will require platelet activation and a corresponding wound healing response that can often accompany a scar. Many other references spend extensive time on the process of wound healing, the formation of granulation tissue, the deconstruction of the wounded site, and the recruitment of new cells to rebuild the connective tissue network where the wound is located. Any device that is installed will be exposed to this cascade and that needs to be accounted for in both device and wound healing.

Increasingly, people are aware that the natural processes that occur at the basement membrane can sometimes go haywire with aging, leading to diseases, the most common to the reader include skin cancers of a variety of different cell types. In Chapter 6, Environmental Effects on Natural Tissues, the formation of tumors is mentioned, those types of cell dysfunctions at the basement membrane are linked to basal and squamous cell carcinoma. Those relating to the dysfunction of the melanocytes are linked with melanoma.

4.4.5 Skin Care as a Business

Of course as time marches on, one is more likely to encounter skin cancers and other skin conditions that are all part of the generally-understood, natural-aging process. Any trip to the personal care section of the grocery store will confirm that there are many different products vetted and sold commercially as cosmetics, skin conditioners, soaps, oils, and other cleaners that are designed to enhance texture or softness, or to or limit the damage to skin structures. Considering the economy of scale, it is worth noting that skin, nail and hair care affects everyone, while a much smaller subset of affected individuals are presenting clinical conditions requiring clinical management. This comment is made not to discount the aspects of dermatological conditions requiring clinical interventions, but there is just as much biomedical engineering and biomaterials development involved in understanding the performance characteristics of cosmetics and creams as in eradicating acne for example. The science of cosmetics could benefit from more formally trained researchers and engineers who have a larger understanding of skin, nail, and hair physiology. There is much that has been learned from prior lessons about formulated additives in commercial skin products and any latent issues relating to contact dermatitis.

It is one thing to be applying creams and moisturizers on skin surfaces. The proliferation of skin inks and tattooing as decorative features for skin is more invasive as opposed to relying on passive absorption and mass transfer to interact with skin, tattoo inks are directly injected bypassing the normal barrier functions of skin to prevent its interaction. There has been an evolution in the types of dyes used moving away from metal and organometallics. An example analysis of skin tattoo pigments included in one type of commercial ink kit is included in Table 4.2. There is an increasing interest in organic inks and the ones that can

Table 4.2: Analysis of tattoo inks supplied in a commercial kit by Huck Spaulding Inc. and determined by X-ray fluorescence [30]

Stock No.	Color	Titanium (22)	Aluminum (13)	Silica (14)	Copper (29)	Chromium (24)	Iron (26)	Chlorine (17)	Sulfur (16)	Carbon (6)	Oxygen (8)	Magnesium (12)
8001	Black	...	0.25	...	...	...	85.95	...	0.29	...	13.51	...
8007	White	98.55	1.45	...	...	...	...	...	...	...	...	...
8016	Fire red	...	26.21	...	...	...	...	9.68	10.76	23.29	30.06	...
8022	Flesh No.1 (tan)	74.27	1.75	...	...	...	23.98	...	...	...	...	...
8031	Indian brown	41.98	0.76	...	...	...	57.26	...	...	...	...	...
9001	Crimson red	...	...	17.2	...	...	...	...	...	49.36	22.25	11.19
9002	Devil's red	27.65	2.6	0.53	...	...	...	...	...	51.67	17.55	...
9008	Lotus (red)	40.17	3.2	...	...	...	...	...	...	17.71	38.92	...
9009	Venetian brown	...	0.38	1.73	...	...	79.85	...	...	...	18.04	...
9014	Florida orange	...	...	...	...	...	...	...	...	84.35	15.65	...
9017	Lemon yellow	53.06	1.86	...	...	...	...	...	...	23.9	21.18	...
9022	White	96.41	3.59	...	...	...	...	...	...	...	...	...
9023	Black	...	...	...	...	...	87.98	...	...	...	12.02	...
9024	Permanent green	...	0.89	...	13.32	...	...	51.55	...	34.24	...	...
9025	Emerald green	5.45	0.49	...	...	72.66	...	4.15	...	...	17.25	...
9026	Pine green	44.34	4.08	...	8.27	...	...	6.71	...	14.64	21.96	...
9029	Parrot green	44.34	4.08	...	8.27	...	...	6.71	...	14.64	21.96	...
9036	Sky blue	37.95	1.9	...	11.06	...	...	2.16	...	35.41	11.52	...
9061	Blue green	...	1.14	...	14.46	...	...	52.24	...	32.16	...	...
9090	Cerise (red)	51.51	2.18	...	...	...	15.34	...	...	9.81	21.16	...
9091	Yukon white	94.98	5.02	...	...	...	...	...	...	...	...	...
9092	Misty green	51.5	2.51	...	...	...	...	3.59	...	18.43	23.97	...
9093	Misty blue	94.82	4.13	...	...	...	...	1.05	...	...	...	...
9094	Tulip yellow	27.29	2.29	0.22	...	...	...	2.29	0.3	37.3	30.31	...
9095	Peony (pink)	63.77	2.38	...	...	...	...	...	...	13.85	20	...
9096	New blue	50.93	2.36	...	8.54	...	...	1.39	...	18.21	18.57	...
9097	Blush (orange)	58.06	2.25	...	...	...	...	2.87	...	14.39	22.43	...
9098	Wild violet	65.29	2.88	...	...	...	...	...	...	9.56	22.27	...
9099	Tulip red	...	0.19	13.4	...	...	...	...	...	52.29	25.12	9
Not applicable	India ink	...	...	...	...	...	...	...	...	92.19	7.81	...

Element

be more easily faded or deconstructed, as the cost of removing tattoos is as much as it costs to perform the initial tattooing procedure.

4.5 Hair

4.5.1 Hair Morphology

Keratinocytes and melanocytes are fully functional at the basement membrane. Other production of keratin occurs in the hair bulb that is found well within dermis and is also known as a dermal papilla, shown in Fig. 4.7.

There are four stages of the hair cycle—the growth phase (anagen), catagen, telegen, and exogen phases. Each bulb is vascularized to nourish the growing cells found there. A similar process of mitosis occurs similar to what is found at the basement membrane where newly divided keratinocytes work to extrude the older cells away from the bulb. Similar to what happens in epidermis, as the cells migrate from its nourishment pathway, the living elements tend to initiate apoptosis. There are equivalent melanocytes that are found in the hair shafts that help to provide color and pigmentation to the growing hair being extruded in the shaft in the lower root sheath. The hair is really made of three different concentric sheaths. The innermost portion of the hair is called the medulla. The role of the medulla is subject to conjecture, but structurally, it contains relatively large cells and is typically devoid of pigment. The annulus formed around the medulla is called the cortex and contains more organized keratinocytes and melanocytes that convey the pigments produced in hair into the cells. The cortex also comprises most of the mass of the actual hair.

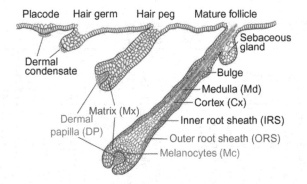

Figure 4.7

The evolving hair follicle, showing that new keratinocytes are added in the dermal papilla and matrix, pigmented by adjacent melanocytes. The process of adding keratinocytes to the cortex tends to extend the fiber length and extrude the fiber through the hair pore. *Reproduced with permission from M. Rendl, L. Lewis, E. Fuchs, Molecular signatures of the developing hair follicle. PLoS Biol. 3 (11) (2005) e366. doi:10.1371/journal.pbio.0030366 [31].*

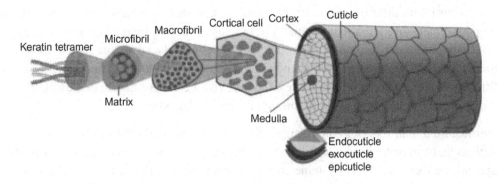

Figure 4.8

Schematic of how an individual hair scales from keratin to a single strand, showing the medulla, cortex, and cuticle. *Reproduced with permission from C.F. Cruz, C. Costa, A.C. Gomes, T. Matama, A. Cavaco-Paulo, Human hair and the impact of cosmetic procedures: a review on cleansing and shape-modulating cosmetics, Cosmetics (3) (2016) 26 [32].*

The presence of more cysteine found in keratin allows for more sulfur-crosslinking between aligned keratin fibers and increased resilience in healthy hair.

The cuticle is a protective wrap that helps to protect the cortex from other environmental interactions. The cuticle is not necessarily an individual protective layer, but an ensemble of integrated fibers that coalesce over the cortex and control the relative water content found in the hair itself. Healthy hair possesses a sharkskin-like morphology, and it can vary in smoothness. More water in the hair will weaken its structure and even wearing longer hair raises the load on the hair shaft just due to gravity. There are instances from heat or other chemical damage that makes the cuticle friable, hence the origin of split ends. The fix for this is to cut the fraying segments to retain cuticle regions that are more integrated and less fractured.

All three layers tend to be coextruded down the hair shaft, shown in Fig. 4.8. Hair tends to grow slowly, with typical growth rates of ~ 1 cm/month. Similar to epidermis, hair is most living near its vascular connections and keratinocytes contained with hair tend to die with hair length. The process of extruding hair fibers out of the upper root sheath would be harder and require higher pressures to push these hairs through the pore regions. Hairs are commonly lubricated by sebaceous oils released from reservoirs into the hair shaft regions that tend to lubricate the fibers as they are being extruded.

4.5.2 Features and Attributes of Hair

A keen observation is that type of pore through which hair is extruded has a keen effect on the relative curliness of hair being expressed. Hair extrusion through a circular pore (aspect ratio of 1, comparing the major and minor axes) as it protrudes from the upper root sheath of skin outward with little torque on it; the resulting hair that protrudes tends to be straight. As the pore dimensions are altered from a circle to an oval with increasing aspect ratio (1.1−1.2 comparing the major and minor axes), torques are placed on the hair shaft as it protrudes. An even larger aspect ratio tends to make hair even curlier. There are hair conditioners that can make curly more relaxed and vice versa, but the inherent torque resolves from extruding circular hairs through a noncircular pore.

Another feature of hair relates to the relative clinginess of hair, derived from electrostatic interactions that can make it more difficult to isolate one hair from others. There are disulfide linkages arising from the higher cysteine content found in keratin that is less prevalent in collagen. As a result, there are instances in dry environments where it is challenging to comb through thick and curly hair. The functionality of dispersions like conditioners are designed with the notion of coating individual hair with surfactant molecules that allow for more effective hair repulsion allowing more easy untangling and combing.

Hair is also peculiar in that one does have a single, continuous growth phase, but undergoes follicle release and regeneration of hair follicles. Each hair cycle has its cycle of growth, dormancy, and regeneration. Hair growth is classified in terms of several specific stages, the longest phase is identified as the anagen phase, a growth phase, which typically lasts several years linked with a 1-cm/month growth rate. Periodically, at the end of the anagen phase, some small fraction of cells can enter the categen phase, a period less than 2 weeks typically where the hair follicle shrinks and decouples from the hair dermal papilla. Hair can progress to either the telogen or exogen phases. The telogen phase is linked with a stable, rest phase where the hair is not growing but not being shed either. The telogen phase can occur over a period of months, typically while a new follicle is being formed. The exogen phase results from shedding of hair follicles that have been displaced close enough to the surface where they can be decoupled from the pore and down the drain during washing. The long cycle of the anagen phase allows one to consider hair analysis as a marker for historical metabolism and physiological health, as discussed in Chapter 15, Special Topics: Assays Applied to Both Health and Sports. If one has stable hair growth, there is a net balance between hairs being lost in the exogen phase and new hair cells being activated in the anagen phase. For those suffering from net hair loss, there are efforts to influence the relative lengths of the different hair growth phases to bias the anagen phase.

Therapies and even clinical procedures can result in altered hair growth. A common side effect of systemic chemotherapy has been temporary hair loss [33]. It is also noted that as an outcome of X-ray fluoroscopy, commonly used for endovascular surgeries where there is no direct line of sight, skin surfaces are under constant fluoroscopic observation during a procedure. Those areas often do not have a lower density of hair cells after the procedure as the anagen phase of many exposed hair cells in the field of view is often destroyed [34]. Fluoroscopy can also burn skin tissues of sufficiently overexposed.

4.5.3 Hair as a Business

The same comments presented earlier relating to the issue of hair being a commodity that affects everyone apply. If one has too much hair in the wrong places, there is a desire to get rid of it. Similarly, there is substantial intellectual property in reversing the evolution of baldness, which requires substantial understanding of hair physiology. A range of products are available to alter the color and texture of hair products, and there is a separate section in the grocery store for the products to interface with skin and hair tissues. Hair, like skin, is one of these egalitarian features we are born with. The care of hair requires each of us to maintain it accordingly, and perhaps some better than others.

4.6 Nails

Nails are also regenerative structures that also produce keratin but in a different way than with hair and epidermal tissues. Schematic of a fingernail is shown in Fig. 4.9 [35]. Keratin is also produced in the nail matrix, which constitutes about 20% of the surface below the nail that is uncovered by the nail fold while the nail bed constitutes the rest. A similar extrusion process to hair and skin also occurs where older keratin is displaced distally by the new nail growth. The process of nail growth is subtly different than with hair, in that there is no identified fluctuation in the keratin nail growth rate and no periods like the exogen phase where an old nail is jettisoned and a new nail is formed from a different growth structure. There can be defects in nail growth and there are instances where a nail is weak and separates new growth from older keratin, but overall, nail growth is a more regular process of keratin synthesis and displacement. Instances of localized damage and capillary rupture in and around the nail matrix is commonly observed as discolorations in the keratin that is produced and it takes time for the nail to extrude the discolored region of the nail accordingly. If there is profound trauma to the nail matrix, it is sometimes difficult to resolve the nail problems that form as a result.

The nail constitutes the integration of three different forms of keratin that are deposited in the nail matrix at the base and below the nail surface [36]. The narrow region of the dorsal nail layer is composed of keratin of intermediate hydration and hardness that is laid down on the roof and the base of the nail bed, and along the lateral nail fold. A second layer, called the intermediate layer, is a harder keratin structure and deposited along the proximal nail fold through the lunula. The third layer is a softer keratin and is deposited near the middle of the nail bed. The keratinocytes in the nail matrix produce ample keratin protein that is glued together and with continuous protein production, there is a continuous production of nail extruded from the nail bed at a growth rate of ~ 1 mm/week [36].

The keratin that is produced within the nail is both tough and relatively stiff. Baden mentions a modulus on the order of 4 GPa [37], which is clearly stiffer than the corresponding skin tissue into which this can apply pressure during ingrown conditions.

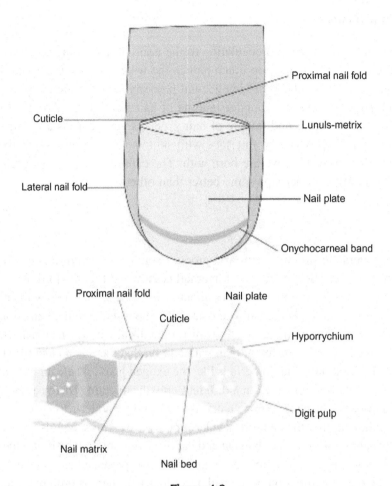

Figure 4.9
The plane and sagittal sections of the nail. *Republished with permission from D. de Barker, Nail anatomy, Clinics Dermatol. (31) (2013) 509—515 [35].*

It is clear that the level of hydration in nails is fairly important to the toughness of the tissues and when decoupled, often-clipped nails become quite stiffer and more brittle once decoupled from the owner.

Of course, nails, like skin and hair, are embellished with nail lacquer and creams that are perceived to tint or otherwise strengthen nails and the liquid components can be sufficiently permeable to interact with the nail bed. Also, people who wear rubber gloves and/or those involved in hand dishwashing typically have rather large transepidermal water loss (TEWL) rates that raise the water content in their nails which can make them both weaker and more apt to fracture. Finally, the presence of surface cracks, and the use of nails in lieu of a real tool can be initiation points for nail fractures.

4.7 Muscle Tissues

SMCs have been mentioned as being integrated into a variety of soft tissues already including both skin and the vasculature and are used to provide both resilience and the tissue closing capacity. There are actually three different types of muscles that are found in connective tissue. Beyond SMCs, both skeletal and cardiac musculature are also found. Cardiac musculature and skeletal muscle are similar, but cardiac muscle has a subtly different architecture and is only found in the heart. All three muscle types allow for actin and myosin overlap as part of contracting and requiring ATP metabolism to maintain the contracted state.

Both smooth muscles and cardiac muscles are considered involuntary muscles in that there is no conscious effort to deform the cells or the muscular network during normal cardiovascular conveyance. There is a functional metabolism, but the stretching and recovery of muscle cells is linked to the coordinated pressurization of the cardiovascular system. Arrhythmias and fibrillation can occur but under normal physiology, the contractions and recoveries are very coordinated.

Skeletal muscle is a voluntary muscle response in that conscious or planned displacements and motions are directed by the muscle movements. The leverage of skeletal muscular tissue derives from their anchoring to bone through tendons. Skeletal muscle tissue is a similarly load-sensitive tissue like bone in that new muscle tissue can be triggered through those loading events.

Functionally, muscle tissue is also self-assembled from smaller building blocks. Skeletal muscles are housed within a tough, connective tissue called the epimysium. Within the epimysium, ensembles of hundreds of muscle fibers called fascicles are self-assembled and isolated from each other by another connective tissue called the perimysium that also contains nerve connections and the vascular supply. The individual fibers are composed of thread-like myocytes (also known as myofibers) that are extended to create aligned regions that can undergo directed compression. The most critical design element of each myofiber or muscle cell is called the sarcomere, where segments of myofibrils organize into distinct regions that are composed of actin and myosin in separate zones.

There is a well-defined, microscopic signature of the sarcomere that is replicated hundreds of time along an individual fascicle. Myofibrils of actin are found tied to a dense layer by interference optical microscopy and is denoted as a "Z" line. The thin actin filaments radiate out on either side of this "Z" line and constitutes the "I" band also noted by microscopy. The thicker myosin filaments form the center region between "I" blocks called the "A" band, which is invariant with muscle firing. Myosin has a globular head and a long tail section. The myosin head also binds to ATP that contributes to the metabolic pathway of muscle contraction and release.

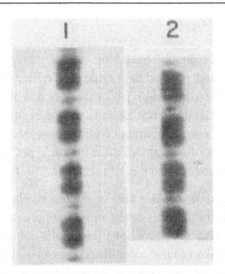

Figure 4.10
4 separate sarcomeres identified by interference microscopy showing the 5 "Z" lines in the rest state (1) and after exposure to ATP (2) which triggers an affine contraction of ∼15%. Further contraction was observed up to 50%. *Reproduced with permission from A.F. Huxley, R. Niedergrove, Structural changes in muscle during contraction: interference microscopy of living muscle fibres, Nature (173) (1954) 971–973 [40].*

There is some rather sophisticated biochemistry and biophysics that involves ATP, the presence of Ca^{2+}, and a structural rearrangement of the myosin filament which pulls the actin filaments into closer proximity with adjacent myosin filaments. There is some variability in terms of the size of both the overall relaxed sarcomere dimension and the length of the A and I bands. Typical sarcomere dimensions are ∼3 μm in length [38] and the A band is typically 1.85 mm in length in human tissue [39]. Upon activation, the actin filaments are ratcheted into the myosin filament environment where they interact more closely, those tissues densify and the length between Z bands shrinks, as shown in Fig. 4.10 [40].

There are thousands of sarcomeres along the length of a single muscle fascicle, and the bulk contraction as one flexes their elbow is the summation of thousands of contraction events all happening in coordinated way to create the appropriate bulk bending force. It is also worth noting that there is continued metabolism required to maintain the flexed state just from the muscle alone. That is one rationale why there is the muscle becomes exhausted under continuous muscle use given the replenishment rate of ATP into the muscle tissue.

4.8 Looking Ahead

There are whole books dedicated to other specialized connective tissues beyond what has been discussed here. What is impressive about these unique hybrid tissues is that nature has incorporated engineering design features to increase specific attributes such as the attachment potential, for example, muscles to bone through tendons. But overall, these structures contain cells, connective tissue proteins, and water. There is certainly continuing interest in understanding the formation and structure of blood vessels, valves, epithelial tissues, and muscular tissues. The presence of muscle cells within other connective tissues means that there are both composition and organizational details regulating mechanical behavior. We know that specific genetic disorders actually produce connective tissues and skin that are statistically different in terms of mechanical behavior than control subjects.

Large swaths of the regenerative medicine community including doctors, scientific researchers, investors, health care companies, private foundations and institutes, and government health institutes are motivated by the broad goal of harnessing the capacity of pluripotent stem cells to regenerate otherwise functionally morbid tissues, whether resulting from infarction, trauma, disease and the need for resection, or other general aging. Any tissue-engineered solution has to resolve how to coculture mixtures of different cell types including myocytes and fibroblasts together in the right proportions and at the right times to produce some shape or function that was lost. The challenge is grand, and well beyond the scope, of this book to have these answers. Future advances might look like pharmaceutical therapy to upregulate natural healing in a specific location, or a tissue implant, designed, perfused, and constructed in a way to replicate the prior function, or perhaps some hybrid solution in between.

4.9 Conclusions

This chapter has been focused on the composition, structure, and attributes of tissues that normally do not mineralize. The examples presented including blood vessels, heart valves, skin, and other elements linked with the integument and muscular tissues. Non-mineralized soft tissues make up a large volume fraction of the average mammal, and if one considers that other organs are perfused with blood as part of each system function and contains some of the same building blocks, we can also consider other organs not discussed here under the notion of soft tissue structures.

It is this unique interplay between fibroblasts that produce colleganous tissues and muscular fibers and cells as they are seamlessly cocultured in vivo directed by nature and allowing for other functional load or vascular structures to be built. Blood vessels need both elastic fibers and muscle fibers to respond to the variations in blood pressure during pulsatile flow and nature designs a higher elastic fiber content near where pulsatile pressures are greatest. It is also evident that the endothelial cells present in blood vessels are critical in presenting a similar surface to blood and activating components, regardless of the muscularity of the structural elements of the vessel in question.

It has also been shown that hardening of these soft structures, whether by arteriosclerosis within blood vessels or by calcifications on heart valves, can affect the normal physiology which can mimic more profound conditions such as congestive heart failure. Proper assessment through diagnostic imaging and signaling can present a clearer picture of the underlying cause.

The composition, structure, and properties of skin, hair, and nails were included in this chapter. These tissues are interesting in that they are devoid of mineral content, soft, viscoelastic, and have some capacity of regeneration. We described about the layers of skin, the protective barrier properties of skin, and how each layer helped in that capacity. Also discussed here was the function of the basement membrane to separate a living cardiovascular system held within dermis and the regenerative piece that allows for exfoliation, and the dislodging of parasites and bacteria that are sloughed off with some regularity, but never completely. Even though there are no blood vessels within the basement membrane, there are still living cells, although the farther away they are, the more likely they are in the process of dying and transforming their structure.

Here also, was a larger description of the regenerative capacity of hair and nails, similar structures produced by keratinocytes also. Included was the interplay between melanocytes that produced pigmentation and keratinocytes that have uptaken the melanin pigment.

Even though the focus was on the medical elements of these tissues, there are many environmental interactions between our outermost tissues, and there is as much interest in producing functional creams, soaps, conditioners, and cosmetics that make skin softer, nails and hair stronger and less prone to breakage, and without creating contact dermatitis with those components interacting with skin.

A brief overview relating to muscular tissue was also presented, the notion of the sarcomere as the building block element replicated hundreds of times down each fascicle. Muscle cells are viable and active in both voluntary and involuntary movement, requiring perfusion to maintain their vitality. Perfusion is easy in the blood running through the vessels can perfuse those elements of the blood vessel wall along the way. For voluntary movement, active metabolism is required to maintain the contracted state of the sarcomere. Pointing forward, it is worth noting that soft connective tissues have been characterized in terms of their mechanical response (Chapter 5: Property Assessments of Tissues) and the effects of aging on soft connective tissues are also included (Chapter 6: Environmental Effects on Natural Tissues). More comprehensively the clinical interventions linked with soft connective tissues are found elsewhere relating to the cerebrovascular (Chapter 12: Neural Interventions), cardiovascular (Chapter 13: Cardiovascular Interventions) system, and artificial organs (Chapter 14: Artificial Organs).

4.10 Problems

1. Explain why density measurements on soft tissues are less an indicator of compositional differences than in bone? In other words, what is difference in the density between components in soft tissue if it was composed of more elastin?

2. Explain the mechanical effect if a thicker layer of collagen was deposited on the outer surface of a blood vessel? In your answer, find reasonable numbers for the thicknesses of the intimal layer, the medial layer, and the adventitia sheath and the fibrous making up an average vessel.

3. From Fig. 4.1, determine the modulus of the vena cava and carotid arteries stretched radially versus being stretched along the axial direction (longitudinally).

4. Explain whether the directional modulus measurements in these tissues be different?

5. From Fig. 4.2, you propose human mammary artery bypass using the human saphenous vein. Explain the impact on the relocation on the graft response

6. Explain why hypertension (high blood pressure) might have a larger impact on mortality based on the mechanical measurements presented in Chapter 4.

7. Describe the impact of Marfan's syndrome on the cardiovascular connective tissue, as presented in Fig. 4.3.

8. Explain why the region of the connective tissue is most likely affected, between the intima, the medial layer, and the adventitial sheath.

9. Explain why duct tape peeled off skin or using a loofah sponge in the shower is a very small, kind of weight loss regimen?

10. Explain how moisturizers affect the corneocyte layer in skin. What is the physical sensation before and after moisturizing and would one expect moisturizers permanently solve dry skin?

11. How is it that skin might be sensed as drier in one location than another?

12. Burns are often graded based on depth of the wound site. Why might a 1st degree burn be easier for wound healing to resolve than a 3rd degree wound of the same surface dimensions?

13. If calcifications (the deposition of inorganic calcium phosphate residues precipitating out of the bloodstream) on a natural heart valve is a concern, explain how might a density measurement of the tissue be an indicator of the severity of the disease?

14. Explain why it might be more painful to remove a bandage from someone who is regularly moisturizing their skin as opposed to someone who never moisturizes?

15. How might a cosmetics company evaluate the product claim that their formulation
    a. softened skin?
    b. reduced wrinkles?
    c. was hypoallergenic?

16. Fig. 4.10 mentions that all of the sarcomeres contract the figure the same amount under ATP activation (affine). Explain whether it might be possible to have nonaffine deformation in a muscle... what regulates the "affine" attribute of the muscle?

References

[1] M.C. Meyers, P.Y. Chen, Biological Materials Science, Cambridge University Press, Cambridge UK, 2014.

[2] J.O. Hollinger, An Introduction to Biomaterials, CRC Press, Boca Raton, FL, 2012.

[3] Y.C. Fung, Biomechanics, Mechanical Properties of Living Tissues, Springer, New York, 1993.

[4] P. Pugliese, Physiology of the Skin, Allured, Carol Stream, IL, 1993.

[5] J. Castro. 11 Surprising Facts About the Circulatory System. Available from: <http://www.livescience.com/39925-circulatory-system-facts-surprising.html>, September 25, 2013.

[6] C.L. Dinardo, G. Venturini, E.H. Zhou, I.S. Watanabe, L.C. Campos, R. Dariolli, et al., Variation of mechanical properties and quantitative proteomics of VSMC along the arterial tree, Am. J. Physiol.-Heart Circ. Physiol. 306 (2014) H505−H516.

[7] Y.C. Fung, Biomechanics: Mechanical Properties of Living Tissues, Springer, New York, 1993.

[8] F.H. Silver, P.B. Snowhill, D.J. Foran, Mechanical behavior of vessel wall: a comparative study of aorta, vena cava, and carotid artery, Ann. Biomed. Eng. 31 (2003) 793−803.

[9] J.E. Wegenseil, R.P. Mecham, Elastin in large artery stiffness and hypertension, J. Cardiovasc. Transl. Res. 5 (2012) 264−273.

[10] P.B. Dobrin, Mechanical behavior of vascular smooth muscle in cylindrical segments of arteries in vitro, Ann. Biomed. Eng. 12 (1984) 497−510.

[11] F.N. Littooy, J. Golan, B. Blakeman, J. Fareed, P.B. Dobrin, Intimal hyperplasia and medial thickening in autogenous vein bypass grafts: influence of anastomoses and platelet-inhibiting drugs, Assoc. Acad. Surg., Abstracts Sci. Papers (1981).

[12] P.B. Dobrin, T. Canfield, J. Moran, H. Sullivan, R. Pifarre, Coronary artery bypass: the physiological basis for differences in flow with internal mammary artery and saphenous vein grafts, J. Thorac. Cardiovasc. Surg. 74 (1977) 445−454.

[13] P.B. Dobrin, A.A. Rovick, Influence of vascular smooth muscle on contractile mechanics and elasticity of arteries, Am. J. Physiol. 217 (1969) 1644−1652.

[14] P.A. Abraham, A.J. Peredja, W.H. Carnes, J. Uitto, Marfan syndrome: demonstration of abnormal elastin in aorta, J. Clin. Invest. 70 (1982) 1245−1252.

[15] A.W. Chung, H.H. Yang, M.W. Radomski, C. van Breeman, Long-term doxycycline is more effective than atenolol to prevent thoracic aoritic aneurysm in Marfan syndrome through the inhibition of the matrix metalloproteinase-2 and -9, Circ. Res. 102 (2008) e73−e85.

[16] A. De Paepe, F. Malfait, Bleeding and bruising in patients with Ehlers−Danlos syndrome and other collagen vascular disorders, British Journal of Haematology 127 (2004) 491−500.

[17] M. Misfeld, H.-H. Sievers, Heart valve macro- and microstructure, Philos. Trans. R. Soc. Lond., B: Biol. Sci. 362 (2007) 1421−1436.

[18] J.D. Hutcheson, E. Alkawa, W.D. Merryman, Potential drug targets for calcific aortic calve disease, Nat. Rev. Cardiol. 11 (2014) 218−231.

[19] M. Krotkiewski, P. Bjorntorp, L. Sjostrom, U. Smith, Impact of obesity on metabolism in men and women, J. Clin. Invest. 72 (1983) 1150−1162.

[20] K. Konishi, Characteristics of blubber distribution and body condition indicators for Antarctic minke whales (*Balaenoptera bonaerensis*), Mammal Study 31 (2006) 15−22.

[21] R.Y. Ha, K. Nojima, W.P. Adams, S.A. Brown, Analysis of facial skin thickness: defining the relative thickness index, Plastic Reconstr. Surg. 115 (2005) 1769−1773.

[22] E. McLafferty, C. Hendry, A. Farley, The integumentary system: anatomy, physiology and function of skin, Nurs. Stand. 27 (2012) 35−42.

[23] R.A. Bergman. Anatomy Atlases: Section 7: Integument. Available from: <http://www.anatomyatlases.org>, 2017.

[24] A.B. Ackerman, A. Boer, B. Bennin, G.J. Gottlieb, Histologial diagnosis of inflammatory skin diseases, Derm101 Website (2017). Available from: <https://www.derm101.com/inflammatory/embryologic-histologic-and-anatomic-aspects/ground-substance/>.

[25] P.G. Agache, C. Monneur, J.L. Leveque, J. De Rigal, Mechanical properties and Young's modulus of human skin in vivo, Arch. Dermatol. Res. 269 (1980) 221−232.

[26] J.M. Sorrell, A.I. Caplan, Fibroblast heterogeneity: more than skin deep, J. Cell Sci. 117 (2004) 667−675.

[27] J. Tigges, J. Krutmann, E. Fritsche, J. Haendeler, H. Schaal, J.W. Fischer, et al., The hallmarks of fibroblast aging, Mech. Ageing Dev. 138 (2014) 26−44.

[28] G.L. Wilkes, I.A. Brown, R.H. Wildnauer, The biomechanical properties of skin, CRC Crit. Rev. Bioeng. 1 (1973) 453−495.

[29] J. Thingnes, T.J. Lavelle, E. Hovig, S.W. Omholt, Understanding the melanocyte distribution in human epidermis: an agent-based computational model approach, PLoS ONE (2012) 7. p. e40377.

[30] A.L. Timko, C.H. Miller, F.B. Johnson, V. Ross, In vitro quantitative chemical analysis of tattoo pigments, Arch. Dermatol. (2001) 143−147.

[31] M. Rendl, L. Lewis, E. Fuchs, Molecular dissection of mesenchymal−epithelial interactions in the hair follicle, PLoS ONE 3 (2005) e331.

[32] C.F. Cruz, C. Costa, A.C. Gomes, T. Matama, A. Cavaco-Paulo, Human hair and the impact of cosmetic procedures: a review on cleansing and shape-modulating cosmetics, Cosmetics 3 (2016) 26.

[33] C.C. Muth, Chemotherapy and hair loss, J. Am. Med. Assoc. 317 (2017) 656.

[34] V. Ounsakul, W. Iamsumang, P. Suchonwanit, Radiation-induced alopecia after endovascular embolization under fluoroscopy, Case Rep. Dermatol. Med. 2016 (2016) Article 8202469.

[35] D. de Barker, Nail anatomy, Clinics Dermatol. 31 (2013) 509−515.

[36] L. Farren, S. Shayler, A.R. Ennos, The fracture properties and mechanical design of human fingernails, J. Exp. Biol. 207 (2004) 735−741.

[37] H.P. Baden, The physical properties of the nail, J. Invest. Dermatol. 55 (1970) 115−122.

[38] R. Horowits, R.J. Podolsky, The positional stability of thick filaments in activated skeletal muscle depends on sarcomere length, evidence for the role of titin filaments, J. Cell Biol. 105 (1987) 2217−2223.

[39] R.L. Lieber, Skeletal Muscle Structure, Function and Plasticity, Lippincott, Williams and Wilkins, Philadelphia, 2002.

[40] A.F. Huxley, R. Niedergerke, Structural changes in muscle during contraction: interference microscopy of living muscle fibres, Nature 173 (1954) 971−973.

CHAPTER 5

Property Assessments of Tissues

Learning Objectives

This chapter is designed to show that tissues have innate properties and that one can establish constitutive relationships to gauge material properties such as modulus and resistivity. The focus is on mechanical behavior, image analysis as might be derived from X-ray or magnetic resonance imaging diagnostics, and electrical and optical properties of natural tissues and select candidate replacement materials. Presented here are schemes to analyze appropriate datasets, and to show some of the complicating factors that arise when treating tissue as material. Living systems may bend and break on some level, and the regenerative capacity of some tissues makes these materials distinct from materials with no regenerative capacity. It is noted that tissues will change composition with age, with disease, and with tissue preparation, therefore in vivo types of experimental tools are probably the most relevant going forward.

5.1 Introduction

In the digital age, it seems both laborious and expensive to replicate long exhaustive analyses in one treatise. The mechanics of extensional load–displacement testing and three-point bending have been solved long ago and have their own wiki sites. The origins of why there is magnetic phase contrast between hydrogen atoms in different chemical environments is the origin of magnetic resonance imaging (MRI) and it has its own wiki site, as does how our status as living semiconductors allows electrical probing of us by electrocardiogram (EKG) and electroencephalogram (EEG) among other diagnostic imaging modalities. But applying the principles discussed here and presenting supplementary information on specific subtopics should allow the reader to not only understand what is generally available in the open literature, but also to apply this information in new and relevant ways. As such, there is more focus on both examples and on quantitative problems that can be used and adapted accordingly.

There are many biophysical assessments that can be performed on biologic solid, fluid, and gaseous products as well as substitute synthetic materials. Failed tendons, ligaments, and bones all yield different biomechanical responses that can be resolved commonly by twisting and bending limbs and articulating one bony segment relative to another. Cell

Biomaterials. DOI: http://dx.doi.org/10.1016/B978-0-12-809478-5.00005-5

blood count and urinalysis are often used as assays of diagnostic health from easily extractable or excreted biofluids. And the breathalyzer assay is essentially an analytical biochemical assay of alcohol partitioned in the gaseous phase during respiration.

At its most basic level the distinction between healthy and diseased tissue can be harnessed as the first line of defense in diagnosis. If the distinction in mechanical stiffness was not sufficiently palpable for example between healthy tissue and cancerous tumors in the breast for example, there would be no reason to perform palpation-based self-exams. With synthetic biomaterials the replication or replacement of mechanical function of often first considered, but replicating mechanical response can only go so far. There is a much more widespread need to replace or augment the repair of partial or more comprehensive organ function which requires a larger understanding of the electrical, optical, and magnetic response of these systems both in vivo and in vitro. Separately, while we think more commonly in terms of biomechanical properties, cells, tissues, and organs also have physical and compositional attributes that allow for these tissues to be probed in terms of heat transfer, electrical and ionic conductivity from the organ level to the cellular level. Furthermore, it is the structural make-up of cells, membranes and their metabolites that create relatively impermeable structures except for specific regulated pathways (sweat, ion channels, etc.). Here we take a broad swipe linking seemingly unrelated topics more directly together.

5.2 Mechanical Properties

We bend and stretch, compress and twist, often within some sort of normal physiological limit unless we are double jointed, contain hyperelastic skin or are otherwise overly limber contortionists hired by the Cirque de Soleil. We rely innately on organ compression by cardiac heart muscle tissue to properly transport blood through the cardiovascular system, and lung tissue expansion upon inhaling a breath to properly perfuse that blood within the pulmonary system. We also rely on our innate compression that results from standing erect to stimulate bone-forming cells called osteoblasts to maintain and regulate bond density within the skeletal structure. At all levels across the continuum of tissue, cells and organized cells composing larger tissue masses possess biophysical attributes related to their structure that regulate how resistant they are to deformation, heat transfer and the like. We often refer to these properties much like we would with other synthetic materials cognizant that the living component of these tissues could alter the composition and the structure of what we would define as tissue, hence older tissue might not have the same composition or the same properties as younger tissue. Discussed here are mechanical, thermal, optical, and mechanical property evaluations of normal natural tissues, cognizant of the fact that we are treating these specimens like synthetic materials. The bottom line is that the same tools we use in materials science to evaluate stiffness of rebar or concrete could applied to probe the behavior in bone. We need a broader understanding the composition and structure different natural tissues and how they compare to other metallic, ceramic, polymeric, and composite materials.

5.2.1 Uniaxial Extension and Compression

The relative stiffness of a material is commonly assessed by uniaxial load-deflection measurements. If the samples are extended, that is considered a tension test, and if compressed, a compression test. In the elastic limit, though they follow Hooke's Law of Elasticity that is often considered invariant regardless of the loading mode or the rate of extension. As a first approximation, it is assumed that there is a *pseudo*-elastic behavior and that there is a linear relationship (Hookean) between the applied stress on a tissue sample and the corresponding strain. It is worth considering that biomechanically, there are instances where tissue is loaded in compression and tension. Consider the simple process of picking up grocery bags with our arms pointed down and holding them indefinitely. The static load of the bags when raised off of the ground creates a gravitational force on the humerus, radius and ulna which cause small extensional strains, the size of which is regulated by the Hookean modulus of elasticity (stiffness) of the extended bones. A stiffer bone with a higher modulus of elasticity has less extension under the same loading and stress conditions. The Hookean modulus of a material (bone in this case) can be determined through uniaxial mechanical measurements schematically shown in Fig. 5.1 by tracking the relationship between load and extension. The modulus is calculated as the slope of the stress (load/cross-sectional area) versus strain (extension/gauge length). Think of it as adding bottles of water to the bags you are holding.

The force applied causes a certain displacement in the length of the segment being loaded if we opt for the easiest direction to test and if we assume that this material is homogeneous. The height and width of this specimen compose the cross-sectional area, with the stress determined in the loading direction is the applied force divided by the cross-sectional area. The strain is defined as the displacement divided by the original length of the specimen between the grips. Hooke's law identifies a linear correspondence between the applied

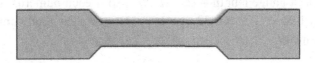

Figure 5.1
Tensile test specimen geometry. This specimen has a thickness, a width in the gauge section and a gauge length. The larger edge regions are more easily gripped and the smaller cross-sectional area concentrates the stress.

stress and the corresponding strain, regulated by the modulus of elasticity, hence materials that behave in this manner are identified as Hookean solids.

While the grocery bags create tensile load and ulnar extension, just the opposite happens if one is standing where legs experience compression. Our legs also sustain the added load carried with our arms, such that a larger gravitational force is experienced compressing them. The relative amount of compression is again regulated by the Hookean modulus of elasticity in the femur, tibia and to a smaller extent, the fibula. Even though the loading requirements on the arm bones are different than those of the leg bones, no obvious structural or compositional distinctions exist, they all have the same general structure and formation characteristics.

Example 5.1 When going to the gym the lifting of free weights is a direct compressive loading if we use a weight bar and place ourselves below it. Assume a 25 kg bar plus weights, the force is 25 kg Xg, the gravitational constant (9.81 ms^{-2}) = ~249 N.

- If the force of the bar compresses the two humerus bones, of axial length, 33 cm, with the outer radial diameter of the bone being 2.5 cm, and an annular cortex thickness of 0.6 cm, *Determine the stress on each bone?*

Stress is force/unit area. Each humerus bone is an annular ring with annular area of $\pi(R^2 - r^2)$. If the cortex thickness is 0.6 cm, then that is the difference between the interior and outer dimensions of the annulus.

$\sigma = 249\ N/[2\ \text{humerus bones}^*[(3.14^*(0.0125\ m)^2 - (0.065\ m)^2)]] = 249\ N/(0.0007\ m^2)$
$= 0.35\ \text{MPa}$

5.3 How Much Does the Humerus Bone Length Shrink Upon Loading With the Bar?

If the modulus of the cortex is 18 GPa, from Hooke's law

$$\text{Strain} = \frac{\sigma}{sE} = \frac{0.35\ \text{MPa}}{18\ \text{GPa}} = 1.94 \times 10^{-6}$$

Strain is displacement $\times$ gauge length $= (L_f - L_o)/L_o$, so if each humerus is 33 cm long, the total displacement is $1.94 \times 10^{-6} \times 0.33\ m = 6.4 \times 10^{-7}\ m$. The total compression of a fraction of a micrometer.

5.3.1 The Tensile Test

Several other material test parameters are identifiable during a tensile test as discussed above. A representative graph is shown in the diagram in Fig. 5.2. The initial slope of the

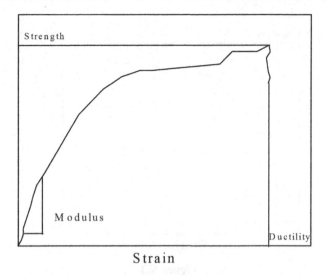

Figure 5.2

Typical stress (tensile load/cross-sectional area) versus strain (displacement/gauge length) curve. The initial linear portion is attributed to the modulus of elasticity.

stress—strain diagram corresponds to the modulus of elasticity. True stress is defined as the load divided by the instantaneous cross-sectional area, an important distinction for highly extended tissues. Engineering stress is the load divided by the initial cross-sectional area. The deviation from elastic behavior is defined as yielding, shown in Fig. 5.3. There are many interpretations of the stress and strain at which yielding occur. Samples can deform and ultimately fracture, the stress and strain at which are defined as the *tensile strength* and the *ductility*.

5.3.2 Hookes Law and Hookean Behavior

Hookean solids respond independently of strain rate. Natural tissues that are extracted before loading deviate in two ways. First, connective tissues like bone, skin, and muscle are strain rate dependent, with a perceived stiffening with increasing strain rate called viscoelasticity. The origins of the time-dependence of the tissue arise from the interactions of the long chain polypeptides composing the proteins. If the rate of loading is faster than the molecular dynamics of chain disentanglement between chains, one achieves a stiff response, and a slower displacement rate allows more disentanglement to occur, sensed as a lower modulus and more compliant behavior. Second, these same connective tissues are usually under some preloading condition in vivo. As such, there is usually an initial nonphysiologically relevant force-deflection relaxation encountered called a *toe region* to regain the physiologically relevant prestrain condition.

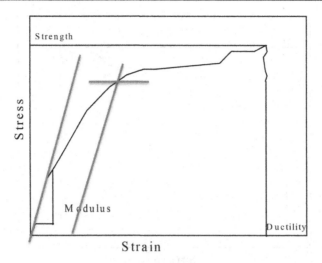

Figure 5.3

An example of the offset yield condition shown schematically. A parallel line is drawn at a specific offset strain and when the stress–strain diagram intersects with this offset line, the yield strength is noted.

5.4 Strength

Determination of stress requires an appropriate assessment of the cross-sectional area that, for solid tissue samples, is relatively straightforward. For bones, most cortical bone segments are actually tubular in geometry, so it is the annular cross-section that regulates the actual stress.

The tensile strength corresponds to the highest stress associated with the true stress-true strain test. Loading the grocery bags with more mass is the equivalent of traversing away from the origin on the stress–strain diagram. There is an equivalent compressive strength and bending strength depending on the loading mode and it is likely these are different values.

5.4.1 Yield Strength

Commonly, the stress–strain response in a pseudo-elastic test of bone or other biological material deviates from a linear, elastic behavior, a phenomenon called yielding. There are several ways to interpret when yielding occurs as a function of loading stress in all loading modes. The simplest is an offset yield condition, the intersection of a parallel line to the modulus curve at a defined offset strain with it. Typical offset strains are 0.002 and 0.02 depending on the relative stiffness of the material. If the material was truly Hookean, the linear response would never intersect with the offset line drawn parallel to the modulus curve. Real materials yield, with plastic deformation, dislocation formation in crystals, cavitation (void formation), and grain boundary dynamics that can render them permanently deformed. Under these conditions, their mechanical response can deviate from Hookean and intersect with the offset line drawn parallel to the original stress–strain diagram. There is no single accepted standard for interpreting yield for biological tissues; many common approaches to considering yield in other synthetic materials seem acceptable to the biological tissue community. It is appropriate to point out that yielding and failure of healthy bone commonly occurs well beyond the normal physiological limit of stress and strain testing. We typically observe pain responses before and during achieving a yield condition. There are instances of impact loading such as falls in elderly patients with osteoporosis where direct bone failures are observed. Many measurements assessing tensile strengths have been performed on cadaver tissue extracted for testing.

5.5 Bending

After carrying the groceries into the house, arm bones bend when the bags are suspended over the counter. Holding the bags suspended by gravity at arms length causes cantilever bending, with a fixed constraint by the shoulder and gravitational point loading by the dead load in the bags. Bending stresses are also common, with compression on the bottom of the loaded bone and tension on the upper segment. Bending modulus measurements can be made using several geometries. They include 3 point, 4 point, and cantilever geometries, shown in Figs. 5.4–5.6, the solutions of which have all been extensively detailed in mechanics of materials books and schematics are shown below. It is noted that 4-point bending is more accurate than 3-point bending.

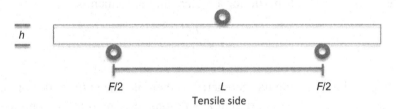

Figure 5.4
3-Point bending geometry with point loadings symmetrically placed with thickness *h* and depth *b*.

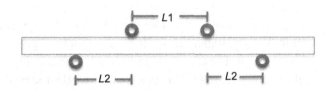

Figure 5.5
4-Point geometry with symmetrically placed loading points, again with thickness *h*, and depth *b*.

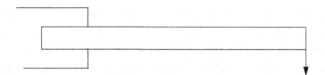

Figure 5.6
Single cantilever bending geometry with a point loading at the end.

The stress for a bending beam varies with the depth of the beam according to the following relation.

$$\sigma = \frac{My}{I_x} \tag{5.1}$$

where M is the bending moment at y, the distance from the neutral axis, x, and I_x is the 2nd moment of inertia around the x dimension which is a function of the cross-section of the beam.

The modulus of elasticity in 3-point bending can be resolved by classical beam theory for rectangular specimens by using the force/deflection curve (P/y), and the geometry of the specimen and testing configuration as shown in Eq. (5.2)

$$E = \frac{L^3}{4bh^3} \frac{P}{y} \tag{5.2}$$

And where the area moment of inertia for a rectangular specimen is

$$I = \frac{bh^3}{12} \tag{5.3}$$

For compact bones, this is an annular geometry so there is a need to work in radial dimensions and to accommodate a different areal moment of inertia. Loading the bone tube causes a deflection, and the corresponding force/deflection curve yields a modulus of ~ 18 GPa, recognizing that deflection rates and geometric considerations can influence what is ultimately measured.

Much like uniaxial testing, one can achieve yielding and fracture by overloading these specimens beyond the normal physiological limit. It is appropriate to point out that if the modulus of elasticity of bony tissue is easier to load in bending than with extension, bending evaluations might be more common. There are an excellent series of texts that go into exhaustive detail to insure the mechanics of these experiments account for an accurate determination of bending modulus, however loaded.

5.6 Torsion

Twisting on one leg can create a torsional force, the size again which is regulated by the stiffness of the bone undergoing the twisting motion as might occur with rotation of the spine. Much like bending the torsional shear stress is a principal stress to consider. The stress is given by the following relation.

$$\tau = \frac{\text{Torque}^* r}{J} \tag{5.4}$$

where M is the polar torsional moment at point r, the radial point around which the torsion is occurring and J is the second moment of inertia in torsion. Recognizing a bony segment as a marrow filled tube in which the center region does not contribute to the stiffness, the moment of inertia, J, is defined as

$$J = \frac{\pi}{2} (r_{\text{outside}}^4 - r_{\text{inside}}^4) \tag{5.5}$$

Again the mechanics of torsional loading has been solved for homogeneous materials with specific loading conditions. Torsion is probably less evaluated from a biomechanics perspective, nevertheless, humans and other animals can load themselves in torsion, and it is worth considering that ways that these tests can be conducted as well.

5.7 Cyclic Loading and Fatigue Resistance

Fatigue is the study of failure of a material under cyclic loading conditions. Biomaterials, like other materials in the design environment, are subjected to loadings, some of which are considered benign and others induce some sort of plastic deformation and damage. We are all used to the concept that materials in use can wear out, and often this is due to both anticipated and unanticipated loadings that induce damage. We also consider that repeated loadings can also damage biological tissues. Overexertion can lead to muscle strains and bone bruises can arise in overused tissues. Bone bruises are related to microcracks that arise in bone often in athletes undergoing training with repeated overloadings and can release fluid into joints that can be sensed as a pain response. Consider marathon runners who whose legs take on average roughly 26 (miles) $\times$ 1875 (steps/mile assuming a 3-foot step) individual compression events during the race. Run while overweight, with heavier clothes or with a water bottle and each step is linked with that much higher compressive loading. Each compression event is magnified as compared to walking, so running is perceived as more damaging on joints are more likely to cause bone bruises and microcracks to form. Luckily, bones heal with time with new bone growth. If the residual strength of the damaged structures was evaluated, its possible that a certain number of steps correspond to a certain amount of damage in bone. For implant type devices, one can more directly measure the characteristics of repeated loadings on materials. This is critical for considering the mechanics of heart valve replacement tissues for example. Replacement valves have to function without failing as they articulate nominally (70 beats/min 60 min/h $\times$ 24 h/day $\times$ 365 days/year) times in 1 year. From a design perspective, its worth considering how load can be reduced or the structure altered to lower the risk if it is a device susceptible to a fatigue-based loading.

The implication of fatigue is that the higher the cyclic loading stress the fewer the number of cycles or exposures are required to create a material failure. Cyclic loading is normally performed between a maximum stress, σ_{max}, and a minimum stress, σ_{min}, and failure can be defined in terms of actual fracture, or some deviation in strain, or stress. The stress ratio, R, is equal to the ratio, $\sigma_{min}/\sigma_{max}$. The general idea is that a single tensile test to failure would be a cycle of 1, with a stress ratio of zero, loaded in a tensile mode. It is possible that in loading experiments above the yield strength and below tensile strength of the material or tissue, failure could still occur, but it might take more loading and unloading events to trigger it. Fatigue loading can be often performed as a constant strain experiment or as a constant stress experiment. Fatigue is worthy of discussion as it relates to biomaterials but remember that in living systems, healing is a viable option and can lead to stress reductions by depositing more bone to an overloaded bone, more muscle to an overloaded muscle. As a result, fatigue evaluations and mechanical interpretations associated with fatigue are much more complicated for living systems. And ideally, from a liability perspective, designed device loadings and strains should be low enough that the material never fails. There have been instances when that has not happened.

The strength of any material may be quite reasonable in its most pristine state, but the overall durability of any material is related to its performance in real usage. The mechanical performance of a compromised material or device can be evaluated by a number of techniques including notched tensile tests, compact tension tests, and other fracture mechanics tests with initiated notches. Using the compact tension specimen and assuming linear fracture mechanics the fracture stress associated with the cracked structure is a function of the original crack length by Eq. (5.6)

$$K_{1c} = \sigma(\pi a)^{0.5} \tag{5.6}$$

where K_{1c} is the plane strain fracture toughness of the material; a is the crack length, and σ_f is the stress at failure for this cracked construction.

Using these tests, one can evaluate the energy needed to extend the already formed crack some further distance. This evaluation can also be done through stress cycles under fatigue loadings.

$da/dN = A(\Delta\square)^m$ where da/dN is the crack extension per cycle, A is a proportionality constant, $\Delta\square$ is the change in stress between high and low stress cycles, and m is a weighting factor relating to how damaging each successive cycle is in propagating an existing crack.

The reality is that the best one can hope for is that the health of tissues around implant materials can be better understood and loadings are such that material and component lifetimes that of loaded components are longer than the anticipated lifetime of the recipients. Fatigue can assess how robust replacement materials are, but understanding the true fatigue resistance of natural tissues is complex and well beyond the scope of both this book and others. It is important to at least consider.

5.8 Relationship to Natural Materials

It is not a given that all ex vivo property determinations of a natural material can be effectively evaluated. Or in other words, nature normally does not make biomaterials in the form of an ASTM test specimen and clearly no guarantee that natural materials are homogeneous and symmetric. There are often some modifications in order to evaluate the properties of a natural tissue specimen. Ideally, one can use a small amount of material during analysis; this way, more than one measurement can be taken. Additionally, there are other concerns such as concerns about storage and the length of time between a sample being obtained and measured. This is especially critical when discussing the material properties of soft tissues that are wildly dependent on the water content. But with reasonable care, proper preparation and adequate documentation, good measurements of natural tissue properties are valid and worth noting. Also, material property characteristics of some common biomaterials are included as well.

5.9 Viscoelasticity

If natural tissues were not viscoelastic, then one would experience the same stress–strain diagram under both impact-loading conditions and under a less rapid loading. It is well known that this is not true and it complicates what is meant by tissue stiffness, because it depends on how its loaded. Examples in bone, tendon, and skin are shown in Figs. 5.7–5.10. These datasets show tissues, while they can be tested as elastic solids, do not behave with a simple elastic response like a spring. Instead, there is a combined effect that leads to a strain rate dependence on loading as well. The time-dependence on mechanical response has been considered in terms of time-dependent mechanical models, where Hookean solids responding elastically and represented by springs, and viscous fluids, represented by fluid filled pistons, are linked together. A higher modulus polymer or tissue will correspond to a stiffer spring. The dashpot in the model represents viscous dissipation and the larger the viscosity of the fluid filling the dashpot, the more sluggish the response to load.

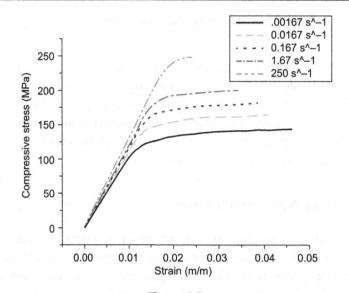

Figure 5.7
Viscoelastic response of bovine compact bone tested longitudinally (along fiber dimension)
in tension as a function of strain rate (s^{-1}) cited in both Lee and Hyman [1] and Crowningshield
and Pope [2].

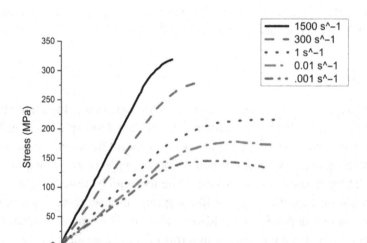

Figure 5.8
Bovine compact bone as a comparison tested as a function of strain rate in compression
from McElhaney [3].

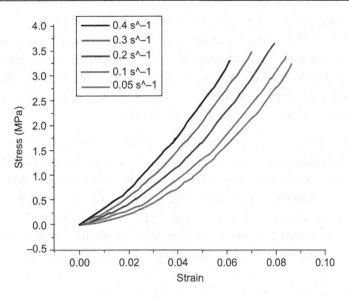

Figure 5.9

Viscoelastic response of anterior cruciate ligaments tested at five different strain rates. From both DeVita and Slaughter [4] who has developed constitute models and Pioletti et al. [5] who has published data on the viscoelasticity of the ACL.

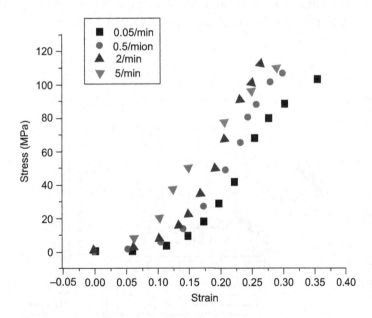

Figure 5.10

Stress—strain diagrams of wet goat skin tissue in its native state tested as a function of strain rate: (squares) 0.05 min^{-1}; (circles) .5 min^{-1}; (diamonds) 2 min^{-1}; (inverted diamonds) 5 min^{-1}.

From V. Arumugam, M.D. Naresh, R. Sanjeevi, Effect of strain rate on the fracture behavior of skin. J. Biosci. 19 (1994) 307–313.

It is the linking of the springs and dashpots together to make solids that exhibit both elastic and viscous responses. The simplest models have only two elements, one elastic and one dynamic. One can connect the mechanical elements together, either in series (a Maxwell model) or in parallel (a Voigt-Kelvin model). More complicated models can contain more elements. Generally, both representations are relevant as the capture pieces of viscoelastic mechanical behavior. Let us consider both of them here.

Viscoelasticity in natural tissues does not have to be evaluated ex vivo. There are other, relatively inexpensive suction-based devices that can be built to track time-dependent strain of skin in situ on a living specimen under reduced pressure, an example of which is shown in Fig. 5.11. The notion is that by tracking skin height under suction with time, one can identify not only an initial strain due to pressure, but also continued suction into the tube. The dynamics of loading and recovery look very similar to those achieved by ex vivo experiments [7]. This is key for assessing living tissue more effectively.

Fast forward to today and there are now developmental devices containing integrated piezoelectric strain sensors that are equipped on conformal, soft patch-like devices that can actually measure in-plane strains and stresses. Calibrations are required, but the overall idea of being able to produce sensory patches that can sense strains under loads allow for much more sophisticated ways to interrogate soft tissue mechanical properties even on a transient basis. Examples of such are included in Figs. 5.12 and 5.13.

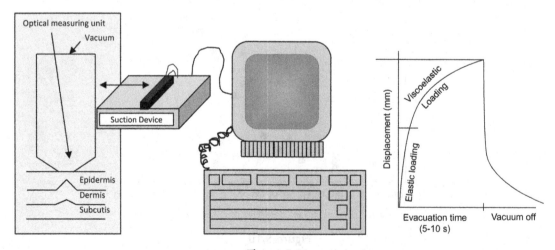

Figure 5.11

Schematic of a skin suction device showing its dynamic mechanical response as a time-dependent displacement upon fixed loading and unloading.

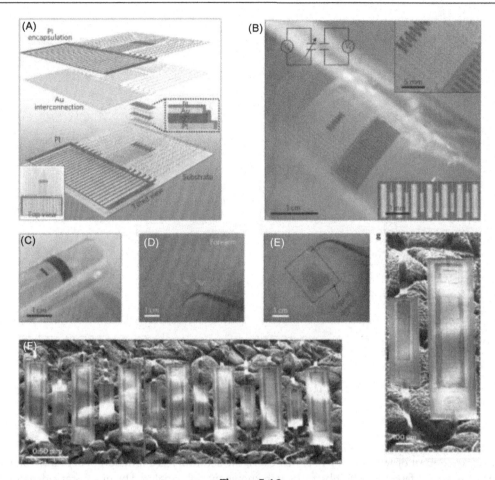

Figure 5.12

A schematic of the construction method for producing conformal piezoelectric sensors that can attach to skin for in vivo testing. (A) Expanded view schematic of the device, with the top view in the lower-left inset, and a section view of the actuator/sensor arrangement in the black-dashed region. (B) Photo of the device on a Si substrate, optical microscopy images of the interconnect region (upper region inset), the actuator/sensor arrays (lower right inset), and a simple electrical circuit diagram of the actuators and sensors (upper left inset). (C) Photograph of the device on a cylindrical glass support. (D and E) Photographs of ta device partially and fully laminated on skin. (F) SEM image of a device on an artificial skin sample. (G) One of the sensor/actuator arrays in (F), where the sensor and actuator are on the left and right sides. *Reproduced from C. Dagdeviren, Y. Shi, P. Joe, R. Ghaffari, G. Balooch, K. Usgaonkar, Conformal piezoelectric systems for clinical and experimental characterization of soft tissue biomechanics. Nat. Mater. 14 (2015) 728–736.*

5.9.1 Maxwell Model

The simplest Maxwell model has one spring and one dashpot connected in series and conceptually shows stress relaxation at constant strain and all polymer books show the

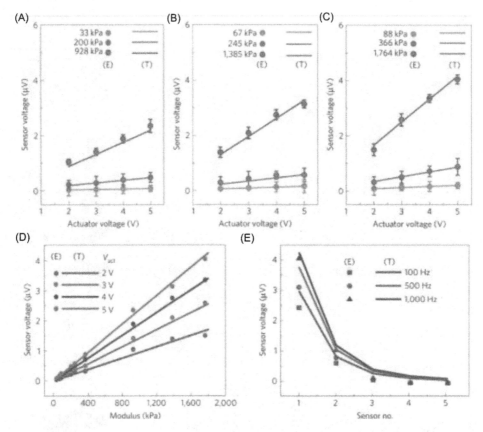

Figure 5.13

(A) Voltage output of sensor #1 (sensor nearest to the actuator) as a function of actuator voltage, measured on different PDMS substrates with known moduli, analyzed by quasi-static dynamic mechanical spectroscopy. Here the symbols and lines correspond to experimental (E) and theoretical (T) results. Error bars correspond to calculated standard error deviation. (B) Output voltage from sensor #1 as a function of the E of the substrate, for four different actuator voltages, V_{act}. (C and D) Output voltages for each of the different sensors in the array (e.g., sensor #1, #2, etc.) measured during use with PDMS results where the substrate E is 1800 kPa (C) and 30 kPa (D), at three different frequencies using an actuation voltage of 5 V, and (E) tangent d, the phase angle for a viscoelastic substrate, as a function of the actuator frequency. For curves (A–C), the slope correlates with the modulus of the substrate. For (D), the higher the voltage, the higher the slope. *Reproduced from C. Dagdeviren, Y. Shi, P. Joe, R. Ghaffari, G. Balooch, K. Usgaonkar, Conformal piezoelectric systems for clinical and experimental characterization of soft tissue biomechanics. Nat. Mater. 14 (2015) 728–736.*

development of different physical models to represent time-dependent mechanical response data [9]. If these two elements are linked together in series, they will sense the same loading, but their individual strains are independent of each other. With instantaneous loading the spring will immediately respond and the dashpot will have zero response. If loaded to a specific strain and held, there is a strain transfer from spring to the dashpot

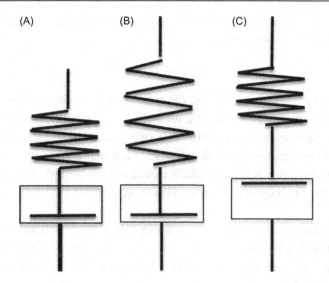

Figure 5.14

Schematic showing a 2-element Maxwell at rest (A), with instantaneous loading (B), and after long time (C). The movement of the piston within the dashpot is regulated by the fluid contained it. The positive extension of the dashpot is equal and opposite the retraction of the spring. The relaxation time corresponds to the ratio of the viscosity of fluid in the dashpot to the modulus of the spring.

and ultimately the stress relaxes due to the displacement of the dashpot. The faster the loading the more the spring is isolated from the dashpot. This interplay between the spring and dashpot under constant strain is what is considered relaxation, shown in Fig. 5.14 and defined by Eq. (5.7).

For stress relaxation: the stress on both the spring and dashpot is the same

$$\sigma = E\varepsilon_{\text{spring}} = \eta \frac{d\varepsilon_{\text{dashpot}}}{dt} \tag{5.7}$$

After instantaneous loading and with constant strain, any change in spring strain is offset by an opposite change in the dashpot

$\frac{d\varepsilon}{dt} = \frac{d\varepsilon_{\text{spring}}}{dt} + \frac{d\varepsilon_{\text{dashpot}}}{dt} = 0$ under stress relaxation conditions with fixed strain

The time-dependent stress can be interpreted as

$$\frac{d\sigma}{dt} = E\frac{d\varepsilon_{\text{spring}}}{dt} \tag{5.8}$$

Substituting for both dynamic strains

$$\frac{1}{E}\frac{d\sigma}{dt} + \frac{\sigma}{\eta} = 0 \tag{5.9}$$

This first order differential equation can be integrated with the initial condition that $\sigma = \sigma_0$ at $t = 0$ and the solution can be rearranged to

$$\sigma = \sigma_0 e^{-tE/\eta} \text{ or } \sigma_0 e^{-t/\tau} \tag{5.10}$$

where t is defined as a relaxation time and the ratio of the viscosity of the dashpot relative to the modulus of the spring. This simple 2-element model would suggest that a single exponential stress response decays to zero stress over time. The example for tendon tissue below clearly shows incomplete stress decay suggesting that a more complex model is needed to represent the tissue response which would require a third element (a second spring) to account for the incomplete stress relaxation.

Example 5.2 : For this specific example, shown in Fig. 5.15, a 3-element model that has a spring in parallel with a Maxwell element can create a mechanical response which at long time reflects the spring in parallel with the Maxwell element that complete relaxes to zero stress. The equation to define the mechanical response is

$$\sigma(t) = (\sigma_0 - \sigma_\infty)(e^{t/\tau}) + \sigma_\infty \tag{5.11}$$

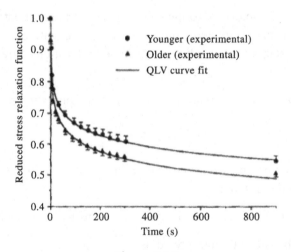

Figure 5.15

Stress relaxation data of both younger and older tissue donors of patellar tendon tissue including model fits of a quantitative linear viscoelastic (QLV) model to fit the data. The dynamics of these types of datasets can be interpreted by creating mechanical models to match the response. This dataset is from Johnson et al. [10]. The takeaway is that older tendons have faster relaxation times and are more completely relaxed. *Figure replicated with permission from the G.A. Johnson, D.M. Tramaglini, R.E. Levine, K. Ohno, N.Y. Choi, S.L.Y. Woo, Tensile and viscoelastic properties of human patellar tendon. J. Orthopaed. Res. 12 (1994) 796–803.*

If one normalizes the equation by the maximum stress, σ_0, the model constants can be extracted.

Conceptually, the additional spring is sensed in this model as a plateau at long time at a stress of σ_∞, which for the example in Fig. 5.13 is between a normalized stress between 0.4 and 0.5. If there is incomplete relaxation, this is better represented as a 3-element model with a second spring than a 2-element model. The time constant, t, relates to the rapidity of the dynamic relaxation to the plateau elastic stress, and the two spring constants comprise the total stress both instantaneously and at long times. As an exercise, one can extract the data of normalized stress with time, and replicate the quantitative linear viscoelastic response as shown in Fig. 5.15.

5.9.1.1 Voigt model: retarded behavior

If one applied a constant stress to a Maxwell model, it would exhibit an initial instantaneous response form the spring and a linear strain with time for the dashpot. This is usually not observed in typical creep loading tests under constant load. The simplest model that captures this retarded strain response is achieved by connecting a spring and dashpot model in parallel, shown schematically in Fig. 5.16. The dashpot shields the spring from sensing the initial load, but with additional time, more of the load is transferred to the spring. Unfortunately, this model is limited in that the implication is that creep only occurs to some maximum level and instantaneous loading exhibits no strain response. What it

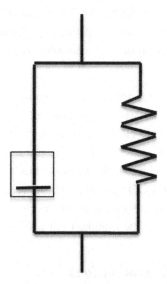

Figure 5.16
Retarded voigt model: The application of instantaneous force to this model yields no instantaneous response. The presence of the dashpot in parallel shields the spring from sensing the load. Its requires time to transfer the load to the spring.

suggests is that viscoelastic tissues and their replacements are often represented by more complex models that possess both an initial instantaneous response and a retarded dynamic response achieved by more than two elements.

5.10 Time-Dependent Stress–Strain Behavior

Both the creep and stress relaxation experiments are different than the loading scheme for a typical tensile test which has a fixed strain rate where loading is neither instantaneous nor controlled. When considering viscoelasticity, molecular models make the most sense to consider. Given that viscoelastic materials have significant molecular mobility when energized to have bulk coordination motion along the chain backbone, it is the relaxation time, τ, associated with molecular mobility that needs to be compared to the overall strain rate for the experiment. Under conditions where the test rate is fast relative to this relaxation time the molecules do not have time to displace during loading. Under conditions where the test rate is very slow the material can relax to the loading. There are finite limits to the response on the slow end and on the fast end of the testing range and overall, this leads to a general stress-strain diagram over the entire range of strain rates that lead to variations in material behavior. This diagram is called the stress–strain or failure envelope and all viscoelastic material behavior is included within this envelope. The modulus is variable and depends on the strain rate and temperature for that matter. The slowest strain rates generate a curve called the equilibrium stress–strain diagram that corresponds to deformation under near equilibrium conditions. There are other tools that can assess this viscoelasticity such as dynamic mechanical spectroscopy that creates a frequency dependent loading scheme and probes the dynamic strain simultaneously which can extract similar information.

Representative data of natural tissues are shown to exemplify how the mechanical response varies depending on how specimens are loaded, and the viscoelasticity is a separate consideration that yields not a single Hookean response but a range of responses due to the molecular structure and composition of these natural tissues. It has been shown how different types of tests can be conducted, the relevant mathematical representations of mechanical behavior and some example datasets. If the goal is to replicate natural connective tissues (tendons, blood vessels, skin, bone, etc.), it is worth considering how not only pseudo-elastic behavior can be matched but also the viscoelastic response as well.

5.11 Physical Property Determinations

The identification of structure in natural tissues in diagnostic medicine is most often associated with finding techniques that distinguish phase contrast. The most common techniques for diagnostics have included the use of X-rays that use variations in density to identify soft versus hard tissue, radioactive tracers in ingested compounds to observe intake, digestion and distribution, the response of nuclei as in MRI, and signal reflection as in acoustic and ultrasonic imaging techniques which are related to the stiffness of materials.

5.11.1 Density

The use of density differences has been the most often used diagnostic imaging tool in medicine. The fact that X-rays interact with materials of varying density with different levels of absorption has led to a substantial amount of work in diagnostic imaging since the days of Röntgen.

5.11.2 Conventional X-ray Measurements

The standard X-ray procedure uses an X-ray source driven by a high voltage source as a cathode and a rotating anode with a target inserted between. There are a number of target materials including aluminum, copper, and tungsten. The target forms X-rays that are then collimated and passed through an X-ray window in one direction. For tissue diagnostics the patient is placed between the X-ray source and an X-ray detector. Years ago, films were developed but new sensory systems allow for digital signal response. The actual phase contrast is generated by the difference in density between the crystallites in bony tissue that scatter, absorb, and diffract more of the X-ray intensity than the corresponding soft tissue. Thus the X-ray is a wonderful tool to identify the anatomy of the hard bony tissue. With the interest in lowering the damaging effects of X-ray exposure, more sensitive X-ray detectors have dramatically lowered the needed dose (intensity times time) of the X-ray beam in order to generate phase contrast. The absorption of X-rays in a material is governed by Beer's law

$$I = I_0 e^{-\alpha x} \tag{5.12}$$

where $I(x)$ is the intensity at depth, x, I_0 is the intensity of the X-ray at the surface, and α is an extinction coefficient. There is a corresponding equation to relate the absorption coefficient which has a similar exponential feature.

By virtue of the higher absorptivity for calcium and phosphorous in the hard segments of the calcium hydroxyapatite than for soft tissues which are essentially transparent to the X-rays, phase contrast is achieved. A table of density characteristics of different materials is given in Table 5.1.

The reason for a compact bone segment to look like two distinct white lines with a hazy interior segment is linked with the observation that the path length through the annular regions of the bone are longer than in the middle of the bone. As such, more scattering occurs near the edges of the bone than in the middle and a lower transmitted X-ray

Table 5.1: Densities of relevant gases, liquids, solids, and gels

Material	Density
Air	0.0013 g/cm^3
Fat	0.94
UHMWPE	0.93–0.95
Water	1.0
Soft tissue	1.01–1.06
Silicone	1.1–1.5
Polymethyl methacrylate	1.2
Compact bone	1.8–2.1
Dentin	2.1
Aluminum	2.7
Enamel	2.8–3
Titanium	4.5
Stainless steel	7.9
Wrought Co–Cr	9.2

intensity is noted at the detector. The absorption coefficient for relatively abundant elements of interest and tissues is shown in Table 5.2.

X-rays diagnostics can identify defects in the bony structure, and other malformations, fractures, etc. in the hard tissue segments. A fracture would be noted as a separation or a mis-registration between bone segments resolved if it is observed in the field of view. Usually fracture diagnostics requires more than one view to image the separation or misalignment. And since most soft tissues are relatively transparent to the X-rays, there is little potential to resolve differences in soft tissue structures by X-ray diagnostics

Table 5.2: X-ray absorption coefficients of different elements and biological tissues

Material	Atomic #	Absorption Coefficient, α (cm^{-1})	Specific Absorption Coefficient, α/ρ (cm^2/g)
Fat	—	0.1788	0.196
Muscle	—	0.2045	0.2045
Brain		0.2061	0.2061
Bone		0.466–0.548	~0.28 cm^2/g since bone ρ correlates with α
Al	13	131	48.7
P	15	132	73
Ca	20	266	172
Cr	24	1.86×10^3	259
Fe	26	2.55×10^3	324
Co	27	3.19×10^3	354
Pb	82	2.73×10^3	241

Source: *Data compiled from J.B. Park, R.S. Lakes, Biomaterials, An Introduction, Plenum Publishing, New York, 1992, chapter 4 and S.A. Kane, Introduction to Physics in Modern Medicine. second ed., CRC Press, Boca Raton, FL, 2009, chapter 5.*

without the use of phase contrast agents. To determine differences between soft tissues, other diagnostic techniques MRI and computer tomography (CT) scanning are more common. In addition, with conventional X-ray diagnostic techniques, more than one X-ray picture is required in order to resolve hairline fractures and other defects that may be resolved with more than one angular X-ray picture. For these problems, X-ray CT is increasingly used.

5.11.3 Computer Tomography Aided X-Ray Analysis

Using a rotating source with an opposite X-ray detector, there is no reason why more than one image can be taken of the patient at a series of angles as shown in Fig. 5.17.

With the advances in computer-aided processing and imaging, these images of the patient at several resolved angles can be reconstructed into a three dimensional picture of the patient. The technique of reconstructing these images is called CT. The technique makes use of rotating sources and detectors. The patient is manipulated in and out of the source using a step length of $1-10$ mm per section with the source rotating around for each slice of the patient. It takes only a couple of seconds for the source to traverse one revolution around the analyzer. Therefore for a large section with a significant amount of detail, it takes minutes to hours for an image to be properly collected. The reconstructions are essentially based on identifying a model form that would recreate the spatial absorption function as a function of radial location and length. The improvements in resolution and increasing

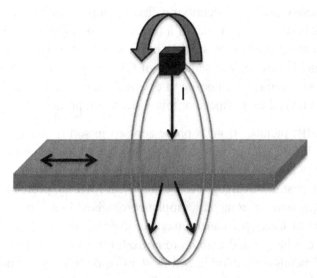

Figure 5.17
Schematic of CT-based imaging modalities. The camera/detector system is rotated around patient allowing 2-D camera images and detector measurements at a range of angles.

detector quality and higher computing speed for analysis has led to closer to real-time imaging. The improved sensitivity in CT is about 100 times the standard X-ray and allows the distinction of fat from other soft tissues, fluid from natural tissue, etc. X-ray CT still is not as sensitive as other imaging modalities like MRI. Common disorders resolved in soft tissue X-ray include fluid accumulation in the lungs and congestive heart failure and ipneumonia which can manifest itself with symptoms of shortness of breath, fatigue, and coughing.

5.11.4 Magnetic Resonance Imaging

This technique is much like X-ray CT scanning except that the source and detectors are different. In this case an orthogonal pulsed magnet is used to alter the alignment of nuclear moments (protons) that are contained in tissues under the presence of a large permanent magnet. This pulsed magnet simply reorients the signals orthogonal to an already active permanent magnetic direction. Shortly after the pulsed signal is turned off, the signal reverts back to the alignment of the original magnet that is still left on during this procedure. The speed with which these nuclear spin states realign with the static field is related to the chemical environment from where these protons reside. Protons in proteins contained in a liquid or gel environment are more mobile than proteins associated with proteins contained in bone mineral deposits. The resolution is quite good, much finer than individual organ level, and coupled with CT quite exquisite maps of images of tissue both normal and diseased can be resolved. Thus MRI is very sensitive to the chemical environment and is generally regarded as much more sensitive in identifying diseased soft tissue relative to normal tissue. One reason why this is so powerful is that if a tumor is more highly vascularized than the tissue around it, it is more likely to be subtlely hotter which alters proton motion in the tumor relative to the surrounding tissue. The same sort of CT reconstruction can also be performed using MRI in order to generate a composite of diseased areas, tumors, vascular blockages, etc. Phase contrast is related to the speed of this realignment process.

The advantages of MRI include stronger phase contrast in soft tissue and avoiding the mutagenic response linked with prolonged X-ray exposure. Protons composing both soft tissue and hard tissues contain hydrogen can be clearly sensed through the image development. The largest disadvantages associated with MRI are probably the risks associated with people who have metallic implants somehow interacting with the beam. With the deployment of larger permanent magnets, even diamagnetic steels, benign to lower field strength MRI, can be torqued with more powerful instruments. The risk could cause the displacement of metals embedded in soft as stents and clips. Hence patients are extensively screened to prevent their exposure if the possess implants, stents, wires, and clips from prior surgical interventions. We are only now at a point where correlations are being made between imaging and actionable therapy and intervention. More is on the horizon and advances in computing power and parallel processing should yield near real-time imaging and analysis.

5.12 Optical Properties

5.12.1 UV/Visible Light Transmission

There are only a few areas where optical properties of materials are important. There are some obvious applications replacement lens materials for corrective vision and lens replacement. The lens itself is a specialized noncrystallizing form of collagen that allows for effective light transmission for focusing on the retina. Cataract formation is a condition in which microcrystalline precipitates form within the lens create their own scattering response due to differences in the index of refraction between the native lens and the precipitates. Light scattering results in light reflection rather than transmission to the retina leading to poor vision. In patients with cataracts the pupil is also much brighter due to its reflection of scattered light rays. A similar Beers law analysis can be done with optical transmission and optimum light transmission results with very small extinction coefficients within the lens. A larger coefficient results in more scattering.

Optical scattering is also important in reflection when matching the color and tone of natural tissues. This is important in dental applications and in matching skin tone in artificial skin. Interestingly, teeth have some translucence particular near the bite zones, and there are gradients in natural tooth coloration, thus a replacement tooth or tooth repair will attempt to match the tooth tinting of the surrounding teeth.

Optical transmission characteristics are measured much in the same way as in X-rays but using a different source (a visible source) and a visible detector. Optical transmission over the visible energy range is done using a spectral analyzer with the sample of interest mounted between. A schematic is shown in Fig. 5.18.

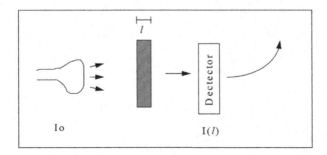

Figure 5.18
Schematic of the visible light transmission experiment through a layer of thickness *l*.

Remember that there are extinction coefficients for both scattering and absorption for these transmission experiments. Ideally the cornea and the lens are transparent in the visible region leading to nearly complete transmission of the visible spectrum to the retina.

If tissue or synthetic replacements are being used as lenses, reasonable transmission is a given requirement as better lens materials won't reflect incoming light away. There is also concern about its optical focusing power linked to its geometry and the corresponding index of refraction of whatever the lens material is. For this, we need to consider Snell's law. The relevant experiment to be performed uses incident waves interacting between two media, one being the incident medium where light originates from, and the other being the sample medium. By comparing the corresponding angles with respect to the incident and refracted waves, one can evaluate the index of refraction in the sample medium if the index of refraction in the incident medium is known, as shown in Fig. 5.19.

$$\text{Snell's law: } n_1 \sin(\theta_1) = n_2 \sin(\theta_2) \tag{5.13}$$

where n_i is the index of refraction of the ith component and $\theta(i)$ is the angle with respect to the ith medium.

The relevant experiment is outlined below and a table of some values of n_i are listed for some typical lens materials. The index of refraction will vary slightly with the wavelength of light, and ideally, this type of information is available for the incident medium (Table 5.3).

In terms of specific lens fabrication the radii of curvature and the index of refraction define its focal length. For this the lens maker equation is used as shown in Eq. (5.14)

$$\text{The lens maker equation} \rightarrow 1/f = (n - n_{\text{incident}})[(1/r_1) - (1/r_2)] \tag{5.14}$$

where f is the focal length and r_1 and r_2 are the radii of curvature.

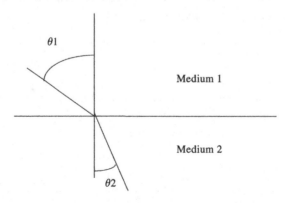

Figure 5.19
Schematic of refraction experiment.

Table 5.3: The index of refraction for various substances, optically transparent materials and tissues

Material	Index of Refraction
Vacuum	1.0
Air	1.003
Water	1.33
Human aqueous humor	1.336
Human vitreous humor	1.338
Human cornea	1.376
Human lens	1.42
Silicone rubber	1.43
Polyhydroxyethyl methacrylate	1.44
Polymethyl methacrylate	1.49
Polyethylene	1.50
Polycarbonate	1.59
Flint glass	1.66

Source: From J.B. Park, R.S. Lakes, Biomaterials, An Introduction, Plenum Publishing, New York, 1992; Physics, Halliday & Resnick, Wiley, 1978.

For a double convex lens, one *r* is positive and one *r* is negative. But the goal is to focus the lens so that the focal length converges onto the retina. A normal functioning eye has a focal length of ~ 1.6 cm with much of the focusing power linked with the curvature of the cornea. The eye normally measures approximately 2.2 cm from the cornea to the retina with the lens sandwiched between. The other point worth noting for a biomaterial application is that the biomaterial lens will have at least one interface with tissue fluid or eye tissue. In terms of cataract surgery the ability to use flexible lenses allows for the replacement lens to be folded prior insertion allowing for a smaller incision in the eye and a faster healing time as a result.

There are other diagnostic evaluations and procedures used in ophthalmology including measurements of high ocular pressure, linked with diabetes, and corneal geometric manipulations through LASIK surgery to adjust the focal length to that required to focus the image on the retina. Interestingly, there is a tool called a optical response analyzer that measures the time required for recover its shape from a pressure impulse, and the scope of displacement relates to the internal pressure of the eye. Here is another example where the mechanical response of corneal tissue yields other understanding about the overall ocular health.

5.13 Electrical Properties of Tissues

We are semiconducting beings, due to the high concentration of soluble ionic salts contained within our tissue and biofluids. Our capacity for some amount of electrical transmission allows electrical diagnostic characterization of physiological events such as cardiac cycling, brain activity, and other neuronal signaling. Our capacity for electrical transport also makes us susceptible to electrocution and electrical shocks. We need to consider here both tissue as a conductor and semiconductor, as well as example conductors that are used, for example, for enhanced cardiac pacing.

Early work highlights the resistivity of various biological tissues, noting upper and lower ranges for anisotropic (fibrous tissues). Resistivity, ρ, is a material property, with units of ohm-cm. If a homogeneous resistor could be made into a cylindrical geometry with an axial length L, and a circular cross-sectional area, πR^2, its resistance (in ohms) is governed by Eq. (5.15)

$$R = \frac{\rho L}{A} \qquad (5.15)$$

Table 5.4 shows the variation in resistivity for a range of different tissues and fluids. Included are also typical resistivity values for other synthetic materials.

The ability to introduce electrical signals to mimic natural impulses such as for a pacemaker, a defibrillator, or a neurotransmitter, requires thin, flexible, wires that freely move with the heart for example. Ideally these wires are diamagnetic rendering them compatible with subsequent MRI imaging. The smaller the resistance, the smaller the power required for signaling, and the more easily the miniaturization of the devices can progress.

From a diagnostics perspective, there is interest in native impulse generation that arises with typical EKG patterns. The rhythmic contractions arising from each heartbeat in addition to forcing blood into the aorta for continued perfusion also generates an electrical charge that can be observed in the patient if electrodes are places across the heart and monitored. The normal cycle is identified as a PQRST wave, with a characteristic normal

Table 5.4: Resistivity of different tissues, fluids, and materials

Material/Element	ρ (Ω-m)
Copper	1.7×10^{-8}
Iron	9.7×10^{-8}
Seawater	0.22
Blood	1.6
Liver	7
Heart	2.6–5.6, depending on directionality
Fat	2.5
Skeletal muscle	1.5–2.3, depending on directionality
Bone (wet)	46
Deionized water	2.4×10^5
SiO_2	10^{10}
PMMA	10^{14}

Source: *Data drawn from CRC Handbook and S. Rush, R. McFee, J.A. Abildskov, Resistivity of body tissues at low frequencies. Circ. Res., 12 (1963) 40–50.*

voltage versus time spectrum. Abnormalities are identified as arrhythmias and are associated with signaling problems at the sino-atrial node, infarction, and other cardiac tissue damage such as congestive heart failure, valvular distortions, and leaflet tears. These different disease states can all be sensed by tracking the EKG and correlating the time response to known conditions (regurgitation and septal defects are discussed in Chapter 13, Cardiovascular Interventions: The Alliteration of Ps Relating to Medicine. Proper Perfusion Prevents Pervasive Procedures Proffered to Improve Cardiovascular Health). One can also perform these diagnostic evaluations while the patient is on the treadmill to perform a stress test under a more demanding cardiac load. It is often under the load of a stress that arrhythmias are more pronounced. The presence of scar tissue on the surface of the electrode can reduce signal quality, as the scar tissue has a different composition, structure, and higher inherent impedance compared to the native chest connective tissue. This suggests that continued monitoring of patients with these implants is needed.

There are other both diagnostic and therapeutic probes that can be implanted with the notion of overriding physiologic signals with a more controlled signaling strategy. The concept of both pacemakers and defibrillators requires electronic impulses and leads to transmit the signal to the appropriate signaling locations. The miniaturization of these devices while maintaining function allows for more facile insertion. Other types of on board analytical instrumentation such as continuous glucose monitoring sensors require large electrode surface area to improve the signal to noise ratio, and lower resistance electrode materials are preferred. A range of neurostimulators also can be implanted into brain tissue to trigger muscular contractions in patients suffering from Parkinson's disease for example. Obviously the conductivity of the probes is most important for proper function. Design constraints are more related to the use of diamagnetic materials to allow for subsequent MRI imaging and the use of conductive electronic probes has evolved.

In considering electrical and optical properties of natural tissues the same types of characterization tools can be used to resolve tissue properties such as the index of refraction, the resistivity, etc. Nature, equipped with the capacity for protein synthesis and groups of amino acid-based building blocks, has an amazing array of structures that can be synthesized robustly. Certain specific tissues such as lenses and corneas perform amazing functions quite distinct from other connective tissues that are primarily mechanical. There are disease states that produce proteins that have different characteristic responses or suboptimum function (cataracts for example), some are brought on by age, some are congenital. But we need this basis to be able to understand how synthetic materials can seamlessly interface with natural tissue to augment or regain functional morbidities.

5.14 Conclusions

In this cursory scan of the literature tied to property evaluations of tissues, there is a wealth of detail that is found and linked to the archives. Digital libraries available through searchable databases and even reputable web links allow for deeper research on any individual topic that is presented here. It has been shown how mechanical, electrical, and optical properties can be assessed, how the mechanics of test modalities can affect property determinations, and the long chain molecular architecture of proteins in both bone and connective tissues leads to viscoelastic responses under mechanical loading that complicate the process of determining how disease and trauma affect protein structure.

An important series of takeaways are worth noting here. First, we are interested in comparing tissue as material as much as biomaterial replacements. There is interest in testing these materials in clinically relevant circumstances and there are some needs to optimize how to actually probe tissue properties. It is also clear that both tissues and materials deform, bend, and twist, and devices to not necessarily designed to fail in service. As a result, synthetic replacement components are overdesigned. Also, there is huge distinction between living and inanimate systems related to repeated cyclic loadings in that living systems can have the capacity to be damaged and repaired, which is less the case in acellular synthetic materials and has a big impact on how we interpret the usage of fatigue in lifetime assessments of materials and tissues. There are efforts to distinguish between normal and excessive loadings, as failure under normal loading conditions of synthetic replacements usually constitutes a design flaw and raises torts issues with product liability. It is also worth noting that functional diagnostic evaluations using magnetics, optics, and conductivity are all gaining in importance as clinicians involved in disease diagnostics are using a wider array of tools to probe health.

5.15 Problems

1. If physiologically viable compact bone can be treated as a pseudo-elastic Hookean Solid and is loaded uniaxially to a strain of 0.004 at a strain rate of 1500/s, using Fig. 5.8, determine the stress on the specimen (in MPa) upon achieving that strain.
2. If the sample was held at a strain of 0.004 for five times as long as it took to strain it to 0.004 at 1500 s^{-1}, determine what should the stress on the sample be if it is allowed to relax (in MPa).
3. A skin sample can be treated as a single Maxwell model (1 spring and 1 dashpot in series), with a spring modulus of 10 MPa at 37°C. If the sample is extended to a strain of 0.1 and held, with a relaxation time of 10 s at 37°C, determine what is the stress after 15 s?

4. If the skin specimen was tested at ambient temperature as opposed to 37°C, what effect does the lower temperature have on both the spring constant and the viscosity of the dashpot in the Maxwell model. Would you expect a longer/shorter/invariant relaxation time?

5. A 3-element model combining a Maxwell (spring + dashpot in series) element linked with a second spring in parallel is better at capturing the dynamics of stress relaxation. Draw the model and also a conceptual stress versus time curve showing a characteristics stress decay indicating how the second spring affects the long time stress response.

6. If a tissue for X-ray transmission analysis contains 80% fat and 20% muscle tissue by volume, and assuming the density differences between them are small, determine how much lower is the intensity of the of the X-ray beam (I/I_o) after passing through a segment of tissue 5 cm thick?

7. X-ray diagnostics are often used to resolve tooth decay. Consider the demineralization of teeth as a step in the pathway for dental caries formation. Explain how might a dentist look at an X-ray of a tooth margin and determine that it could be demineralized?

8. When you go in for these X-rays the dental hygienists often lay a lead (Pb) filled blanket over your chest while installing the X-ray film in your mouth. If the X-ray source is targeted at your tooth, why might being covered by the blanket be safer to you?

9. Explain why might hairline fractures (small fractures) be difficult to resolve by 1-D X-ray diagnostics?

10. If a compact bone segment is imaged as an annular tube section for a 1D X-ray, explain the variance in X-ray intensity (phase contrast) as X-rays are transmitted through the annulus near the edge versus through the center of the tube. In both instances the X-rays are traversing through the bone.

11. If titanium-based metallic implants are installed in bone, explain what bearing that has on subsequent imaging of the surrounding bone stock after installation.

12. Dubbleman and Van der Heijde [14], indicate that for a model myopic eye system that the convex intraocular lens has a posterior radius of curvature is 25 mm and that of the anterior is 15 mm. Calculate the focal length of this myopic double convex lens, f. Would one expect problems focusing with this lens in a viable eye?

13. Obviously the cornea is a concave/convex, calculate the focal length of the cornea assuming similar geometries of the posterior and anterior and compare that with that of the lens in Problem 12.

14. What role if any do the precipitates when forming cataracts have on the focusing power and light transmission of the lens?

15. Scar tissue commonly forms around implantation locations at the sino-atrial node for pacemaker recipients. How would the increased impedance affect signal transmission?

16. If a resistor was formed from muscle tissue, of dimensions 10 μm in diameter and 4 cm long, what is the resistance of this natural resistor?

References

[1] M. Lee, W. Hyman, Modeling the faiure mode in knee ligaments depending on the strain rate, BMC Musculoskelet. Disord. 3 (2002) 3 Article 3.

[2] R.D. Crowningshield, M.H. Pope, Response to compact bone in tension at various strain rates, Annal. Biomed. Eng. 2 (1974) 217–225.

[3] J.H. McElhaney, Dynamic response of bone and muscle tissue, J. Appl. Physiol. 21 (1966) 1231–1236.

[4] R. DeVita, W.S. Slaughter, A structural constitutive model for the strain rate dependent behavior of anterior cruciate ligaments, Int. J. Solids Struct. 43 (2006) 1561–1570.

[5] D.P. Pioletti, L.R. Rakotomanana, P.K. Leyvraz, Strain rate effect on the mechanical behavior of the anterior cruciate ligament-bone complex, Med. Eng. Phys. 21 (1999) 95–100.

[6] V. Arumugam, M.D. Naresh, R. Sanjeevi, Effect of strain rate on the fracture behavior of skin, J. Biosci. (India) 19 (1994) 307–313.

[7] A.B. Cua, K.P. Wilhelm, H.I. Maibach, Elastic properties of human skin: relation to age, sex, and anatomical region, Arch. Dermatol. Res. 282 (1990) 283–288.

[8] C. Dagdeviren, Y. Shi, P. Joe, R. Ghaffari, G. Balooch, K. Usgaonkar, Conformal piezoelectric systems for clinical and experimental characterization of soft tissue biomechanics, Nat. Mater. (2015) 14, 728.

[9] I.M. Ward, J. Sweeney, The Mechanical Properties of Solid Polymers, Wiley, Hoboken, NJ, 2004.

[10] G.A. Johnson, D.M. Tramaglini, R.E. Levine, K. Ohno, N.Y. Choi, S.L.Y. Woo, Tensile and viscoelastic properties of human patellar tendon, J. Orthopaed. Res. 12 (1994) 796–803.

[11] J.B. Park, R.S. Lakes, Biomaterials, an Introduction, Plenum Publishing, New York, 1992.

[12] S.A. Kane, Introduction to Physics in Modern Medicine, second ed, CRC Press, Boca Raton, FL, 2009.

[13] S. Rush, R. McFee, J.A. Abildskov, Resistivity of body tissues at low frequencies, Circ. Res. 12 (1963) 40–50.

[14] M. Dubbelman, G.L. Van der Heijde, The shape of the aging human lens: curvature, equivalent refractive index, and the lens paradox, Vision Res. 41 (2001) 1867–1877.

CHAPTER 6

Environmental Effects on Natural Tissues

> **Learning Objectives**
>
> From the first several chapters, one comes away with an understanding of normal cell functions, normal protein expression, how tissues are constructed in vivo and some ideas of how structure is characterization in terms of diagnostic evaluations. Physiology, though, is dynamic, and that there are well-known aging and disease processes that alter tissue, composition, cellular expression, and response. As the clinical disciplines interact with patients in a grand effort to improve their overall health, we, as engineers with a stronger sense of systems function, should also consider how aging perturbs structure and composition not only of natural tissue but engineered repairs and haptics.
>
> In this chapter, we dedicate time on the "physics" of diseases, and strive to understand how these aging responses are manifested. Included are descriptions of the state of the art and presentations of some misconceptions that might help explain that we only learn by understanding what we do not know as well can we consider material replacement in the right context. This is important for early interventions where tissue repairs need to accommodate growth for example. It might also help explain how physical evaluations are used to probe disease and to gauge the success of repair.
>
> As result of reading this chapter one should be able to:
>
> - Describe the physical attributes of several different age-related diseases
> - Describe how certain age-related diseases manifest themselves
> - Describe the nuances between well-characterized interventional needs versus those medical conditions lacking in a generally agreed upon playbook. The goal is not to produce a physiology book within a book, but more to at least how one can perform the deep dive necessary to characterize potential engineered therapies.

6.1 Introduction

The aging of several tissues is discussed in more detail. The focus here is on several age-related diseases (arteriosclerosis, valvular disease, and cancer) that have identified defensive playbooks to lessen the consequences of disease and manage symptoms. Also presented are diseases that are either less publicized or more rare. These types of ailments are just as

Biomaterials. DOI: http://dx.doi.org/10.1016/B978-0-12-809478-5.00006-7

important and perhaps more so given that these diseases lack a consensus on how to respond. Orphan diseases also present an opportunity to consider how engineered solutions can be design, built, and tested accordingly without so many other competitive financial pressures at the outset. The takeaway is that to offer credible alternatives to improve health, we need to understand disease and aging much more comprehensively.

6.2 Arteriosclerosis

In populations >30, identified subsets of the population show the formation of vessels that are biomechanically altered in terms of their pressure-dilatational response. A large fraction of these hardening events arise from fatty lipid and cholesterol deposits on and within the connective tissue lining of blood vessels. Diets higher in concentrations of saturated fats likely correlate with higher concentrations of low-density lipoproteins (LDL) within blood and within the connective tissue. LDL is not the only factor though luminal shrinkage can arise due to the precipitation of these deposits (the pipe gets thicker), and functionally, the blood vessels are less compliant and appear stiffer, hence the term "artery hardening."

With the etiology and epidemiology of arteriosclerosis the challenges are daunting. Baseline diagnostics can resolve age-related changes in blood pressure for example a hypertensive population needing more regular monitoring and drug therapy interventions. But early diagnostics to identify changes are not done on a compulsory level and before electronic medical records; these sorts of diagnostic evaluations were often lost. With e-records more common, there is a better chance that baseline electrocardiograms or EKGs will be a part of someone's traveling e-record.

Arteriosclerosis is a systemic problem and it is difficult to envision a successful replacement material that could be substituted wholesale for compromised arteries. Fractional blockages in critical areas are commonly dealt with by interventional balloon angioplasty to compress the fatty deposits and reopen these regions and by stents that have been installed to extend specific regions that are too small. These procedures can be done by catheterization and are treated essentially as outpatient procedures. Cardiologists have commonly used more invasive coronary bypass surgery to reroute blood flow around cardiac blockages. There is limited donor tissue available for autograft strategies, and these are complicated and involved surgeries that are often very expensive. But there is a need for specific, reasonably sized simulated blood vessels to replicate critical small and medium diameter grafts.

Synthetics that have been used as replacement vessels have included expanded polytetrafluoroethylene foam-like structures and other types of endothelial cell-seeded prosthetic surfaces with a larger discussion in Chapter 9, Polymeric Biomaterials. One can clearly see that there are many more diagnostic procedures relative to the actual ones involved directly in the intervention. Hence, catheters, balloons, deployment structures, and phase contrast imaging agents are much more in demand relative to each prosthetic blood vessel that gets installed. There are other stopgap measures for single vessels that are partially obstructed, and with stenosis of carotid arteries, there is increasing usage of titanium stents that can be unfurled in conjunction with balloon angioplasty. The efficacy of these interventions is continually being assessed, restenosis of initially blocked and opened vessels remains a challenge, and refinements are being made to resolve which patients should receive stents in the event that blockage is not complete and ischemia is not imminent.

As was noted earlier, arteriosclerosis is a systemic disease, which means that if there is a motivation to clear blockages in one or just a few critical vessels, there is probably similar interest in opening up more and smaller vessels. This drive is the basis for the biased focus on development of small diameter vascular grafts and drug therapies to control cholesterol and lipid composition in the vasculature. Drug-based therapy is preferred to reverse systemic cardiovascular fatty lipid deposits but when presenting in the ER as a crisis case, materials-based bypass schemes, coupled with clot-busting drug therapy is common. Diet, metabolism, and exercise all reduce the need for intervention. Nonetheless, there are runners with superior metabolic health but are also rife with plaques and also victims of heart attacks. No one is immune.

A common misconception is that the plaques are actually a separate concentric layer with a smaller radius than the original intima. There may be some amount deposited on the intimal lining, but larger fractions of the deposits are actually found in the vessel, as shown in Fig. 6.1. The accumulation can be quite large and block a significant fraction of the lumen

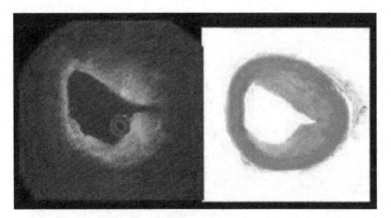

Figure 6.1

Optical coherence tomography looking axially down a blood vessel showing a diffusively occlusive plaque on the left and the corresponding histology on the right. *From F. Prati, E. Regar, G.S. Mintz, E. Arbustini, C. Di Mario, I.K. Jang et al., Expert review document on methodology, terminology, and clinical applications of optical coherence tomography: physical principles, methodology of image acquisition, and clinical application for assessment of coronary arteries and atherosclerosis. Eur. Heart J. 31 (2010) 401–415.*

area as represented as a stenosis, shown in Fig. 6.2. Thus melting and scraping strategies that are only focused on the wall are probably incomplete in eradicating the change in the biomechanical properties of the vessel walls. These plaques can be dislodged from walls by shear flow and conveyed downstream and can result in ischemic stroke if the plaques clog the vessel or activate platelets to form a clot.

More than half the adult population (likely 1 in 2) is hypertensive, has high cholesterol, plaque build-up, and other heart and arterial disease. Inexpensive screenings (LDL, e.g., in a blood test) and other diagnostic assessment can identify the populations most in need to continued observation and screening. And as we age, these deposits can add up. Disruptive technologies that yield substantially better cardiovascular transport outcomes might be worthy of investigation, but there is an inertial challenge to change the common strategy for managing chronic cases and dealing with the crises as they are encountered.

6.3 Kidney Disease

Proper renal function is critical as kidneys are the primary filters for purifying blood. Their continuous operation coupled a high perfusion (a strong blood supply fed by the renal arteries) and appropriate selectivity yields a purified blood composition that is almost invariant with time. The renal system is an amazing and robust filtration system. As such, it is important to see just how expensive and how much impact kidney disorders have on the medical health care system in general.

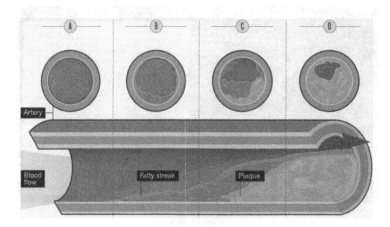

Figure 6.2

In A, healthy blood flow is occurring, in region B, the presence of a fatty sheath around the intimal wall is observed, in regions C and D, there is an creasing amount of plaque build-up within the vessel and the open region in the middle is compressed. *From B. Cannon, Biochemistry to behavior, Nature, 493 (2013) S2–S3.*

It is accepted that young adults in their 20s have the most robust renal system function, in terms of both efficiency and what is measured as a glomerular filtration rate. The functional transport of blood impurities, excess salts, proteins, and fluids, and other metabolized by-products occurs in the nephron. The anatomists have identified a range of structures the form in the normal kidney and the key features include the glomerulus, a sac-like structure that is at the beginning of the nephron and then a tubular structure called the nephron. Together, these form a blood/urine transport membrane and blood from the renal artery is directed to smaller and smaller vessels until reaching individual glomeruli. There is an axial blood flow to continue perfusion downstream, and there is a radial flow of the metabolites and water across this nephronic membrane where they are collected and conveyed to the bladder for subsequent excretion, as shown conceptually in Fig. 6.3.

The origin of how kidneys age is the realm of pathology and it remains of interest how metabolism, vascular health, and kidney health are interlinked [4]. From an initial paper by Darmady et al., who autopsied donor kidneys from 105 people who died suddenly from something other than kidney failure over a range of ages from birth to 101 years [5], comparisons of tissue structure, size, and weight were made. They found a general shrinking of nephron volume past age 30 but the ratio of the glomular surface to the tube volume in the nephron was conserved [5]. They also found increases in the connective tissue content in the small vessels of the nephron [5]. Later autopsy-based studies focused on quantifying the number and size of functional glomeruli in individuals also not apparently compromised by kidney disease at death [6]. A gradual loss in the number of

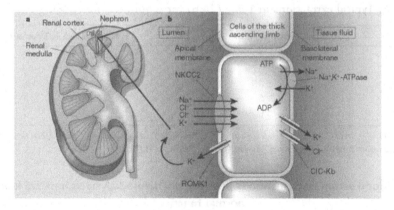

Figure 6.3

Schematic of kidney transport. Blood is routed through the nephrons of the gross kidney (a) where blood passes into renal cortex and renal medulla, which contain a larger number of replicated nephrons represented as a membrane (b) across which water, ions, and other small molecules permeate and are transported to the ureter. *From M. Hunter, Ion channels: accessory to kidney disease, Nature 414 (2001) 502—503.*

glomeruli after age 60 and glomerular volume (the number of functional glomeruli * the volume of each one) were noted, proportional to a reduction in kidney weight [6].

The kidneys work remarkably well, continuously purifying blood day and night. There are fluctuations in performance, but it is a finely tuned system that works exceedingly well. A functional kidney removes a fraction of each metabolites and with continued filtration, steady state can be achieved balancing metabolism and extraction to the bladder. An example of a normal kidney's extraction potential is shown in Table 6.1 and typical serum concentrations of metabolites found pre- and post- dialysis compared with a volunteer with a normal functioning kidney is shown in Table 6.2.

Rule et al. [8] have studied more closely what they define as nephrosclerosis and there is a perceptible hardening of tube segments within the nephron suggesting that the same type of atherosclerotic activity occurring in the general vasculature is also occurring in renal vasculature as well. It is understood that toxic exposure to renal cells has some consequences on cell viability there, and progressive cell death will damage organ function. It is speculation but perhaps it is these sclerotic precipitates clog pores in the nephron, they can reduce kidney efficiency without necessarily killing off renal cells. This physical hardening mechanism also reinforces the notion that addressing could have a positive effect on extending renal clearance.

In terms of function the glomerular filtration, this measure of efficiency drops by about 10% per decade of life past about age 30. The reasons for these drops in efficiency are due to acute infection, but other diseases such as hypertension, diabetes, atherosclerosis, and other cardiovascular anomalies (sickle cell anemia, for example) damage the number of

Table 6.1: Typical extractions in 1 day (24 h) for a normally functioning renal system

Compound	Normal Adult Man	Normal Adult Woman
Water	2.15 ± 1 L	2.22 ± 0.9
Na + (mequiv.)	226.3 ± 79	205 ± 63
K + (mequiv.)	60.2 ± 19	56.1 ± 18
Urea (g)	21 g ± 6	18.7 ± 6
Creatinine (g)	1.48 ± 0.3	1.02 ± 0.3

Source: From A. B. da Silva, M.D.C. Molina Mdel, S.L. Rodrigues, E.B. Pimentel, M.P. Baldo, et al., Correlation between the creatinine clearance in the urine collected during 24 hours and 12 hours. Braz. J. Nefrol. 32 (2010) 165–172.

Table 6.2: Blood serum concentrations pre- and posthemodialysis vs a native kidney under normal function

Metabolite	Predialysis	Postdialysis	Normal Kidney Under SS
Urea	42.2 mg/dL ± 22	10.33 mg/dL	13 mg/dL
Creatinine	8.9 mg/dL ± 2.2	2.93 mg/cl	0.84 mg/dL

Source: From T.L. Sirich, B.A. Funk, N.S. Plummer, T.H. Hostetter, W.M. Meyer, Prominent accumulation in hemodialysis patients of solutes normally cleared by tubular secretion, Am. J. Nephrol. 25 (2014) 615–622.

effective glomeruli thus affecting the rate of filtration. The rapid rise in the number of people suffering from Type II diabetes and the relative obesity epidemic are stark factors that are increasing the number of potentially affected people with some fraction of kidney failure. Kidney disease can also initiated by secondary side effects of drug therapy, infections, and chemotherapy, and the infections are often difficult to eradicate. The reduced efficiency is normally not acutely noticeable until 75–85% reduction. By then, its normally too late to regenerate improved renal function, although diet and conditioning lower the subsequent damage on glomeruli.

There are anomalies such as the ability to extract water but not metabolites. Internists, nephrologists, and general practitioners monitor the urine density to insure that the urine contains metabolites, and when the density drops from 1.2 toward 1, that is an indicator that fluid extraction is on-going but the kidneys are challenged in purifying the blood, and as the rise in vascular concentration of the normally clearable metabolites is essentially poisoning the blood.

The mathematics of renal function have been worked out elegantly by Depner [9]. Consider a mass balance around the kidney as a functional separator. Blood flows into the kidney with known concentrations of cells, proteins, metabolites, and water. When everything is working correctly, there is a general balance between the inputs and outputs in such a way that blood leaves the kidney with fewer contaminants, which are extracted and directed, into the urine for excretion. The renal system has some variable rate of extraction (depending on water intake and exercise for example) but day-by-day, functional systems should have something approaching an average extraction rate.

6.3.1 Models of Kidney Transport

There is certain volumetric flow rate through the kidney and with one metabolite, urea for example, any fluctuations in concentration can be established, and the urine can be collected and measured for dynamic extraction rates. The functional kidney is always operational, so a material balance considers bloodstream concentration, and knowing that there are sources of urea (metabolism) and sinks (renal clearance). A material balance on urea in blood is shown in Eq. (6.1)

$$\frac{D(CV)}{dt} = k_0 - k_1 C \tag{6.1}$$

where C is the concentration of urea, V is the blood volume, k_0 is the urea generation rate from metabolism, and k_1 is the clearance rate, which is first order relative to the urea concentration in blood. As the concentration gradient rises across the membrane, the larger the effective clearance.

There are some special cases to consider. For example, at steady state, the left side of the equation is zero, and clearance is directly related to generation. We might also consider when the volume is increasing linearly with respect to time:

$$V = V_o + \beta t \tag{6.2}$$

Under instances when k_1 is 0 (no clearance) and $\beta = 0$ (kidneys clear only water), the dynamic concentration $C(t)$ is represented as

$$C(t) = C_0 + k_0{}^*t/V_0 \tag{6.3}$$

where urea concentration rises linearly with time from an initial concentration.

Removing the constraint on constant volume ($\beta > 0$) leads to rising urea concentration, but one that is diluted by the increasing blood volume.

$$C(t) = C_0 + k_0{}^*t/V(t) \tag{6.4}$$

Under iso-volume constraints, and $k_1 > 0$, the following exponential expression represents the dynamic metabolite concentration

$$C(t) = C_0 e^{-k1t/V_0} + (k_0/k_1)(1 - e^{-k1t/V_0}) \tag{6.5}$$

This same type of analytical expression could be used for all metabolites with the understanding that they all have different k_1 values, and some could rise while others could be cleared.

Kidney failure is linked with a number of symptoms including weight gain, nausea, fatigue, and others. Kidney failure is a quick diagnosis given what is observed. Patients presenting with compromised kidney function are directed for dialysis. In 2009 The National Kidney Fund [10] in the United States reported that there were nearly 400,000 patients undergoing dialysis on a regular basis, about 95% of those were undergoing hemodialysis, and the remainder were doing peritoneal dialysis. There are about 100,000 new cases per year identified, and transplants account for roughly 1/3 of all patients who have kidney failure. In any given year, there are 90,000 people on the transplant list, and about 15,000 kidney transplants per year. As a result, there is a large, unmet need.

Hemodialysis is performed typically every 2 or 3 days depending on metabolism and it requires transportation to a clinic or hospital. The acute hemodialysis is done by needle injection and the blood is routed through an ex vivo dialysis membrane called a hemodialyzer, shown in Fig. 6.4.

Hemodialysis is essentially a bypass procedure where a fraction of the blood is extracted by needle incision and rerouted through a porous separations membrane and then redirected into an adjacent vein. The prosthetic dialyzer is a porous, tubular construction that under counter-current flow conditions bathes the outsides of a large number of porous fibers on one

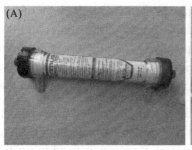 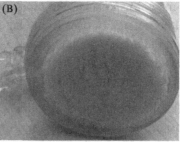

Figure 6.4

A typical hemodialyzer. (A) Pressurized blood flow is axial with radial extraction of metabolites and water into the dialysate fluid in the outer chambers. The hollow fibers are observed and again aligned axially on edge in (B).

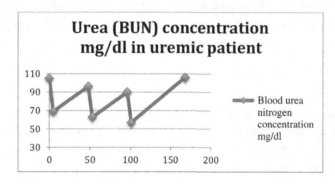

Figure 6.5

Example dataset of the BUN concentration over time as the drops coincide with each dialysis procedure. *Reproduced From A. Dhondt, R. Vanholder, W. Van Biesen, N. Lameire, The removal of uremic toxins. Kid. Int. 58 (2000) S47–S59.*

fluid (the dialysate) and allows blood flow through the interior segments of the fibers. There are 1000s of fibers nominally composing a single dialyzer, typically of ~ 200 μm in diameter and with submicron sized pores to allow for radial transport. Blood and its metabolites are conveyed down the axial fiber length and a radial concentration gradient serves as a driving force to push metabolites through the fiber radius and back into the. Metabolites and other small molecules are conveyed into the dialysate and the longer the dialyzer operates, the larger the accumulation of the filtered metabolites. By control of the chemistry of the dialysate the dialyzer pore size, and the pressure drop across the membrane, one can control the extraction rate from blood; for a single dialysis procedure a complete dialysis takes several hours. Metabolites and water are isolated from purified blood and collected in a counter fluid called dialysate and the blood is returned for reperfusion [11].

It is critical to maintain access to the dialysis clinic as blood metabolites will rise quickly in instances of kidney failure [12]. An example dataset of one metabolite blood urea nitrogen (BUN) as a function of two dialysis treatments and missing 1 day, as shown in Fig. 6.5.

The filtration time corresponds to the rapid drops in the saw tooth curve of serum BUN concentration. It systemically rises following departure from the clinic, and BUN concentrations in the uremic population are typically two–three times normal even under conditions of adequate dialysis. Missing a clinic apt as which happens in this dataset at 100 h causes a BUN concentration rise to almost what was before going on dialysis.

The length of flexible tubing (usually silicone resins or plasticized polyvinyl chloride) required to transport the blood to and from the dialyzer to the patient constitutes the largest linear distance of temporary, disposable, vascular graft materials used in medicine, and the need is staggering. With an aging population the demand for chronic management of an increasingly needy population for hemodialysis is a significant drain on the health care system. And while kidney transplants are highly successful, the donor database is small relative to the need list and immunosuppressant, antirejection drugs are still needed to maintain the donor kidney in the recipient. The diabetes crisis is also a dialysis crisis, as more people needing dialysis tie up a larger segment of the clinics on a regular basis.

6.4 Obesity

The obesity epidemic is a growing and pervasive problem that impacts many other metabolic diseases and more than just older people, and by solving the obesity challenge, the overall rate of related diseases could be impacted as well. Table 6.3 represents data showing recent obesity statistics presented by the US NIH.

Functionally, it is known that with aging and with the onset of menopause, there are metabolic changes that alter energy storage within what is consumed. By not adjusting caloric intake when these metabolic changes commence, often an energy imbalance arises with increasing energy storage as fat. The general problem is simply an energy balance problem, and with more attention to foods and diet control, there is a sense that one can alter the caloric intake as these changes arise with aging. It is easier said than done though.

Table 6.3: Weight statistics amongst adults above age 20 in the United States based on body mass index (BMI)

Normal or underweight: BMI <24.9	31.2%
Overweight: 25 < BMI < 29.9	33.1%
Obese 30 < BMI	35.7%

Source: From K.M. Flegel, M.D. Carroll, B.K. Kit, C.L. Ogden, Prevalence of obesity and trends in the distribution of body mass index among US adults, 1999–2010. J. Am. Med. Assoc. 307 (2012) 491–497.

In addition to the issue of aging and metabolic dynamics, there is a more daunting challenge of obesity that is occurring in youth that has a more dramatic impact on what is defined as average weight, height, and body mass. Changes in the dietary patterns of families relating to processed foods, what is available at schools for lunches and snacks, and exercise patterns is altering the baseline health of children growing up in large segments of the developing world. And if adequate health diet and exercise regimens are not established early for kids, it will be more difficult to empower these people to maintain their health in general.

Heavier people will be more susceptible to the age-related diseases as mentioned earlier in this chapter. It is known that caloric restriction is an effective tool at promoting longevity at least in other mammalian populations. It is not just the extra body weight as there are a host of metabolic diseases that accompany an imbalance in glucose management, type II diabetes, and hypertension in youth today, and these diseases will likely be with them earlier in life as well. This is not a book directly about diet and nutrition, but adequate oversight of dietary quality has the potential to reduce the need for later interventions if the average pool of clients is healthier to begin with.

6.5 Osteoporosis

Geriatric doctors are also focused on how both menopause and aging affect bone synthesis, bone remodeling, posture, gait, and instability. Falls of the elderly are arguably, one of the most prevalent pathways where independent ambulatory people suddenly become much reliant on the health care network to sustain them. The mechanisms of bone loss can be readily evaluated through diagnostic imaging. Peak bone density is normally found in females by age 18, and in men, by age 20. Biochemically, it is understood that an increasing imbalance arises between osteoclasts, cells involved in deconstructing bony tissues, and the osteoblasts, the number of cells that are involved in reprecipitating minerals are reduced leading to a lower bone density with age. There is an equivalent drop in bone density in men, although the link with a specific event like menopause is more ambiguous [14].

And at least for traumatic fracture with falls and other trauma events, there is a correlation between residual bone density and the incidence of bone fracture as noted in the work by DeLaet et al. [15] (see Figs. 6.6 and 6.7). Clearly, these events are easy to document as they are linked often with visits to the ER.

The mechanics of aging bone structures is a large topic of discussion emphasizing hard tissue engineering and rehabilitation. It is perhaps more important to consider other areas

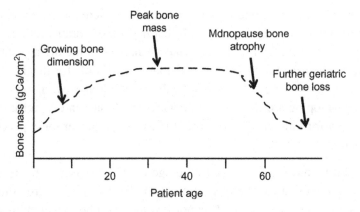

Figure 6.6
Relative bone density as a function of patient lifetime.

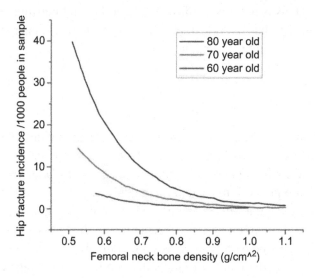

Figure 6.7
Correlates between bone density, age at fracture, and bone density with cumulative fracture potential in 1 year for a given age group. Clearly more fractures occur in older populations with lower bone density. *Data replotted from DeLaet et al., BMJ (1997) 315, 221.*

relating to lumbar support and spinal compression that are just as important in maintaining proper skeletal health.

The primary biomechanical observable associated with osteoporosis is an increasing spinal fulcrum that arises from spinal compression fractures [16], as shown schematically in Fig. 6.8. Osteoporosis thins the bone in cancellous vertebrae, often to the point that they cannot sustain normal pressure in exaggerated cases. The thinned bones can collapse during normal activity (bending over, lifting, and overexertion), leading to a spinal compression

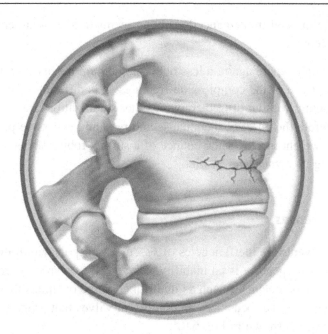

Figure 6.8
Example of a vertebral compression fracture, Republished with permission from Getty Images.

fracture and can herniate the corresponding cartilage causing pain, nerve sensitivity, and numbness down the legs to the point of instability. It is reported that 40% of all aged reach 80 will have at least one compression fracture [16]. And just to consider the link with other sections of this chapter, a more obese person will have more mass on top of the fulcrum, and as deterioration initiates, overload conditions will happen in heavier people first. Vertebral compression fractures can permanently alter the shape and strength of the surviving spinal segments. The fractures often heal without medical intervention (there is not much one can do) and the pain with a single event can often subside. However, sometimes the pain can persist if the crushed bone fails to heal adequately.

Compression fractures are one type of vertebral fracture that results in spinal height loss and a humped back, especially in elderly women. This disorder (called kyphosis or a "dowager's hump") is an exaggerated forward curvature of the spine that causes the shoulders to slump forward and causing the back to look enlarged and humped. There are interventions such as kyphopasty that stabilize these types of degenerative conditions by installing a balloon in the anterior segment of the compression fracture, followed by the injection of bone cement to extend the crushed bone and stabilize the remaining vertebral segments composing the spine. This type of intervention lowers the chance of subsequent compression fracture as the fulcrum of is reduced. Mineral loss from cancellous bone is much more of a crisis than in the cortical bone, the content is lower to begin with and the reinforcement of the mineral in the cancellous bone seems to have a larger role in mechanical reinforcement.

Here is another example where again, a less obese population results in lower skeletal load and reduces the incidence of the compression fractures. It is difficult to resolve how to arrest continued fracture without drug therapy or other stabilization. But improving one's skeletal structure before the onset of menopause and reducing excessive passive loading just by one's own body weight increases the chance of a strong, robust skeletal structure capable of sustaining its owner later in life.

6.6 Valvular Diseases

Other cardiac aging events are inefficiencies of vascular transport within the heart. What is defined as valvular incompetence is an inability to seat valve openings correctly. While there are congenital incompetencies such as malformed valve openings that can cause similar outcomes innately, we focus here on competent valves that progressively function more poorly over time, as shown in Fig. 6.9.

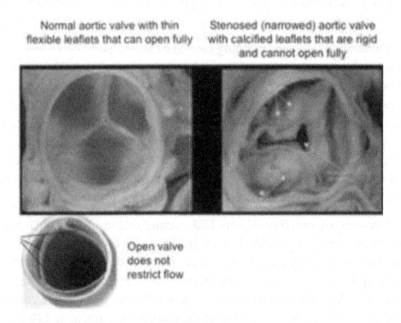

Figure 6.9

An example of a normal aortic valve and one that has calcified leaflets and stenosis preventing a complete opening. *From Transcatheter Aortic Valve Replacement. (2014). Published with permission from http://www.heartgroup.co.nz/Patient + Information/Therapeutic + Procedures/ Transcatheter + Aortic + Valve + Implantation + TAVI.html.*

The diagnostic determination of incompetence is through EKG and other catheter-based diagnostic evaluations. It is a routine determination now for proper valve function, as regurgitation is easily identifiable. The larger question is the underlying reason for the incompetence. There can be a similar hardening of these tissues from calcification or a degeneration of the tissues making up the leaflets identified as degenerative valve disease.

Calcification of leaflets from components dispersed in blood has a rather dramatic effect on the mechanical response of the leaflets and can cause the free opening of the valve to be blocked in larger ways. First in terms of the mechanics the leaflets are designed to be highly flexible and extendable. The presence of inorganic deposits on these surfaces tends to make them much harder, much less extendable, and more retarded in the instantaneous viscoelastic mechanical response. A separate issue arising from deposition is the deposits can affect the fluid dynamics around the valve entry, and there can be more hemolysis arising from either higher velocities entering through the valve or issue with stagnant flow patterns due to where the calcifications are situated.

Why the deposition occurs is somewhat unknown. Too much calcium in the diet in one origin, and there was a recent spate of valvular calcification events as a side effect that occurred by the ingestion of Cox II type inhibitors to address rheumatoid arthritis. Calcified valves can be replaced and the mitral valve stenosis replaced at the same time that a new ascending aorta is installed. Other valves have been replaced on an as needed basis but mitral valve disease has been with us for quite a while and its replacement has dramatically improved cardiac output accordingly. There are many other repairs that can be accomplished by cardiologists for example suturing of torn leaflets.

6.7 Cancer

As humans age, there are many types of disruptions in the cell cycle that if not auto-corrected, can remain unchecked leading to the formation of tumors. Cancer diagnosis and more importantly treatment using chemotherapeutic cocktails, resection and radiation therapy have led to remission and cure of many different types of cancers. The story remains incomplete as there are many types of cancers that if found at a later stage has eluded successful treatment strategies. From a materials perspective, there are hybrid systems such as magnetically or RF sensitive tags which allow for binding to tumors and can be either radiated or absorbed into the tumor as at higher rates than into surrounding tissue to generate selectivity.

Advancing age is a common factor in more likely diagnosis with cancer, and these are diseases of the aged. But there are many more options and in terms of functional morbidities associated with being diagnosed and treated, there is an on-going need for rehabilitative devices to help augment function for affected populations.

The National Cancer Institute publishes statistics on the prevalence of specific cancer types, and environmental triggers including air and water pollution, smoking, alcohol consumption, correlations with red meat, carbon residues from grilling, etc. Each disease has its own pathway and its own designated clinical experts, and we are learning more about subclassifying individual cancers at present, which helps in terms of pharmaceutical targeting. The ability to link cancer to genetic typing has led to a larger understanding of risk factors someone might possess to generate a cancer, and family history is already a screen. Cancer of specific organs can be classified as relatively benign or aggressive, and treatment strategies can include the deployment of chemotherapeutics directly adjacent to tumors that occurs with prostate cancers, to the generation of tissue-engineered constructs to replace the lost tissue and function that can happen with oral cancers. To those affected by bladder cancer, there is a loss of the resected organ and there is a need replicate the voiding function as might arise in Chapter 14, Artificial Organs. What is beyond conjecture is that the older the patient, the more likely that they are living with or have survived one or more cancers.

6.8 Amyloid Diseases

If the playbook is established in treating cancer and heart disease as diseases of the aged, the same cannot be said in terms of amyloid diseases. The term amyloid relates to the expression of misfolded protein that is either synthesized without the appropriate hierarchical structure, or are somehow environmentally conditioned or coerced to create a errant and misfolded structure. There are both reversible and irreversible misfolding events and the longer a protein is misfolded, the more likely this is a permanent structure. And misfolding results in structures that are in energetically unfavorable conformations, do not present the same receptors, and do not have the same solubility characteristics as the native functional proteins with the same sequences. It suggests that there is both a cellular pathway leading to amyloid structures in the first place and an environmental pathway that may drive these proteins into aberrant conformations. There is a rationale to consider both options.

There are nominally 20 + disorders that are lumped under the term amyloid diseases and there is usually at least one key protein that is identified as part of the disorder. The diseases that have the largest impact at least in terms of numbers include Alzheimer's disease, Parkinson's disease, Huntington's disease, and Prion disease. There are a number of so-called tissue amyloidoses that arise in the end stages of terminal disease as amyloid proteins are precipitated out in the connective tissue. The ones that harbor much more concern are the proteins directly linked with dementias that are found in the cerebrospinal fluid (CSF), as these proteins resist breakdown and are not clearable in any effective way. Amyloid proteins and fragments tend to aggregate into what are defined as amyloid plaques and during their residence, and they can be toxic to adjacent cell structures. What is affected (memory, neuromuscular control, etc.) is more a function of where within the brain these plaques form and why.

It is generally known how amyloid disease progress, but the realm of diagnostics is incomplete. A confirming diagnosis of AD, for example, usually is only complete at autopsy so better and more effective diagnostics earlier have more potential to treat symptoms early.

Functional MRI and PET scanning has been used to probe activity in the Alzheimer's brain, and it appears that the first regions to turn off are near the hippocampus as noted in Fig. 6.10 and Fig 6.11.

In limited instances, it is also known how amyloid diseases originate. For example, some amyloid diseases are genetic disorders (Huntington (HD) and Familiar Alzheimer's disease

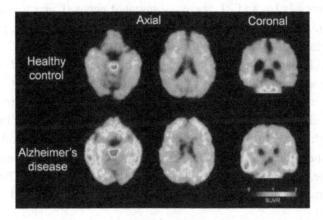

Figure 6.10

^{18}F PET images from 60–80 min post-injection in a healthy control subject (72-years-old) and a patient with Alzheimer's disease (68-years-old), using 2 axial cuts and one coronal cut. *Image with permission From Okamura et al., Brain 137 (6) 1762–1777.*

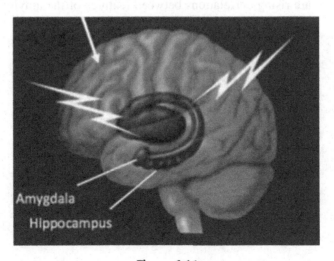

Figure 6.11

It is thought that the horns of the hippocampus, denoted in red (darker grey in print edition) are the earliest diagnostic reference to the onset of Alzheimer's disease. *Printed with permission from McEwen et al., Nature Neuroscience, 18 (2015), September 25, 2015.*

(AFD)). In the case of HD the huntintin gene is found on chromosome 4 and within it, there are normally a number of CAG codons that repeat within the structure. In the wild type (normal) sequence, there are usually between 5 and 27 repeats of this codon that codes for glutamine. People who have more CAG linkages (over 35 repeat units) are more likely to produce an amyloid form of huntingtin, the amyloid protein linked with HD.

In Familiar Alzheimer's disease (FAD), β amyloid formation is regulated by more players [17]. On chromosomes 1, 14, and 21, there are mutated genes (Chromosome 1: presenilin 1 (PSEN-1)) that regulates the expression of γ secretase (Chromosome 14, presenilin 2 (PSEN-2) that regulates the expression of β secretase and Chromosome 21: amyloid precursor protein (APP) that regulates how much protein can be directed into an amyloids). Upregulation of these genes either adds to the potential source material (APP) capable for forming amyloids, or increases the efficiency with which APP is converted to β amyloid through enzymatic cleavage by the secretases, to form clusters, as noted in Fig. 6.12. What we know about Alzheimer's grows every day, by studying susceptible and less susceptible populations about their lifestyle, their local environment, in addition to understanding more about both the nucleation of the disease and managing its progression. There is an intense, on-going drug discovery campaign to resolve how to tackle any one of these mechanisms in fighting disease.

There is a general consensus that disease commences much earlier than when observable symptoms become apparent, and correlations between one or more physically stressful events such as an earlier traumatic brain injury could be an early trigger for the nucleation. Diagnostically, there are rising correlations between features of the amyloid brain and

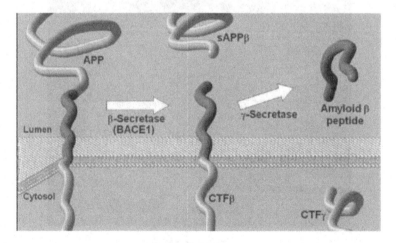

Figure 6.12

Schematic on how extracellular proteins are cleaved by secretases in the progression of amyloid plaques formed in the CSF. *From Y. Hamada, Drug discovery of β-secretase inhibitors based on quantum chemical interactions for the treatment of Alzheimer's disease. SOJ Pharm. Pharmaceut. Sci. 1 (2014) 1—8.*

normal healthy brains of the same age in terms of functional activity. The feature that gives pause to focusing on the genetic front is that FAD strikes affected families very early (typically before age 50) and only accounts for about 4% of the AD cases. AD-based amyloid diseases must contain an environmental element as well.

For the nonfamilial AD cases and perhaps for other amyloid diseases, there must be something about blood chemistry that changes over time that makes geriatric patients more susceptible to plaque formation. There is great attention spent on describing the physics of amyloid protein plaque build-up as a milestone in the progression of the disease and potentially a marker to show its eradication. There are studies to show that the plaque aggregates are toxic to adjacent neurons and the pore size of the blood–brain barrier is very small suggesting that perhaps some fraction of disease progression is a clearance problem, that plaques that are formed cannot be effectively cleared from the CSF and that as the slosh around, they are toxic to the surrounding neurons. There are others who have asserted that the observation of the plaques is just a sideshow, an unrelated observation that is an effect but not a reason why the aggregates are there. In epidemiology, subgroups of people have been studied who seem to have a slightly lower incidence of affliction than average populations including the Cherokee nations [19,20] in the United States among others and some who have higher incidence (e.g., American Football Players) [21]. The murky surroundings about who is affected, what events expose the population to amyloid formation and the origins and biochemical progression of the disease are of great conjecture. Perhaps the synthesis of natural antioxidants is suppressed with age and upregulating these might work. Perhaps proper diet and more exercise can make a difference. Perhaps we can all start drinking red wine and green tea. Perhaps plaque-busting drugs can be developed. Perhaps we can purify and isolate aggregated plaques in the CSF by a similar dialysis technique for blood. There are all so many unanswered questions; we are all left to our own devices in adapting accordingly.

There is hyperawareness of these diseases for several reasons, one is that the overall quality of life is highly compromised in the stages of these diseases; these are neurological diseases affecting memory, neuromuscular control, and thresholds of social acceptance. The afflicted change who they are before our eyes. Second, there is a huge financial impact to caring for affected individuals that often require day/night care and the needs only increase over time. This cost consideration is a much larger financial and resource undertaking than for kidney disease given that as amyloid diseases progress, the need increases. Affected patients are going to be users of any potential therapy, and much like any other lifetime regimen. Third the diagnoses of these conditions continue to be on the rise, in part due to better and earlier diagnosis, but also due to skewed demographics. As the size of the geriatric population relative to the population rises, the prevalence of these disorders will only increase. It is thought that with current diagnosis, about 3% of the population in the United States is suffering from an amyloid condition, that number is slated to rise within two decades.

We are very early in understanding how these conditions form, and the general playbook on how to manage symptoms and reverse the conditions has not been fully developed. And finally, these diseases form and progress is the realm of the specific clinics dealing with symptoms, but the physics of the different diseases is similar, and the grand hops is that strategies to combat one condition might be conserved in fighting others. Drugs and therapies to either counteract the progression of amyloid diseases are the holy grails of therapeutics so to speak.

From materials standpoint, there are already devices such as deep brain stimulators that are approved for insertion to address neuromuscular modulation for Parkinson's patients [22,23]. An example schematic is shown in Fig. 6.13. Rather than the innate expression of L-dopamine (L-DOPA), neuromuscular stimulators are inserted deep within the muscular control centers of the brain to override electrical discharges in patients devoid of the capacity manage and discharge spurious signaling. The outcomes have been promising.

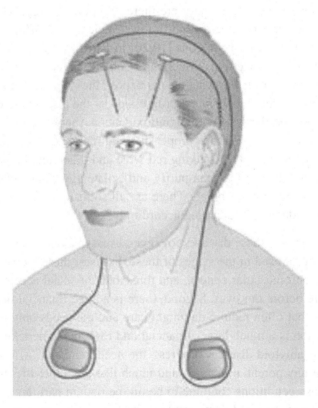

Figure 6.13
Schematic of how deep brain stimulators are positioned and energized by a signal generator(s) linked by electrical leads leading to brain. *Republished with permission from K. Kingwell, Nat. Rev. Neurol. (2012) (8) 119.*

Better diagnostic phase contrast agents will allow for more comprehensive diagnostic and functional imaging. And if drug therapy is ultimately the systemic route to manage afflicted patients, there have to be better packaging strategies to help deploy maintenance drugs that have lead to fewer side effects, have a longer window of effectiveness, etc.

6.9 Skin: How is Aging Manifested?

Skin, the integument, our largest organ, performs a range of functions. Skin is a layered structure, composed of the connective tissue fibers collagen and elastin, and swollen in a proteoglycan gel matrix called ground substance, and covered with a range of probiotic and pathogenic bacteria on the outer surfaces as represented in Fig. 6.14 by Grice and Segre [24]. Each layer of skin, the epidermis, the dermis, and the hypodermis deserve their own chapters in physiology texts focused only on skin. Even within the epidermis, there are easily resolvable sublayers such as the stratum corneum and the basement membrane by histology. The epidermis is the primary regenerative skin tissue. Keratinocytes undergo mitosis at the basement membrane and as new layers of cells form, they displace already formed keratinocytes, pushing them away from the membrane and its nutrients. As these cells are further pushed away, there are a cascade of other changes, including the

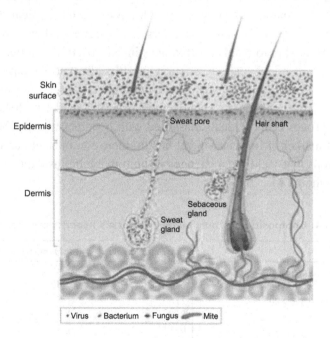

Figure 6.14

Anatomical section of skin showing the epidermis including the stratum corneum, and the corresponding adipocytes found in the fat layer. *Reproduced from E.A. Grice, J.A. Segre, The skin microbiome. Nat. Rev. Microbiol. 9 (2011) 244–253.*

precipitation of keratin within the cells, morphological changes as their nucleus becomes distorted as does the whole cell with further displacement, flattening into plate-like disks, and exuding oils that complicate intercellular transport. These cells are ultimately removed with exfoliation and abrasion sloughing them off while retaining more fluid filled and viable keratinocytes closer to the membrane.

There is a preferred orientation of collagenous fibers composing dermis skin during development, and this is the origin of Langer's lines that direct how to make incisions that have the least scar potential. We also know that collagen I is formed most commonly in connective tissue like skin during development, although there are other collagens that are also produced which we know are critical in the maintaining skin health.

Comparing the composition and structure of the connective tissue in normal and burned tissue [25], there is more type III collagen formed as part of the hypertrophic scar compared to collagen I, as noted in Table 6.4. There are other structural features that can distinguished the attributes in the fibers in these two regions.

We know the general composition of normal skin both swollen and in a dehydrated state. The mechanical behavior of the skin has been resolved for normal people using in vitro biopsies, and more comprehensively using in vivo-type suction devices discussed in Chapter 3, Bones and Mineralized Tissues. In addition to the mechanical response, there is also tremendous interest from the cosmetics, personal hygiene, and care industries to link testing methodology of skin to resolve differences in skin friction, pigmentation, and homogeneity before creaming, soaping, or spraying. It is also known that some people express skin structures and collagen/elastin ratios that are statistically different than the normal population (those with Ehlers Danlos and Cushing's syndrome for example) and there are separate groups of individuals classified with hyperelastic skin. With the skin being a prominent marker of immunological health, there can be acute and chronically sensitive skin regions that yield local changes in immunoglobulins expressed into and within dermis and the ECM.

Table 6.4: Composition of normal dermis versus hypertrophic scar tissue

	Normal Dermis	Hypertrophic Scar Tissue
Water content (%)	64	82
Collagen: % of fat free dry weight	77	77
Collagen fraction	90%	90%
Soluble fraction	0.49	0.67
Ratio of collagen type III/type I	0.25	0.50
Fibril shape	Round	Irregular
Elastin: % of fat free dry weight (FFDW)	4	<0.1

Source: From M.G. Dunn, F.H. Silver, D.A. Swann, Mechanical analysis of hypertrophic scar tissue: structural basis for apparent increased rigidity, J. Investig. Dermatol. 85 (1985) 9–13.

There is a generic disorder in rare cases called epidermolysis bellosa (EB) where young kids and infants are encountered who are not capable of producing collagen VII, and without it, skin layers are not effectively interlinked (like individual sheets of paper as opposed to one continuous organ) causing bleeding events just from rubbing one's eyes in shear for example [26]. There are differences in how much skin oil is produced, pigmentation, sun and wind exposure, and clothing sensitivity even in a single individual.

Skin performs so many functions, protecting internal organs from mechanical insult, as a barrier layer to thermal excursions and bacteria and viruses, and as a marker of immune health and response. The job here is not to necessarily write a treatise here on the broader physiology of skin, but to explain the origins of aging, and to recognize that it is also a dynamic structure. Let us focus first on aging healthy skin and then consider skin from prior traumas.

While it is clear that subsets of the population have distinct differences in connective tissue protein structure and properties, the focus here is on how aging affects a single individual. The most profound effects of aging of normal skin relate to cellular mutations and tumor formation, texture differences, and wrinkle formation. There other secondary effects such as wound healing and neuropathies that become more problematic with aging, but that may be more a function of cardiovascular health and less about the tissue aging itself.

The most common types of cancers that form are skin cancers. Carcinomas are among the most treatable forms of cancers, they are often superficial and relatively easy to access and remove, do not regularly metastasize and often do not require subsequent other follow-up. Skin pigmentation from melanin production derived from melanocytes also in skin is effective at attenuating UV penetration. Some populations with very light skin pigmentation are more susceptible to skin cancers as UV exposure from sunlight permeates a deeper region of the skin surface. Broadband sunlight exposure or through tanning booths is sufficiently energetic to trigger mutations in cells of the basement membrane over time. The sensitivity of a single individual varies suggesting both a local tissue as well as a dose dependence. This is not to say that people with dark pigmentation are immune from skin cancers, just that they possess more natural attenuation. Other types of precancerous lesions can also be triggered by excessive sun exposure creating a related condition called actinic keratosis. Resection and chemical peels are common outpatient procedures for those affected, and patient education is generally increasing sunscreen, hat, and other protective clothing methods to prevent overexposure. Melanomas, derived from mutations of the melanocytes, which are much larger cells and much closer to the bloodstream, allowing for easier pathways for metastasis to arise.

The risk of generating skin cancer is increasing. More prevalent use of sunscreens and UV absorbing fabrics are effective at further attenuating UV exposure, but there are just as many sun worshipers out there as ever, and with an aging population, those who have accumulated exposure are more likely to present with lesions. The same types of preventative measures function for both carcinomas and melanoma. We know what works, but that is not the entire story. It is hard to change lifestyles.

In terms of morphological changes in skin structure with age the most common is wrinkling. Wrinkles originate from essentially a subcutaneous fat redistribution that occurs on the skull, neck, and around joints. Skin is essentially a stretched internally pressurized canvas, and when the pressure is reduced because subcutaneous fat stored subsurface near the eyes, on the forehead, and in the jowl region, are lost over time, there is a viscoelastic relaxation of the stretched collagenous layers. The origin of the face lift as a plastic surgery procedure is essentially the known issue that restretching the skin will lead to fewer wrinkles observed after intervention.

Similarly within the cosmetics community, creams, emollients, and other cosmetics such as vitamin A, nicianamide, and retinol (Retin A), that are readily absorbed into skin structures and if they are capable of swelling the hypodermis, there is an apparent reduction in wrinkling that is noticeable when topically applied over time. An example of such a study where a prescription skin cream was assessed for its efficacy over a period of 8−24 weeks compared to an over the counter regimen of commercial creams, as shown in Fig. 6.15 [27,28]. Not all skin cream constituents are readily absorbed into

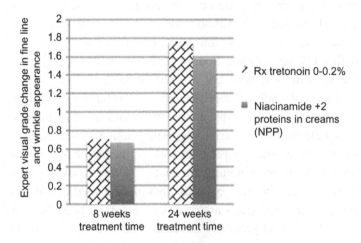

Figure 6.15

A comparison study showing the change in a subjective visual wrinkle reduction by a calibrated expert observer where cohorts of volunteers were distinguished into two groups, one receiving a prescription cream to reduce peri-orbital wrinkles or crows feet (in brick pattern) versus an over the counter concoction of vitamins and proteins in an array of creams, as assessed by on a 10-point scale. A positive visual grade change was interpreted as a smaller wrinkle profile.

skin and not all skin has the same absorption characteristics but cosmetics designers are looking for a functional response (absorption) and an observed response (fewer wrinkles). With absorbable components contained within creams and cosmetics, there are questions of residence time, efficacy, and whether absorbed species are safe in their own right, triggering some other sort of immunological reaction. There are also questions about how extensively cosmetics are tested for safety and efficacy as compared to drugs and devices.

6.10 Burns and Prior Connective Tissue Trauma

There are much larger abrupt changes that result from prior trauma and burns in particular. Wound healing is covered extensively in other treatments, but our effort here is to simply understand behavior of damaged and burned skin relative to passively aging skin. Burns and other wounds are graded based on depth and what is defined as eloquence. Not all skin real estate has the same value, areas around the face, extremities, and joints are more valuable, than on the torso, the back of the legs. When autografting is performed, the less valuable areas are potential donor sites and grafted onto higher value areas after collection.

First, would healing initiates a large cascade where a limited number of colocated fibroblasts near wound sites are coerced to express more connective tissue over what they would normally produce if not signaled. The small number of active cells involved in connective tissue reconstruction suggests that the selection rules of what is functional protein are somewhat more liberal than for collagen 1. It is observed that usually in scar tissue, there is a preponderance of collagen III formed, which has more crosslinks and less directional organization than collagen 1 and is often reported as hypertrophic scarring.

Burns and other types of resolved wounds are what are defined as hypertrophic scarring and are often observed with granulation tissue, an overperfusion of the wound area, and generally less organization to the connective tissue as it is expressed. Comparisons between hypertrophic scar tissue and normal skin have been done on excised graft tissue, the results are shown in Fig. 6.16. Three distinct regions of mechanical response are noted for the natural tissue. There is a relatively low resistance initial phase called the toe or lag region, followed by a linear rise in stiffness followed by a further rise in mechanical resistance as physical crosslinks in the structure are stretched. The initial region is not observed in the hypertrophic scarred tissue. It is perceived that regions 2 and 3 are physiologically relevant and region 1 is only observed due to the relaxation for the tissue not being pressurized internally following excision. So the takeaway is that the natural tissue relaxes upon excision while the scarred tissue is not capable of relaxing suggesting some additional crosslinks in the structure and a stiffer force-deflection in the physiologic region. Clearly the structural organization of the two tissues is different yielding different responses.

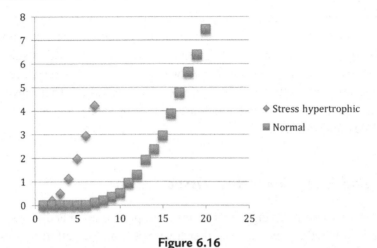

Figure 6.16

Stress–strain test results of normal skin (boxes) and hypertrophic scar tissue (diamonds) excised and evaluated in PBS solution at ambient temperature at a strain rate of 0.1/min. *Reprinted by permission from Macmillan Publishers Ltd.: E.A. Grice, J.A. Segre, The skin microbiome, Nat. Rev. Microbiol. (1 April 2011) (9) 244–253.*

With continued remodeling, muscular tissue and cells will help to reform the connections across the wound site, and continued muscular contraction will pull the mating surfaces together. With continued wound age, there is an effort to remodel wound sites and to redeposit new collagen in an attempt to make the scar tissue more organized and in more harmony with the rest of the surrounding tissue. The larger and deeper the burn location, the more involved will be the clinical management of the burn to an acceptable resolution. The acute issue is to survive the initial insult, and assuming that is a success, there is a coordinated effort of initially dressings followed by both autografts and xenografts to reestablish the barrier properties.

Recently, there has been new clinical research in allograft skin transplants for high value real estate locations such as whole face transplants for severely disfigured individuals. These types of transplants are treated like other transplants and require immune suppression to maintain the tissue after transplant [32]. While the number of whole face transplants has been very small to date, there may more justification for using allograft skin tissues more permanently as opposed to stop gap measures before eventual auto grafting. The expectation is that transplanted tissue should be of a similar structure and mechanical performance compared to what is being replaced.

6.11 Conclusions and Final Thoughts

What the attempt has been made to give the reader some insights on how as engineers, we might consider how to broaden the design environment to consider the age of the tissue or patient as another variable in biomaterials design as the aim for the future is more personalized medicine. I have highlighted very briefly how physiology can change with age within refined constraints. Some examples the reader should be perfectly comfortable with. It is perfectly natural to diseases of the aged as unique to populations above age 70, but in fact, certain diseases progress rather innately regardless of our awareness of them or not. The problem here is not that we do not know how aging affects physiology, but that singular books have been written just on aging of the cardiovascular system, for example. The goal here is to portray disease more in terms of biophysics and to compare and contrast areas of medicine that are well defined versus areas that need more clinical understanding. It is clear that if biomaterials scientists and engineers can make synthetic or even cellular-based therapies to counteract disease, our credibility rises as we understand the clinical dilemmas facing doctors who are invested at the front line of care.

Comparing osteoporosis versus amyloid diseases, for example. We understand that postmenopausal women over a very short period of time trigger relatively precipitous drops in bone density, and there are calcium-fortified foods and vitamins, and estrogen-based pharma therapies that can counteract some of the dramatic consequences of bone loss. Schemes to protect vulnerable locations of the skeletal structure have been studied (hip contusion pads), and exercise programs have been organized and established within the health promotions community to augment weight bearing exercises to counteract these losses. We have built shows with altered skid surfaces, learned how gait and balance alter stability and sensation relating to falls, and efforts to build models of feedback loops are the realm of orthopedic biomechanics. And if vertebral compression fractures arise, or falls trigger an immediate need for hip replacement surgery, the playbook is relatively well established.

Consider that the playbook is a lot thinner for neurologists, gerontologists, and GPs who have patients afflicted with Parkinson's disease or Alzheimer's disease. Billions of dollars are being spent just to establish testing diagnostics to confirm the clinical diagnoses of these disorders. We are still vexed with the dilemma that we cannot establish what is the cause and what are the effects of Alzheimer's disease, and it is more likely that there is more than one trigger to initiate the disease cascade. Billions are also spent in drug pharma to either more effectively clear amyloid plaques or somehow sustain proper neuronal function longer in patients noted with mild or moderate cases. A safe bet is that there will be more venture capital invested in new drugs and devices for Alzheimer's and Parkinson's disease than on a new revolutionary hip implant designs.

This similar clearance problem to Amyloid diseases also exists with kidney disease, although the fluid and the residues are both different. We can clearly consider that the blood–brain barrier and the glomerulus are regulating barriers and perhaps this thickening of walls in the vasculature is also tied to reduced clearance potential over time in these membranes. It is interesting to consider. It is important to consider the impact on the health care community with these age-related diseases. Patients with complete renal failure are going to be severely poisoned just within a few days without dialysis to intervene. And dialysis is a stopgap measure to sustain people, but the current mode to cure is the transplant list. Dialysis is expensive, invasive, and taxing on the health care system. We need some better answers even though we understand what works.

It has also been pointed out where physiological changes in connective tissue are noted in the vasculature and to the integument with age and with disease. It is important to recognize the origin of these aging processes and the allure that drugs and permeating topical creams could have immediate and lasting impact in personalized health care. Its perhaps more daunting to note that skin is not homogeneous and average across the population in all instances, there can be genetic differences that are noted and that can have profound impact on tissue structure, composition, and other related physiology. The takeaway is that simply producing integrated components, structures, functional liquids, and dispersions to supply an industry is not sufficient in biomaterials. The engagement with the clinicians requires a much larger investment of engineers and researchers to understand both who is a user of devices and components, when they become users, and how their own physiology is influenced as they age with synthetic and tissue-engineered graft structures within them.

6.12 Problems

1. If a vascular segment is embedded with fatty lipid plaques with a smaller internal diameter of the lumen as a result, describe the impact on vascular velocity.
2. Explain why it might be difficult to consider widespread vascular grafting of smaller vessels and capillaries as a solution to arteriosclerosis.
3. Describe how obesity and osteoporosis are linked with regard to vertebral compression fractures.
4. Describe the impact of obesity on cardiovascular health. Consider normal activities as well as challenges associated with proper exercise.
5. There are all of these accommodations for obese and physically challenged people in large grocery stores for example using motorized carts. Consider why this accommodation is increasingly common in the United States and less so in other places?
6. Explain which condition is more toxic for patient generating metabolite with a fixed generation rate. Case 1: There is water excretion to maintain fluid volume, or Case 2: There is no water excretion.
7. At this point, do you consider amyloid diseases like Alziheimer's and Parkinsons's to be more or less taxing on families than dialysis?

8. Look up examples of Parkinson's deep brain stimulators. How different are they in terms of construction compared to other electrical devices such as a pacemaker.

9. Some age-related issues are interlinked. There are people who have a genetic defect that suffer amyloid formation of a connective tissue fiber called Fibrillin 1. The condition called Marfan's syndrome and is most commonly manifested as weak valvular structures in the heart. The valves can be easily torn and patients with Marfan's are also more predisposed to Aortic dissection, an unzippering of the lining of the intima from the mulscular wall of the Aorta. Simply replacing valves has not led to as many successful outcomes as simply trying to repair what is innate. Do your own interrogation of Marfan's syndrome, identify what you consider a cause and effect, and how you would determine someone coming in for valvular replacement was not also afflicted by Marfan's syndrome.

References

[1] F. Prati, E. Regar, G.S. Mintz, E. Arbustini, C. Di Mario, I.K. Jang, et al., Expert review document on methodology, terminology, and clinical applications of optical coherence tomography: physical principles, methodology of image acquisition, and clinical application for assessment of coronary arteries and atherosclerosis, Eur. Heart J. 31 (2010) 401−415.

[2] B. Cannon, Biochemistry to behavior, Nature 493 (2013) S2−S3.

[3] M. Hunter, Ion channels: accessory to kidney disease, Nature 414 (2001) 502−503.

[4] R.J. Glassock, The aging kidney: more pieces to the puzzle, Mayo Clin. Proc. 86 (2011) 271−272.

[5] E.M. Darmady, J. Offer, M.A. Woodhouse, The parameters of the kidney aging, J. Pathol. 109 (1973) 195−207.

[6] J.R. Nyengaard, T.F. Bendtsen, Glomerular number and size in relation to age, kidney weight and body surface area in normal man, Anat. Rec. 232 (1992) 194−201.

[7] A.B. da Silva, C. Molina Mdel, S.L. Rodrigues, E.B. Pimentel, M.P. Baldo, et al., Correlation between the creatinine clearance in the urine collected during 24 hours and 12 hours, Braz. J. Nefrol. 32 (2010) 165−172.

[8] A.D. Rule, H. Amer, L.D. Cornell, S.K. Taler, R.G. Cosio, W.K. Kramers, et al., The association between age and nephrosclerosis on renal biopsy among health adults, Ann. Intern. Med. 152 (2010) 561−567.

[9] T.A. Depner, Hemodialysis adequacy: basic essentials and practical points for the nephrologist, Hemodialysis Int. 9 (2005) 241−254.

[10] National Kidney Foundation. Kidney Disease Statistics, 2012. Available from: http://www.kidneyfund.org/about-us/assets/pdfs/akf-kidneydiseasestatistics-2012.pdf.

[11] U. Elbaz, C. Shen, A. Lichtinger, N.A. Zauberman, Y. Goldich, C.C. Chan, A.R. Slomovic, D.S. Rootman, Accelerated (9 mW/cm^2) corneal collagen crosslinking for keratoconus—a 1 year follow-up, Cornea 33 (2014) 769−773.

[12] A. Dhondt, R. Vanholder, W. Van Biesen, N. Lameire, The removal of uremic toxins, Kid. Int. 76 (2000) S47−S59.

[13] K.M. Flegel, M.D. Carroll, B.D. Kit, C.L. Ogden, Prevalence of obesity and trends in the distribution of body mass index among US adults, 1999−2010, J. Am. Med. Assoc. 307 (2012) 491−497.

[14] S.A. Wiggins, H. Cranston, S. Bhattacharya, Osteoporosis; lecture notes from the Landon Center for Aging, 2014.

[15] C.E. De Laet, B.A. van Hout, H. Burger, A. Hofman, H.A.P. Pols, Bone density and risk of hip fracture in men and women: cross-sectional analysis, BMJ (1997) 315. p. 221.

[16] A.K. Kaushik, S.K. Vareed, S. Basu, V. Putluri, N. Putluri, K. Panzitt, et al., Metabolomic profiling identifies biochemical pathways associated with castration-resistant prostate cancer, J. Proteome Res. 13 (2014) 1088–1100.

[17] J. Williamson, J. Goldman, K.S. Marder, Genetic aspects of Alzheimer's disease, Neurologist 15 (2009) 80–86.

[18] Y. Hamada, Drug discovery of β-secretase inhibitors based on quantum chemical interactions for the treatment of Alzheimer's disease, SOJ Pharm. Pharmaceut. Sci. 1 (2014) 1–8.

[19] R.W. Richter, M.F. Weiner, D. Persson, K.E. Taubman, D.B. Dean, R.N. Rosenberg, The first study of dementia within the cherokee nation of Oklahoma, Neurobiol. Aging 15 (1994). p. S41-S41.

[20] R.N. Rosenberg, R.W. Richter, R.C. Risser, K. Taubman, I. Prado-Farmer, E. Ebalo, et al., Genetic factors for the development of Alzheimer disease in the Cherokee Indian, Arch. Neurol. 53 (10) (1996) 997–1000.

[21] E.J. Lehman, M.J. Hein, S.L. Baron, C.M. Gersic, Neurodegenerative causes of dealth among retired National Football League players, Neurology 79 (2012) p. 1970–1974.

[22] M.C. Rodriguez-Oroz, J.A. Obeso, A.E. Lang, J.L. Houeto, P. Pollak, S. Rehncrona, et al., Bilateral deep brain stimulation in Parkinson's disease: a multicentre study with 4 years follow-up, Brain 128 (2005) 2240–2249.

[23] K. Kingwell, Parkinson disease: constant-current deep brain stimulation improves symptoms in Parkinson disease, Nat. Rev. Neurol. 8 (2012) 119.

[24] E.A. Grice, J.A. Segre, The skin microbiome, Nat. Rev. Microbiol. 9 (2011) 244–253.

[25] M.G. Dunn, F.H. Silver, D.A. Swann, Mechanical analysis of hypertrophic scar tissue: structural basis for apparent increased rigidity, J. Investig. Dermatol. 84 (1985) 9–13.

[26] R. Varki, S. Sadowski, J. Uitto, E. Pfendner, Epidermolysis bullosa. II. Type VII collagen mutations and phenotype–genotype correlations in the dystrophic subtypes, J. Med. Genet. 44 (2007) 181–192.

[27] J.J.J. Fu, G.G. Hillebrand, P. Raleigh, J. Li, M.J. Marmor, V. Bertucci, P.E. Grimes, et al., A randomized, controlled comparative study of the wrinkle reduction benefits of a cosmetic niacinamide/peptide/retinyl propionate product regimen vs. a prescription 0–.02% tretinoin product regimen, Br. J. Dermatol. 162 (2010) 647–654.

[28] R. Kafi, H.S. Kwak, W.E. Schumacher, S. Cho, V.N. Hanft, T.A. Hamilton, et al., Improvement of naturally aged skin with Vitamin A (Retinol), Arch. Dermatol. 143 (2007) 606–612.

[29] Transcatheter Aortic Valve Replacement. 2014. Available from: http://www.heartgroup.co.nz/ Patient + Information/Therapeutic + Procedures/Transcatheter + Aortic + Valve + Implantation + TAVI. html.

[30] Alzheimer's expert Doraiswamy answers your questions, in: USA Today. Gannett, Washington, DC, 2008.

[31] T.L. Sirich, B.A. Funk, N.S. Plummer, T.H. Hostetter, T.M. Meyer, Prominent accumulation in hemodialysis patients of solutes normally cleared by tubular secretion, Am. J. Nephrol. 25 (2014) 615–622.

[32] B. Pomahac, J. Pribaz, E. Eriksson, E.M. Bueno, J.R. Diaz-Siso, F.J. Rybicki, et al. Three patients with full facial trnsplantataion, New England Journal of Medicine. 366 (2012) 715–722.

CHAPTER 7

Metallic Biomaterials

Learning Objectives

There are several learning objectives for this chapter. Presented is some of the alchemy leading to pure and mixed metal alloy structures that yield useful combinations of properties that are, in general, both safe and effective. We design and use a range of metals and alloys to make structural components as well as electrical components such as pacemaker leads and electrodes for both active control and diagnosis. It is important to recognize their potential design usage. The latent magnetic potential of metals has lowered their more broad-scale use as screening procedures are in place to isolate patient populations from larger magnet exposure as a health risk in the radiology unit. And finally, it is clear that while we have learned a lot about cellular response to metals and metal ions produced from corrosion reactions, there may still be open design space for new and better alloy design with better haptic interfaces and properties more matched to the natural tissues they replace and surrounding tissues they encounter. In some instances, we remain quite far away from an optimum solution and the regulatory requirements to qualify a new material are impediments to advancement.

7.1 Introduction

Select grades of metallic and metal alloy biomaterials have commonly been used as monoliths in a range of medical implants, functional prosthetics, instruments, and temporary and removable devices. Even in particulate form, specific forms of magnetic nanoparticles and other hybrid, layered structures may be useful in advanced functional diagnostics. It is also commonly understood that we need trace amounts of zinc selenium, copper, and magnesium to sustain ourselves. Consolidated metallic monoliths have been commonly used as components in orthopedics, dental and craniofacial surgery, and cardiovascular devices.

Linked with both temporary and permanent devices, metallic components are also used as surgical instruments because they can be easily reconditioned for reuse without degrading their performance. Overall, it is important to recognize the mechanical, ionic, and electrical response of these components in vivo, the sterilization capacity of these types of alloys, and the ability to produce net-shape or near-net-shape type constructions are key attributes facilitating metallic biomaterial use in vivo. Those attributes are regulated by the composition of the metals composing the alloy, the structure of what forms, and processing schemes to achieve specifically designed shapes and functions.

On a smaller scale, more specialized devices such as stents are integrated devices that also contain metals and metal alloys which are integrated to yield substantially more compliant structures which can be actively expanded by pressure or thermal exposure. Integrated components such as electronic circuitry, pacemaker leads and electrodes also require materials with high conductivity achieved by metallic bonding and that resist oxidation. And on an even smaller scale, dispersions of more potent organometallic phase contrast agents are part of the enhanced diagnostic revolution tied to diagnosing disease earlier and providing more exquisite display of the vascular network, usually in some sort of diseased state, a blockage, a stenosis, etc. Newer repair strategies use a wider array of metallic alloys that may also expand the breadth of material compositions available for therapeutic intervention. Metallic materials, while on the decline in terms of whole-scale use, are increasingly used in niches where specific material advantages exist.

This chapter includes a basic description of grades of typical metallic biomaterial alloys commonly accepted for use in medicine, a description of how alloy composition and processing technique affect both structure and mechanical properties, and several directions for the future. Typical design and processing issues for biomaterial alloy use in orthopedics and cardiovascular engineering are included later in the chapter. The salinity of the aqueous environment in vivo is a major consideration in focusing on alloys that retard active corrosion and undergo passivation. This chapter is not meant as a history lesson but to give the impetus for the current state of the art for integrated components and direction for the future of the subdiscipline.

7.1.1 Metals and Phase Equilibria

Before discussing specific steel types, metallurgy has a defined nomenclature which helps describe different alloy forms, part of which is the basis in an introductory materials science curriculum. If one starts with a pure typical transition metal element like copper, iron, or titanium, under equilibrium conditions, the element transforms from solid to liquid at its elemental melting temperature with a certain enthalpy of melting the crystal; it possesses a certain elemental density and crystallizes in certain preferred orders that are called crystal structures. The element might exist in one or more different crystal unit cells as a function of temperature before ultimately melting at that elemental melting point. By adding trace amounts of other elements (tin, nickel, or zinc for example for copper, nickel, manganese, molybdenum, and titanium for iron) to the pure elemental metal chosen, the impure mixture can also be melted but usually at a range of temperatures lower than the elemental melting point. The enthalpy of melting and the alloy melting point of the mixture is also altered by adding the impurities as alloying elements. Different microstructures can also evolve as a function of composition. The process of adding other elements together is called alloying and the product of this formation in the solid state is a solid crystallizable alloy.

7.1.2 Features of Solid Solutions and Those of Limited Solubility

There are several types of binary alloys or simple systems containing two metals to consider. On one extreme, consider the chances that both elements used in a binary alloy are mutually soluble in each other and have the same crystal structure as shown in 7.1. The alloying of copper and nickel is one such combination. Both elements melt at the left-hand and right-hand sides of the compositional map and everywhere in between, a range of temperatures exist where a two-phase region of A and B combine to form solid AB alloy of one composition and a liquid zone of AB with another composition. The amount of each of these is regulated by the lever rule and there is a continuous solidus and liquidus line. Some other textbooks might go through a detailed presentation of crystal structures, crystal density measurements, Bravais lattices, and the like. But for the purposes here, it is noted that mutual solubility is enhanced when both alloying elements are face-centered cubic (FCC) or body-centered cubic (BCC) for example (Fig. 7.1).

Another conceptually common binary alloy is one in which A and B are not mutually soluble in each other. It is conceivable that A and B could also have different crystal structures as shown in Fig. 7.2. These mixtures tend to form what are called binary eutectic alloys. Two-phase regions arise where A-rich and B-rich zones undergo phase separation regulated by the thermodynamic energetics of mixing. There can be regions of limited solid solubility of element B in A (defined as α) + A in B (defined as β) for example. The eutectic reaction is defined at the eutectic

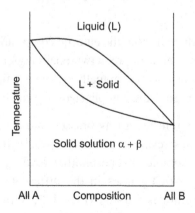

Figure 7.1
A mutually soluble A—B alloy.

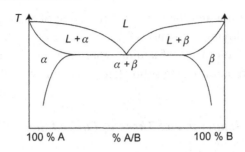

Figure 7.2
An A–B alloy with limited solid solubility.

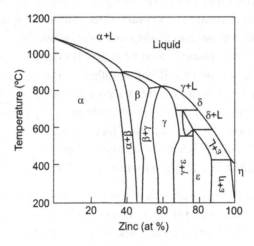

Figure 7.3
The copper–zinc binary phase diagram with copper on the left and zinc on the right. *Reproduced from the Copper Development Association, http://www.copper.org/publications/newsletters/innovations/2006/ 03/images/cuzn_phase.jpg.*

composition and temperature, where heating the eutectic composition raises it directly into a single-phase liquid and below that temperature, a two-phase region lamellar region of α and β form. With these examples presented as conceptually simple examples, it is worth looking at other types of binary alloys just to see how complicated they can be.

Alloys of copper and zinc are referred to as brasses and those of copper and tin as bronzes. Some alloying schemes result in structures where for example zinc and copper (Fig. 7.3A) are only partially soluble in one another leading to the formation of phase-segregated zinc-rich and copper-rich phases in the different crystalline regions.
A simpler example phase diagram is Cu–Ni (Fig. 7.4). With Cu–Zn, there are many different stable intermediate phases that form as the composition of copper and zinc varies, each with a different composition, density, and crystal structure. For Cu–Ni, the

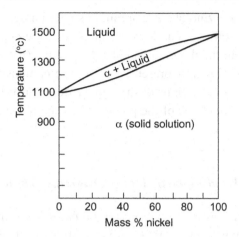

Figure 7.4
Copper–nickel phase diagram constructed from the Copper Development Association [2].

same crystal structure forms over all compositions, and it is just that nickel and copper are mutually soluble in each other, leading to one crystal structure.

Metal alloys, depending on processing conditions and composition, can crystallize into one or multiple zones across a sample. With a two-element alloy (copper–zinc or copper–nickel), the driving force for crystallizing one element is higher than for the other. As a result, the initially solidified product may preferentially include one element, it is all regulated by the thermodynamics.

7.1.3 Attributes of the Binary Phase Diagram

There are certain characteristics of typical phase diagrams presented earlier. Alloys at one composition melt over a range of temperatures as opposed to the elemental base metal that melts at one temperature at atmospheric pressure, as defined by the Gibbs phase rule. The liquidus line denotes at what temperature and composition solidification initiates. Thus, above the liquidus line at equilibrium, the alloy mixture is fully melted and below, there is some solid that forms. In between, there is what is defined as a two-phase region, Liquid + a crystalline solid. Similarly, there is a solidus line below which indicates when the metal fluid or slurry is completely solidified. The copper–zinc phase diagram also highlights an array of single-phase and two-phase regions. Delving into phase equilibria allows one to resolve the microstructure of the phases that preferentially form under equilibrium conditions based on where one is situated on the phase diagram in terms of composition and temperature.

Example 7.1 For the copper–zinc phase diagram, a single phase, γ, should exist for a 60 at % Zn/40 at % Cu alloy at 700°C at equilibrium. Increasing the copper content is the equivalent of moving left on the diagram and at 50% atomic Zn at 700°C, it is observed that there should be two solid phases present, $\beta + \gamma$. The compositions of the phases are regulated by the boundary compositions of the copper-rich phase (to the left) and zinc-rich phase (to the right) and the fractions of the phases would be resolved by what is called the lever rule.

7.1.4 More Complicated and Realistic Phase Diagrams: Three or More Components

Binary alloy phase diagrams are easy to represent on paper but refined alloys used commercially as biomaterials such as 304 L or 316 L stainless steel are often more complicated and contain a lot more than one coalloying element in addition to the base metal. This inclusion of trace elements in an alloy is more often a result of what is not extracted from a metallic liquid as slag since alloys are refined from metal ore. Trace impurities are often included unless specifically removed. As such, there is some alchemy in alloy design, although much has been learned from phenomenology to resolve the role of ternary alloying elements in controlling structure, grain size, corrosion potential, and other features. Most commonly used metallic biomaterial elements are titanium, iron, cobalt, and chromium. Iron alloys form steels with carbon being a coalloyed with other elements to increase corrosion resistance. In dental materials, there is a richer array of precious metals as base metals, including gold and silver that can be coalloyed with copper and nickel among others. Example ternary phase diagram is shown in Fig. 7.5 for stainless steel compositions found traversing the phase map between iron, chromium, and steel at one temperature and Fig. 7.9 showing the immiscibility gap as the temperature is changed in a three-phase alloy of gold, silver, and copper.

7.2 Characterizing Phase Structure

Phase structure can be identified both by microscopy and by X-ray diffraction and the temperature-dependent phase response can be achieved by doing in situ measurements varying temperature. Microstructure is used to describe the phase structure and organization within a specimen and is often quite complicated. Metallic phase diagrams can often be very useful in terms of defining equilibrium structure but are less useful as the complexity of the alloy (number of alloying elements) increases and as nonequilibrium processing yields microstructures that are metastable and absent in the equilibrium phase diagram. Nevertheless, these terms are commonly encountered and it is appropriate to at least introduce these concepts and topics as a brief introduction before encountering the different biomaterial metal compositions most commonly found.

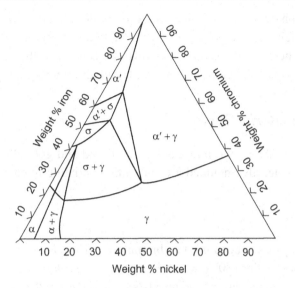

Figure 7.5

The iron—chromium—nickel ternary phase diagram showing the phases in equilibrium at 650°C. The presence of larger amounts of nickel and chromium favor the preferential formation of γ phase austenite, the predominant phase in stainless steels [5].

EXAMPLE: One can use variable temperature microscopy and X-ray diffraction to resolve characteristics of phase structure. Based on the equilibrium phase diagram in Fig. 7.4, if a liquid mixture of 50 wt% copper and 50 wt% nickel is equilibrated at 1400°C and one could analyze this mixture both by microscopy and by X-ray diffraction at 1400°C, no solid structure in the melt would be observable and no coherent scattering linked with the formation of crystals at this high temperature would be noted by X-ray diffraction (XRD), just a broad amorphous halo associated with random scattering. If mixture was cooled to 1300°C and held this at equilibrium, the formation of solid particles forming in the otherwise liquid matrix would be observed and coherent X-ray scattering of moving crystals would lead to some preferred scattering directions, indicative of the unit cells in these crystals. And more convection in the mixture will lead to a lower signal to noise (S/N) ratio due to the mobility of the crystals in the slurry. The slurry fraction is related to how close this mixture is at equilibrium to the liquidus and solidus lines. If the spot in the two-phase region is closer to the solidus, there is a larger fraction of particles in the slush. And as the temperature is lowered to 1200°C and held, the specimen should be completely solid with the observation of grain boundaries in this polycrystalline specimen and using X-ray diffraction, the coherent scattering of the crystals should lead to a stronger S/N ratio, indicative of the crystal structure of the single solid phase forming in Cu—Ni at 50 wt%. Lowering temperature is the process of marching down the phase diagram in a line at 50 wt% in this example.

To learn more about phase structure, microstructure evolution, alloy design, and processing, comprehensive materials science books are more detailed sources of background material beyond the treatment here. The bottom line is that one can use tools like temperature-dependent XRD to resolve how composition and temperature affect the phase equilibrium.

7.3 Metallic Biomaterial Types

Steels, titanium alloys, cobalt—chromium alloys, and gold and gold alloys are the most common metallic biomaterials. Included are subsections relating to each material class.

7.3.1 Steels

Iron—carbon steel alloys have been used as biomaterials for many years as surgical instruments dating back to the 1800s. Much like other tools, steels of that day were designed to be hard, to shape, cut, and excise tissue on an as-needed basis. For amputations, anything sharp would probably work and it was only after more sterile practice progressed to the point that the thought of mending fractures through internal fixation was considered possible. As surgical tools and instruments evolved, the range of steels used in both instruments and as implant materials also evolved, particularly as corrosion became more apparent as a latent risk factor postinstallation.

The development of stainless steels has eclipsed the use of simpler iron—carbon alloys. Stainless steels are compositionally more complex alloys than carbon steels as nickel, chromium, and molybdenum are added in tight compositional ranges as alloying elements. Typical compositions of medical-grade stainless steels are found in Table 7.1. As mixtures of these constituents are melted and cooled into plates, rods, or other shapes, chromium is

Table 7.1: Compositions of various grades of stainless steels acceptable as metallic grade surgical steel

Steel Type	Cr	Ni	Mo	Mn	Si	P	N	C	Other Trace	Iron
316 L[a]	16%–18% max	10%–14% max	2%–3% max	2.0% max	0.75% max	0.45% max	0.1% max	0.03% max	S: 0.03% max	Balance 60% +
F745[b]	17–19	11–14	2–3	2	1.0% max	0.45		0.06% max	S: 0.03% max	Balance 60% +
REX–734[c]	19.5%–22%	9–11	2–3	2–4.25	0.75 max	0.025 max	0.25%–0.5%	0.08% max	Nb 0.25–0.8%	Balance, 60% +
F138[b]	17–19	13–15	2.25%–3.5%	2% max	0.75 max	0.25%	0.1%		S:0.01% max	Balance 60% +

[a]ASTM F-138: A to Z Materials.com [19]
[b]Matweb.com [3]
[c]Reclaru et al. [4]

often expelled to the surface as part of the driving force for crystallizing the alloy, thus increasing Cr composition on the surface. When chromium is at a sufficiently high concentration on the surface, its active reaction with airborne oxygen forms a passivation layer which suppresses further oxidation and ionic release once the oxide is firmly established which can happen long before installation.

With the number of coalloying constituents noted, it is clear why a comprehensive phase diagram of stainless steel is not included here. It is possible to consider limited diagrams that vary only one element, keeping the composition of the rest of the mixture constant at one temperature. With sufficient chromium concentrations (>12 at%) on the surface of the construct, chromium oxidizes preferentially compared to the other alloying elements forming a passivated layer. Without enough chromium on the surface, the chromium still oxidizes but passivation is incomplete and further oxidation of other alloy can occur. Nickel is added as a microstructural control element reducing the potential of carbon-rich carbides from precipitating at grain boundaries that can also affect corrosion potential and strength. Grain structure refinement toughens these alloys and raises their ductility. The presence of molybdenum in surgical steels is thought to reduce the potential for a specific type of corrosion called pitting corrosion deep within the crevices of the alloy surface if produced in a mold for example. Compared with other iron–carbon alloys, surgical stainless steels contain a lot more of chromium and nickel than carbon, the main alloying element in ferritic steels. As carbon content rises in stainless steels, the same coalloying elements do not have the potency on controlled grain structure and passivation and the temperatures at which phase transformations occur also change.

Simpler, binary iron–carbon alloys are usually ferrite-based or α-iron crystals at room temperature. Ferritic phases form magnetic dipoles making these alloy forms viable permanent magnets. Ferrite is a BCC crystal structure with carbon as an alloying element positioned as interstitial defects within the unit cell. The presence of much larger concentrations of chromium and nickel in iron favors the formation of an FCC microstructure (γ) called austenite which does not have the same magnetization potential as BCC ferrite. The relevant phase diagram for the Fe–Ni–Cr system at 650°C is shown in Fig. 7.5 [5]. With the advent of magnetic resonance imaging (MRI) diagnostic devices and larger and larger magnets being used for more objective tissue diagnostics, there is an obvious need to screen people for the presence of ferritic forms of steels as embedded implants before they are exposed near the large permanent magnets of each MRI diagnostic unit. It is part of any protocol for screening patients for jewelry, etc. prior to MRI facility use. One can find stories of construction equipment and other metal objects impacting the magnets of the MRI units when these units were energized with magnetic objects too close. And even small amounts of magnetic phases present in a stainless steel implants (clips, coils, and stents) could be enough to cause their migration or torque during MRI imaging and this potential rises as the size of permanent magnets used in diagnostics increases. This is a larger concern as the size of magnetic field strength increases from 2.3 to 7 T for example. Objects that were inert at 2.3 might not be as transparent to a larger magnet.

The most common medical steel grades being used instruments and implants (e.g.: fracture fixation plates, rods, and screws) are austenitic stainless steels, most of the form 316, 316, and 304 L. There are many compositions that would qualify as stainless steels though, and the American Society for Materials (ASM) has standards based on microstructure that would qualify as stainless steels. New compositions of stainless steel (so-called REX alloys) have been developed recently [4], but these are really variants of the other originally developed alloys. Any new alloy developed and used within the United States would require a more comprehensive characterization by the US Food and Drug Administration (FDA) and other regulatory agencies in other countries. The additional work and expense needed to qualify a new steel alloy formulation is a disincentive to develop alternative alloys to compete with these already established compositions. It is also clear that there are a wide range of alloy composition that still qualify as a specific stainless alloy form.

The most common sites for stainless steel for internal biomaterial use today are focused on fracture fixation plates, femoral intramedullary stabilization rods, screws, and other integrated fixtures tied to primarily orthopedic structures. In terms of removable devices, there is also a viable use of stainless steel as sutures and staples used for closure of large abdominal incisions (tummy tucks, c-section deliveries) and orthodontic bonding appliances to teeth. The surgical stapling procedures are alluring as they allow for rapid wound closure and can do an effective binding of wound sites for a period sufficient to create innate wound strength. For all of these removable devices, there are alternatives. With the passivation (controlled oxidation by Chromium to form a strong adherent oxide) of steels, there is no viable mechanism for biodegradation and ion transport prior to passivation will likely create ions of the metals composing the steel that are conveyed into the surrounding tissue. Separately, the use of steel for instruments dwarfs the use for implants because of their capacity to be resterilized and reused.

Overall, steel alloys, in fully consolidated forms, have a much higher modulus of elasticity (stiffness) than the surrounding bone stock (250 GPa vs 18 GPa for cortical bone, more like 1−3 GPa for cancellous bone), and thus installation of these components also leads to larger stress shielding of the surrounding bone tissue and larger chances for local bone demineralization near steel implant installations. More open questions relate to whether passivated surfaces still release a sufficiently large concentration of metallic ions that surrounding tissues are negatively affected.

7.3.2 Co−Cr Alloys

Co−Cr alloys have supplanted steels in orthopedics particularly as bearing surfaces associated with total joint replacement. These alloys are comparable in terms of mechanical properties to steels so there is no great driving force for opting for Co−Cr over steel but there may be differences in terms of surface finish, hardness, potentially wear and abrasion resistance, and machining complexity.

Co–Cr alloys are nominally equal in chromium and cobalt content, yielding alloys in the middle of the Co–Cr phase diagram shown in Fig. 7.6 [6]. Co–Cr and alloys of Co–Cr typically have hexagonal close-packed (HCP) crystal structures with both chromium and cobalt taking positions as substitutional defects in the other crystal. The alloying of Co–Cr with molybdenum and nickel create other substitutional defects that strengthen the alloy and reduce the machining capacity of cast alloy forms. Medical grades of Co–Cr alloys identified by the FDA are shown in Table 7.2.

Like stainless steels, the presence of sufficient chromium content on the outside surface passivates the surface. The main distinctions between the different alloy forms are either the

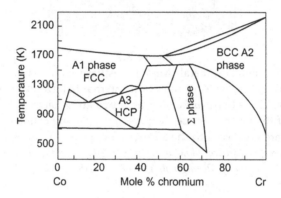

Figure 7.6

Co–Cr phase diagram. *From J.-H.C. Lin, C.P. Ju, C.M. Lee, Medical implant made of biocompatible low modulus high strength titanium-niobium alloy and method of using the same. US Patent Publication #US 6752882, 2004.*

Table 7.2: Co–Cr compositions

	F75	F799	F90	F562
Co	59.9%–69.5%	58%–59%	45%–56.2%	29–38.8
Cr	27%–30%	26%–30%	19%–21%	19–21%
Mo	5%–7%	5%–7%	–	9%–10.5%
Mn	1% max	1% max	1%–2%	0.15% max
Ni	1% max	1% max	9%–11%	33%–37%
Fe	0.75% max	1.5% max	3% max	1% max
Si	1% max	1% max	0.4% max	0.15% max
C	0.25% max	0.35% max	0.1% nominally	–
Other		N: 0/25% max	P: max 0.04%	Ti: 1% max
				S: 0.01% max
W	–	–	14%–16%	–

From J. Black, 1999. Biological performance of materials, fundamentals of biocompatibility, Marcel Dekker, New York.

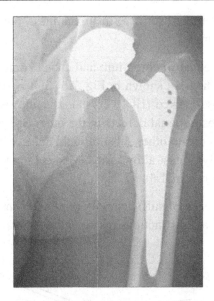

Figure 7.7

A radiographic image of a metal on metal (MoM) prosthesis with a large diameter femoral head. Regular articulation such as walking allows the internal ball to rotate and encounter the surrounding socket. While both surfaces in an articulating joint are highly polished, the compressive loading of the interface once the person is standing can cause local abrasive wear, the residues of which are expelled into the surrounding tissue. An example of a MoM total hip implant in question. *From S. Ostlere, How to image metal-on-metal prostheses and their complications, Am. J. Roentgenol. 197 (2011) 558–567.*

casting method or the postprocessing methods such as forging, annealing, or other hot-working procedures. The F75 is a cast form and the F799 and the F562 are usually forged constructions. All of these can be subsequently annealed to raise workability without dramatically affecting ductility.

Common for bearing surfaces such as knees, hips, and shoulders, the initial surface finish and roughness correlate to rate of erosion of these synthetic counter-surfaces. There has been a recent flurry of regulatory activity tied to concerns of so-called metal on metal (MoM) total hip replacements using Co−Cr due to the significant ionic release that occurs in a fretting mode, where metal surfaces articulate against one another, an example of which is shown in Fig. 7.7. Particles eroded from either side of the MoM implant can invade surrounding areas of the joints creating tissue reactions. Separately, the presence of Cr^{2+} and Co^{2+} ions in higher concentration could be triggers for other diseases, particularly for long-term implant recipients. Beyond these uses, Co−Cr alloys can be competitively substituted for steel, although wider usage is not anticipated.

The modular components are seated and typical walking imparts a shear during articulation. If they are both made out of the same material, one will eventually abrade way, creating both ions and particulates that can corrode in and around where they are expelled.

7.3.3 Titanium and Titanium Alloys

Titanium and titanium alloys are increasingly being used as viable alternatives to steels and Co−Cr alloys for several reasons. First, bulk titanium is about half the density and half the modulus of elasticity of steels and Co−Cr alloy meaning that for a volumetric replacement, the same-sized titanium implant is only about half the mass of the corresponding steel or Co−Cr implant. The titanium also creates a smaller stress shielding response that retains a larger fraction of loading on adjacent cells, at least more than with steel or Co−Cr. Also, titanium also forms a very strong and adherent oxide on its surface like chromium and also passivates. The passivation occurs so rapidly before biomaterial installation that it increases titanium's chemical inertness and avoids ionic transport to neighboring cells that occurs with stainless steels and fretting MoM implants produced from Co−Cr. Bone integration is found to be also more favorable given that titanium and its alloys can be processed into porous forms allowing bone infiltration. Both the lower crystal density and potential to include porosity increase the compliance of titanium-based implants allowing more load transfer to the natural tissue and more bony ingrowth. All of these features increase the viability of native tissues interfacing with Ti-based implants.

Nearly-pure, commercially pure or CP-grade titanium (F-67) is also a HCP crystal structure with trace alloying elements including iron which can oxidize in the alloy increasing oxygen content as well. More specific alloying elements for titanium in higher concentration include vanadium, iron, and aluminum. The presence of substitutional defects in Ti harden the alloy. Separately, alloys of titanium mixed with vanadium and aluminum have been tested sufficiently to be also allowable as biomedical implants. Common titanium-based alloy grades and compositions are shown in Table 7.3.

Titanium has been eclipsing other metals as larger monolithic components in many orthopedic uses. This biochemical inertness of titanium and its alloys is due to its rapid

Table 7.3: Maximum allowable compositions of trace wt% of contaminants in a range of titanium alloys. Grade 4 & Ti6Al4V are the most common orthopedic grades of titanium, as expressed by Ti (commercially pure CP) (ASTM F67) and Ti6Al4V alloy (ASTM F136)

	Grade 1	Grade 2	Grade 3	Grade 4	Ti6Al4V
N	0.03	0.03	0.05	0.05	0.05
C	0.1	0.1	0.1	0.1	0.08
H	0.015	0.015	0.015	0.015	0.015
Fe	0.2	0.3	0.3	0.5	0.25
O	0.18	0.25	0.35	0.4	0.13

passivation which dramatically lowers ionic release. Passivation is often rapid enough to occur long before component installation. The capacity of titanium to passivate and seal itself from ionic release raises its potential in cardiovascular medicine as valves and seals for valvular disease and with heart assist devices, and stents.

Ti has been also developed for bone substructures linked with dental implants that require two surgeries for complete installation. Depending on the size of the intervention, single posts at one end of the spectrum to an ensemble of Ti posts are inserted into the mandible and maxilla and allowed to integrate and heal in the native bone structure. Once integrated, these post regions can be reexposed allowing the anchoring of tooth superstructures for both individual teeth and for larger tooth segments up to whole dentures that can be permanently attached to these posts following the initial installation. The primary metal−bone interface with these devices is Ti.

7.3.4 NiTi Shape Memory Alloys

As alloying content is increased, the phase structure is altered and some specific types of temperature-responsive devices have been developed as a result. Ti alloyed with Ni in nearly equivalent stoichiometry creates alloys that undergo a martensitic phase transformation that is reversible around room temperature depending on the exact composition. The NiTi phase diagram is included in Fig. 7.8.

On the phase diagram is found a single-phase martensite region NiTi but note that its transformation temperature is strongly affected by composition and even a 2% variance of composition is sufficient to prevent its formation. NiTi with its functional and reversible

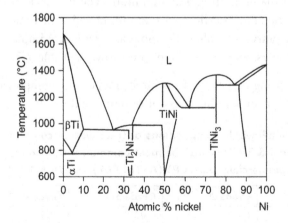

Figure 7.8
The NiTi phase diagram. The intermetallic region at ~50 at% Ni is the phase that undergoes a reversible martensitic phase change near body temperature, redrawn from T. B. Massalski, H. Okamato, P. R. Subrumanian, and L. Kacprzak, Binary alloy phase diagrams, vol. 3, ASM International, Materials Park (OH) (1990) p. 2874.

phase change allows the design of devices for stents, valve templates, and other devices like orthodontic archwires that are soft and flexible at cold temperatures and stiffen as the warming triggers the phase transition as the wire responds to body temperature at 37°C. Reversible expanding catheter stents made from NiTi allow the stent to warm at body temperature that can cause stent expansion. Once the procedure is completed, cold blood can be reintroduced causing the stent to reversibly shrink allowing retrieval. Other, more permanent devices can be installed and deployed without the cold temperature reversion.

Most metallic biomaterials, being so stiff, are so overdesigned from a bulk mechanical behavior standpoint when they are used as substitutes to replace damaged and diseased bone. The resulting structure is often much stronger than the surrounding bone tissue and with time, the loads on the device shield the adjacent bone stock from its physiologic loading over time. As bony tissue is shielded from compressive loading, bone resorption can result, which can compromise the metallic biomaterial installation over time, usually leading to an implant torque that is sensed as a loosening or an instability. To reduce stress shielding, one can lower the modulus of the metallic component or introduce voids or porosity that would contribute to an increased compliance. Since a volumetric replacement is occurring, perhaps a less consolidated metallic component could be considered for the same volume. Alternatively, perhaps the crystal structure of the biomaterial could be altered to one that is less rigid.

Future designs may incorporate hollow sections or other void regions that lower the overall stiffness of the device with a fixed elastic modulus of elasticity. There are open questions about whether it is a desirable goal to ultimately match the stiffness of bony tissue as adding voids may have negative consequences on stress concentrations, and fracture toughness which can further limit ductility and fatigue behavior.

7.3.5 Gold, Gold Alloys, and Other Precious Metal Alloys

Gold, gold alloys, and other precious metals have been extensively used as dental crowns, bridges and inlays. Elemental gold leaf is extremely soft and has been deployed on its own by forging or deforming the leaf on the surfaces of tooth structures as superficial fillings. The foil can be pressed into the crevice or cavity formed and the mechanical deformation causes dislocations in the foil by a process called "work hardening" that strengthens the foil as it is pressed into place. The use of gold leaf in cavity repair is more rarely performed, but it is a nice example of how gold can be used even in its elemental form.

More importantly, Au alloys have been developed that are harder and stronger and can be integrated into permanent structures for tooth loss and replacement. Examples of typical gold and Au alloys and their corresponding compositions and properties are included in Table 7.4. Typical alloying elements for Au include Ni, Cu, Fe, rhodium, and palladium.

A ternary phase diagram mapped to room temperature for gold alloyed with Cu and Ag is included in Fig. 7.9 [9].

Used in dentistry for crowns and bridges, gold alloys are often cast or sintered from prior impressions to more adequately replicate the original tooth structure. More complicated structures such as bridges often require ample alloy engineering to satisfy strength and stiffness requirements. Dental bridges are designed to accommodate elastic flexure with each compressive loading event associated with chewing and higher fractions of alloying elements are added for these implants to accommodate the higher design loading requirement for chewing. The loading schemes for dental bridges can often be quite complicated as those designed to fill the gap where a missing tooth is located undergo

Table 7.4: Mechanical properties of dental Au and Au alloys from [10]. Commercial alloy designations are included in [11]

Type	Au	Cu	Ag	Pd	Vickers Hardness (MPa)	Elongation (%)	Uses
Type 1	83	6	10	0.5	60–90	30	Small inlays
Type 2	77	7	14	1	90–120	25	Inlays
Type 3	75	9	11	3.5	120–150	10–20	Crowns and bridges
Type 4	70	10	11	3.5	150–200	5–10	Partial dentures
Medium Au	46	8	50	6	180–200	5–10	Crowns and bridges
Low Au	15	14	45	25	170–200	5–10	Crowns and bridges
Ag-Pd		-	70	25	150	5–10	Crowns and bridges

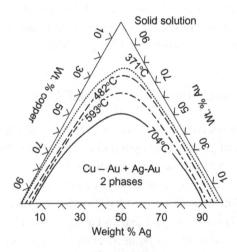

Figure 7.9

Au–Cu–Ag phase diagram projected to room temperature phases identified as a single solid solution and a broad immiscibility gap with Cu and Ag-rich phases. *From A.S. McDonald, G.H. Sistare, 1978. The metallurgy of some carat gold jewellery alloys, Pt 1. Colored gold alloys. Gold Bull., 11 (1978) 66–73.*

flexure, while other bridges to accommodate a missing molar undergo cantilevered bending from more proximal adjacent teeth that are still viable. Bridges are designed to survive thousands of flexure and compression cycles as would be required for any normal tooth.

Porous gold is one scheme being exploited by device manufacturers to further miniaturize electrodes for both sensors and actuators. The process for making these porous devices is by coalloying with extractable metals such as Cu or Au and then immersing the alloy in acids to selectively extract the more corrosive alloying element [12−15]. These resulting porous Au regions have much more surface area than plated Au with a much higher surface to volume ratio, a key feature in enhanced S/N ratio in advanced sensors. Obviously, the process for making these devices and any thermal postprocessing will affect the overall pore density of the final electrode. Thus, the reproducibility of any design is key to more predictable performance.

7.3.6 Other Precious Metals: Pt/ Rh/Pd

Other precious metals including Au can also be used as electrodes for pacemaker leads and other sensory probes. Typical properties linked with these Au and Au alloys are included in Table 7.5. While platinum, rhodium and palladium in bulk can be prohibitively expensive, there are often instances where, in very small quantities of these precious metals can be processed into unique microstructures can make sensor profiles smaller and smaller. Consider the level of surface area available to a disk as opposed to a porous blob of the same metal. The potential to make 3D sensors and leads has the capacity to shrink the current size of alternative signaling and sensory leads.

Table 7.5: Mechanical properties of metallic orthopedic biomaterials

Metal Alloy	Condition	Young's Modulus (GPa)	Yield Strength (MPa)	Tensile Strength (MPa)	Ductility	Density (g/cm^3)
Steels						
F138	Annealed	200	170−205	480−515	40	7.9
F138	Cold worked	200	310−690	655−860	12−28	7.9
F745	Annealed	200	205	480	30	
Co−Cr						
F75	Cast	210	450	655	8	8−9 nominally
F90	Annealed	210	380	900	30	
F562	Solution annealed	230	240−450	790−1000	50	
F562	Cold worked	230	1590	1790	8	
Titanium						
F67	Cold worked	110−120	485	760	15	4.4−4.5
F136	Forged	110−120	896	965	10	4.4−4.5

Based on [3,7,18−21].

Pt is commonly used as an embolism former in and near aneurysms as deposited by catheters. Platelets, exposed to platinum in a rod or coil form, activate which triggers the coagulation cascade creating local emboli near where the coils are deposited. By locally filling berry aneurysms with well-defined geometries with coils, it is possible that the clot will strengthen and help to reduce wall pressure on the aneurysm region which, if it works, will reduce the risk for aneurysm rupture. Rhodium and Palladium can be coalloyed with these but the raw material costs are sufficiently prohibitive that these materials will not be part of any large-scale effort to displace the use of other metals except in niche areas like sensors.

7.3.7 Amalgam

Dental amalgam has been around for hundreds of years and is still used extensively even today, despite potential concerns to both patient and clinical staff associated with mercury processing. Amalgamation constitutes the reaction with liquid mercury with any reactive metal. Mercury reacts with a range of metal powders that have been ground (using mortar and pestle) to expose the metal surfaces. The ease of processing and robustness of the material to compositional and processer variations makes this an ideal filling material for cavities and regularly used today. The most common components in dental amalgam reactions are included in equation 7.1, listed below. Silver–tin and silver–copper intermetallics are pulverized and mixed into the slurry with Hg that reacts with all three metals to form two new compounds. One starting component, γ, is added in excess to insure near complete amalgamation [16].

$$Ag_3Sn(\gamma) + AgCu + Hg(l) \rightarrow Cu_6Sn_5 + \gamma + Ag_2Hg_3(\gamma_1)$$

In dental offices, amalgamation reactions are routine as Hg(l) is usually reacted with alloy powders of copper and tin. The amalgamation reaction is initiated by breaking up the metal powders into fine grains, then mixing vigorously with the liquid mercury into a slurry. As amalgamation progresses, the balance between solid and liquid shifts to more of the solid form. The reaction occurs very quickly, over a period of minutes, and the resulting slurry can be pressed into a cavity (drilled) that is prepared beforehand. Once the prepared cavity is filled, the patient bites down on wax paper, a self-forging process occurs where the amalgam is plastically deformed and hardening while at the same time creating the bite countersurface. Amalgamation (more reactions with Hg and powder surfaces) continues over a period of up to a week following installation. Residual free Hg is collected by wicking excess slurry after subsequent pressings in the chair. By the time the patient leaves the office, the form is solid and hardening. This is one of the rare incidents where liquid metal processing occurs in vivo. There are several variants in terms of the metallic powders used for the amalgamation reaction but higher copper content alloys tend to have less galvanic corrosion between tin-rich and silver-rich phases and overall higher strength overall.

Dental amalgam is much softer than steels and other metals used for orthopedics. Overall performance in terms of compression performance from mastication is excellent, as fillings can last for decades. The larger concern with amalgam fillings is the fate and transport of labile mercury. A number of studies have looked at the corrosion rates and abrasion resistance of these formed alloys as a function of processing and environment. Attributes that could be tracked include ions into a corrosion medium, solution conductivity dynamics with exposure time, or gravimetric determinations at discrete time points following exposure. Overall, the general perception of amalgamation as a viable filling approach is still positive. Alternative filling materials are resin-based composites that are esthetically more pleasing although they are not as robust and fatigue resistant as amalgam.

7.4 Mechanical Properties

From a design standpoint, one relevant comparison is how these metals and alloys behave under mechanical loading, as compared to normal bone stock. Relevant mechanical properties include the modulus of elasticity, the ductility, and the strength, with various modes of testing (tension compression, torsion, etc.). A related presentation of mechanical behavior as a function of titanium alloy porosity is shown in Fig. 7.10.

The Young's modulus of elasticity is identified as the initial slope of the stress (force per unit area)−strain (displacement per gauge length) diagram and has units of Pa. Yield point is commonly interpreted where an offset slope parallel to the modulus curve intersects the stress−strain diagram. Depending on the modulus of the material being tested, there are several offset conditions to distinguish between fully elastic behavior and more permanent deformation, which for metals is commonly a 0.2% or 0.02% offset yield. The stress and strain at this intersection point can be identified as the yield stress and yield strain. There are other interpretations for the yield point but the offset approach is most common. The ductility is referred to as the elongation at some defined failure condition, whether that is gross failure or some other failure criterion. One can integrate the area under the stress−strain curve and interpret some sort of fracture energy per unit volume of sample.

Overall, the mechanical properties of metallic biomaterials are much stiffer and stronger than the natural tissues that they are replacing. Tabulated results for the mechanical properties of metallic biomaterials are included in Table 7.5.

Stretching a metallic alloy creates an elastic and recoverable deformation up to the yield point and then undergoes plastic deformation beyond the yield condition. Stiffness, yield

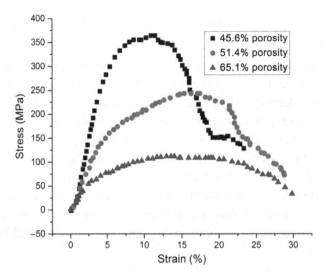

Figure 7.10

Mechanical response of porous titanium alloy composites at room temperature under compression. As expected, more porosity yields more compliance and a lower modulus of elasticity, a lower yield strength, and a larger ductility. *From X. Li, C. Wang, W. Zhang, Y. Li, 2010. Fabrication and compressive properties of Ti6Al4V implant with honeycomb-like structure for biomedical applications, Rapid. Prototyp. J. 16 (2010) 44–49.*

stress, and strain of these metallic biomaterials are controlled both by subtle changes in composition, processing as subtleties in processing can manipulate phase structure.

7.5 Schemes to Stress Shielding Further?

7.5.1 β Phase Titanium Alloys

The mechanical behavior of crystalline metals depends on the modulus of the crystals making up the bulk of the test specimen. Most cast structures yield crystals that are randomly organized, thus diminishing any subtle differences in the mechanical behavior of the crystalline biomaterial based on crystal direction.

Earlier, it was pointed out that besides producing metallic foams, manipulations to the crystal structure by adding other alloying elements could reduce compressive modulus form without voids to something closer to natural bone stock. An example of crystal structure modifications has been done by alloying titanium with niobium, another transition metal element, in relatively high concentration as shown in Table 7.6.

Table 7.6: Phase structure determined by adding varying amounts of niobium to base metal titanium. Single-phase regions are denoted below 25%Nb, with a new BCC β phase forming at higher Nb content

Composition	Phase	Crystal Structure
Ti	α'	Hexagonal
Ti–5%Nb	α'	Hexagonal
Ti–10%Nb	α'	Hexagonal
Ti–15%Nb	α',α''	Hexagonal/orthorhombic
Ti–17.5%Nb	α''	Orthorhombic
Ti–20%Nb	α''	Orthorhombic
Ti–22.5%Nb	α''	Orthorhombic
Ti–25%Nb	α''	Orthorhombic
Ti–27.5%Nb	α'',β	Orthorhombic/BCC
Ti–30%Nb	α'',β	Orthorhombic/BCC
Ti–35%Nb	β	BCC

From J.-H.C. Lin, C.P. Ju, C.M. Lee, Medical implant made of biocompatible low modulus high strength titanium-niobium alloy and method of using the same. US Patent Publication #US 6752882, 2004.

Table 7.7: Mechanical behavior of Ti—Nb alloys

Alloy	Hardness (HV)	Strength	Modulus
Ti–Grade 4		1.315 GPa	110 GPa
Ti–6Al–4V	307	1.857	105
Ti–15%Nb	307	1.56	62
Ti–20%Nb	292	1.46	60
Ti–25%Nb	327	1.65	77

From J.-H.C. Lin, C.P. Ju, C.M. Lee, Medical implant made of biocompatible low modulus high strength titanium-niobium alloy and method of using the same. US Patent Publication #US 6752882, 2004.

Adding Nb to a bulk Ti structure altered the crystal structure with an observed reduction in the mechanical modulus (E) of the resulting alloy [22] as shown in Table 7.7. There was a defined minimum in strength and modulus at 20%Nb.

More work is needed to gauge how an alternative alloy might perform in a wider battery of in vitro and in vivo evaluations. It is also important to not cede so many of the positive benefits of using Ti that have been widely touted. Reducing the modulus of a cortical bone (E- $\sim$ 18 GPa) bone replacement with something less than that for titanium (E- $\sim$ 110 GPa) leaves a wide range of physical phase space to be evaluated overall. This approach has probably been overlooked mainly because of the cost of all of the qualification testing required to make an adequate comparison with steels, cobalt—chrome, and native titanium alloys, and the inherent cost of adding Nb to Ti in such large alloying amounts.

7.5.2 Magnesium-Based Biodegradable Alloys

Other options to consider for orthopedic biomaterials would include Mg-based alloys which have moduli of 45 GPa but with the added feature that they undergo active corrosion in saline environments [23]. Coalloying elements for Mg include rare earth elements like neodymium, lanthanum, and cerium that have a modest impact on the rates of corrosion in vivo. The optimistic perspective would consider the release of Mg ions as nothing extraordinary as we are naturally composed of some Mg and there appears to be some potential for probiotic cell proliferation near where Mg is released [23,24]. This active corrosion response seems to also have potential as a bioresorbable structure but careful consideration is needed to maintain adequate strength to allow for adequate bone ingrowth.

It is also important to recognize the biomechanical schemes for loading that are possible. The world is not uniaxial. Crossing one's legs imparts torsional loading around the hip, turning a key in a lock also imparts a torsional load around the wrist. Carrying luggage is essentially an extensional exercise in the ulna, humerus, and radius of the arm, while doing push-ups imparts both bending and compression in different regions of those bones as well. It needs to be recognized that these bony biomaterial replacement devices are also going to be loaded alternatively as well. This could explain why uniaxial composites that could be designed to match bone mechanical behavior might not perform as a hip implant in the same robust way.

Overall, many of these attributes can be measured for biomaterials as well and these can be used to track issues relating to quality control of processing sequences and formulation efforts designed to yield a specific series of properties with a specific shape.

7.6 Processing

A key factor in understanding biometallic form and structure is that processing can affect structure as much as composition. We consider here cast forms, quench and annealed forms, and plastically deformed or wrought forms.

Casting is common for steels, titanium alloys, and to a lesser extent, Co−Cr. In these instances, the powders are mixed and heated above the melt temperature based on the composition in the phase diagram. They are poured or cast into molds for subsequent use or processing. Slow-cooled shapes often yield the equilibrium structure based on the phase diagram than quench and annealed forms. Quenching is a casting process by which metastable microstructures are achieved due to rapid cooling under nonequilibrium processing. These structures are often stabilized by annealing or heat treating at elevated temperatures but nowhere near temperatures in which the equilibrium phase structure would displace the nonequilibrium phases.

Stronger alloys are made by deformation processing, including calendaring, rolling, and forging. All of these can be performed both at room temperature (cold working and warmer temperatures (so-called hot working). The process of deforming the solidified structures introduces dislocations and other crystalline defects that retard subsequent crystal plane movement, usually coinciding with lower ductility and higher strength. These deformation-induced processing methods can be performed in conjunction with already cast structures. The net result of forging is that the resulting forms are often much harder, of similar density, and reduced ductility, with similar moduli.

Other schemes for making components like screws and pins use subtractive processing schemes such as drilling, cutting, and lathe-based operations. Here, the removal of material creates new surfaces that can expose bare metal and trigger oxidation all over again. All of the features of having compositions of material sufficiently robust as to survive the subtractive processing apply. This is how bone screws, pins, and holes in plates are often made.

7.7 Conclusion

Metallic biomaterials are commonly used both now and for the foreseeable future. Clearly, for hard tissue applications and for some specific soft tissue needs, metallic biomaterials will continue to be the likely standard for the future. With an eye for the future, tissue-engineered solutions for some orthopedics problems will likely displace some need and the National Institutes for Health (NIH) roadmap shows a trend to earlier intervention before the condition is not sufficiently chronic that a more drastic repair is needed. Both of these trends will tend to lower the upside potential for widely expanded options for bulk metallic biomaterials.

7.8 Problems

1. BCC iron has a unit cell lattice parameter, a, one length along the cube dimension = 0.286 nm. With two atoms fully contained within the unit cell and knowing the molar mass of iron to be 55.8 g/mole, determine the theoretical density of the crystal.
2. Explain whether you would expect FCC iron to have a different density than BCC iron? One should be able to quantitatively assess this problem.
3. One might consider whether a similar scheme of crystal structure analysis could be used to identify the density of bone. Explain why the objective determination of a theoretical density of bone is not possible?

4. A titanium rod (E = 110 GPa) is designed to represent the femoral stem of a total hip replacement. The rod is 1.5 cm in diameter and 22 cm long. Calculate the force, strain, and displacement, if elastically compressed with a stress of 8 MPa.

5. The iron–carbon phase diagram shown below shows the presence of both a eutectic and a eutectoid reaction. Identify both the temperature of these reactions and what phases transform under both of these conditions.

6. With a 1.8 weight % alloy of carbon in steel being reduced in temperature from the melt, identify at what temperature solid starts forming and at what temperature is it fully solidified under equilibrium conditions.

7. What crystal structure is most energetically favorable to first form from the melt at 0.85% carbon from the alloy in problem 6? Show on the phase diagram.

8. For the alloy in problem 6, as the temperature is further lowered, a new two-phase eutectoid form is energetically more favorable. Write down the equation to represent this reaction?

9. For the TiNi phase diagram, define the equilibrium phases present at 24 atomic % nickel at 850°C and at what temperature that composition will melt.

10. For the porous titanium composite being compressed in Fig. 7.10, identify the 2% offset yield strength under compression as a function of porosity for the three different samples.

11. Calculate the modulus of elasticity for the titanium composites shown in Fig. 7.10.

12. Determine what volume fraction of pores is needed in stainless steel to match the modulus of both cancellous (@ = 2.5 GPa) and cortical bone (18 GPa). Use a rule of mixtures assessment. The density of the fully consolidated metal is 7800 kg/m^3 and its modulus is approximately 210 GPa. Report your number as a volume fraction.
    Assume a volumetric contribution of stainless steel and air.

13. Describe the corrosion potential for stainless steels, Co–Cr, and titanium. Describe the difference between corrosion and passivation and its influence on mass flux

14. How does the interpretation of a 0.2% yield compare with a 0.02% offset yield? Are they both yield conditions?

15. For the titanium–niobium alloys being produced in Table 7.6, explain how is the identification of a new change in the crystal structure tracked as a function of composition?

16. About 10% of the population has a more pronounced allergic reaction to nickel used in jewelry and also in nickel bases used for dental crowns. Explain how having a larger comprehensive medical history might reduce the chance for chronic immunological response when the allergic patient is a candidate for prosthodontic crown installation.

17. Gold seems a more promising candidate for joint replacement structures than steel based on mechanical tissue matching and relatively little cellular bioincompatibility. Explain whether there a reason why gold might not be ideal?

18. Explain what makes the biomaterials industry different from the electronics industry which has seen tremendous technological advancement in 30 years or the pharma industry that has seen drugs convert from highly priced monopolies to cheaper generics and over the counter medicines? When are patent protections lifted for these producers?

References

[1] Copper Development Association, 2008. Copper-Zinc Phase Diagram. Available from: <http://www. copper.org/publications/newsletters/innovations/2006/03/images/cuzn_phase.jpg >.

[2] Copper Development Association, 2014. DKI German Copper Institute Booklet: Copper nickel alloys; Properties, Processing, Application. [English translation]. Available from: <http://www.copper.org/ applications/marine/cuni/txt_DKI.html > accessed 4/1/2017.

[3] Carpenter BioDur™ 316LS Stainless Medical Implant Alloy, 52% Cold Worked 2008. Available from: <http://www.matweb.com/search/DataSheet.aspx?MatGUID = 04e7d8af93ad440eab7326482e922bc8 >, accessed 2/4/2017.

[4] L. Reclaru, R. Lerf, P.Y. Eschler, J.M. Meyer, Corrosion behavior of metallic surgical implant Rex734-CoCr: Pitting, crevice and galvanic corrosion evaluation, Eur Cell Mater 1 (Supple 1) (2001) 29−30.

[5] G.V., Raynor, V.G. Rivlin, Phase equlibria in iron ternary alloys, Institute of Metals, London, 1988.

[6] A. Kosoffsky, B. Jansson, A thermodynamic evaluation of the Co-Cr and the C-Co-Cr systems, Calphad 21 (3) (1997) 321−333.

[7] J. Black, Biological performance of materials, fundamentals of biocompatibility, Marcel Dekker, New York, 1999.

[8] S. Ostlere, How to image metal-on-metal prostheses and their complications, Am. J. Roentgenol 197 (2011) 558−567.

[9] A.S. McDonald, G.H. Sistare, The metallurgy of some carat gold jewellery alloys, Pt 1. Colored gold alloys, Gold Bull 11 (1978) 66−73.

[10] J.L. Ferracane, Materials in dentistry, Lippincott, Williams and Wilkins, New York, 2001.

[11] R.P. Kusy, K.F. Leinfelder, Age-hardening and tensile properties of low gold (10-14kt) alloys, J Biomed Mater Res 15 (1981) 117−135.

[12] A. Dursun, D.V. Pugh, S.G. Corcoran, A steady-state method for determining the dealloying critical potential, ESL 6 (8) (2003) B32−B34.

[13] A. Dursun, D.V. Pugh, S.G. Corcoran, Dealloying of Ag-Au alloys in halide-containing electrolytes: Affect on critical potential and pore size, J Electrochem Soc 150 (7) (2003) B355−B360.

[14] D.V. Pugh, A. Dursun, S.G. Corcoran, Electrochemical and morphological characterization of Pt-Cu dealloying, J Electrochem Soc 152 (11) (2005) B455−B459.

[15] D.V. Pugh, A. Dursun, S.G. Corcoran, Formation of nanoporous platinum by selective dissolution of Cu from Cu0.75Pt0.25, J Mater Res 18 (1) (2003) 216−221.

[16] Mackert, J.R., 2006.Dental Amalgam and Other Restorative Materials. Available from: <http://www.fda. gov/ohrms/dockets/ac/06/slides/2006-4218s1-03.pdf > accessed 5/18/2017.

[17] X. Li, C. Wang, W. Zhang, Y. Li, Fabrication and compressive properties of Ti6Al4V implant with honeycomb-like structure for biomedical applications, Rapid Prototyp J 16 (2010) 44−49.

[18] J. Chen, M. Rodig, F. Carsughi, Y. Dai, G.S. Bauer, H. Ullmaier, The tensile properties of AISI 316L and OPTIFER in various conditions irradiated in a spallation environment, J Nucl Mater 343 (2005) 236−240.

[19] Azo materials. 2005. Stainless steel−grade 316L—Properties, fabrication and applications. Available from: <http://www.azom.com/details.asp?ArticleID = 2382 >.

[20] J.B. Park, R.S. Lakes, Biomaterials, an Introduction, Plenum, New York, 1990.

[21] D. Williams, Concise encyclopedia of medical and dental materials, Pergamon Press, Oxford, England, 1990.

[22] J.-H.C. Lin, C.P. Ju, C.M. Lee, Medical implant made of biocompatible low modulus high strength titanium-niobium alloy and method of using the same. US Patent Publication #US 6752882, 2004.

[23] M.P. Staiger, A.M. Pietak, J. Huadmai, G. Dias, Magnesium and its alloys as orthopedic biomaterials: A review, Biomaterials 27 (2006) 1728−1734.

[24] F. Witte, V. Kaese, H. Haferkamp, E. Switzer, A. Meyer-Lindernberg, C.J. Wirth, et al., In vivo corrosion of four magnesium alloys and the associated bone response, Biomaterials 26 (2005) 3557−3563.

CHAPTER 8

Ceramic Biomaterials

Learning Objectives

The reader by completing this chapter should be

- Able to recognize that heteroatom structures of cations and anions can also form ceramic crystal structures similar to metals.
- Exposed to examples of ceramic crystals commonly used as biomaterials and how shapes and forms of these materials are produced
- Aware of the range of properties (mechanical and optical) that are produced with common choices
- Capable of comparing properties of ceramics vs. other material classes and natural tissue. Properties of ceramics are functions of defect structure and porosity as regulator flaws which usually propagate and fail under mechanical loading.
- Aware of the fact that ceramics can be deployed as consolidated forms as particulates, as porous structures, and as bioactive glasses.

8.1 Introduction

Hard tissue repairs for fracture fixation, bone augmentation, and implant integration require thoughtful schemes for structural stabilization. Bone implant interfaces can be formed not only with cast and forged metals but using rigid consolidated ceramics as well. Stoichiometric ionic ceramics are produced when groups of cations and anions are combined to often produce crystals with a regular repeating structure and unit cell shape and dimension. So-called nonstoichiometric ionic ceramics can form when a participating cation or anion has more than one stable oxidation state leaving holes in the crystal. There are also defective structures that are sufficiently disorganized that rather than crystallize, they form a glass instead.

Nature does not produce monolithic ceramic structures. Enamel is as close as it comes and even that has some significant organic content (2–3% by mass) contained within it. Bone, whether cortical, cancellous, or as part of dental structures, is composed of microcrystalline or nanocrystalline deposits of inorganic calcium phosphate residues. Thus, monolithic structures (porcelain teeth for example) are quite different both in their organization and composition compared with native structures. Ceramic monoliths are used, but it is worth considering bone and bone minerals composed of calcium phosphate first just so that a larger understanding of the compositional environment for minerals is achieved.

The biomaterials industry has used a range of different ceramics for some time. Some nomenclature is required to classify how these biomaterials are partitioned. First, there are distinctions drawn between calcium-based ceramics and other synthetic ceramic structures as some are soluble and some not. Calcium-based materials are typically soluble or ionisable before ultimately being incorporated or dissolved and reprecipitated into growing bone stock. It is possible that the presence of the ions affects the physiology of those adjacent cells and they would be considered osteoinductive materials. There are also calcium-based materials that are so insoluble that they do not alter cellular responses adjacent to the implant surface. We consider those as osteoconductive surfaces and they can be very useful as potential scaffolds onto which bone cells attach.

Tremendous effort is placed on using calcium hydroxyapatite as the standard reference relating to bone reconstruction and mineralization. Calcium hydroxyapatite has a crystal structure, density, substitutional defects in the structure that alter its surface energy, its hardness, and it is embedded in the pores of an organized collagen matrix. Compositionally, bone mineral deposits have a similar Ca/P ratio to calcium hydroxyapatite (CaHAP), similar broad diffraction peaks where sharper CaHAP diffractions are normally found using X-ray diffraction. It is very difficult to make a direct comparison between nanocrystalline mineral deposits and larger calcium phosphate crystals.

8.2 CaHAP

CaHAP is a hexagonal packed structure with unit cell dimensions a = 9.41 Angstroms and c = 6.88 Angstroms. The mechanical response has been evaluated along the axial c direction and the modulus of elasticity is ~ 35 GPa. Testing off axis to the axial direction will yield a different mechanical response. CaHAP is not homogeneous like more simple cubic structures. Of course, there are many different forms of calcium-based ceramic salts in the form of phosphates, carbonates, and sulfates, and examples of such as shown in Table 8.1. If calcium phosphates are soluble in vivo, there is the chance that these minerals could be sources for the ultimate reprecipitation of new bone mineral deposits. Somehow in the context of bone mineralization and issues relating to both diseases relating to bone density and bone remodeling that occurs following fracture, there is an increasing solubility of many calcium with lower pH shown in Fig. 8.1. It is described that the bone mineral crystal is slightly deficient in the calcium in the crystal, suggesting a slightly lower Ca/P ratio than 1.67 if all calcium sites in the crystal are filled. It is possible that the nanocrystals of CaHAP that would otherwise be rather insoluble to pH above four are actually more soluble at the nanoscale. It is also possible that the number of defects is sufficient to allow for larger mineral dissolution and subsequent reprecipitation.

Table 8.1: Names, chemical formulae, and crystal structures of representative calcium phosphates

Formula Name	Chemical Structure	Density	Ca/P Ratio	Solubility in Neutral H_2O
Monocalcium phosphate	$Ca(H_2PO_4)_2$ Mw = 245 g/mol	2.22 g/cm^3	0.5	20 g/L
Dicalcium phosphate (DCPD)	$CaHPO_4$ Mw = 136 g/mol dehydrated, 172 g/mol as a dihydrate	2.92 g/cm^3 anhydrous, 2.31 as dihydrate	1	0.2 g/L
Tricalcium phosphate (TCP)	$Ca_3(PO_4)_2$, Mw = 310 g/mol	3.14 g/cm^3	1.5	0.02 g/L
Calcium Pyrophosphate	CaP_2O_7, Mw = 254 g/mole		0.5	insoluble
Amorphous calcium phosphate	$Ca_9(HPO_4)(PO_4)_5(OH)$	variable	~1.5	variable
Calcium hydroxyapatite (HAP)	$Ca_{10}(PO_4)_6(OH)_2$, Mw = 502 g/mol	3.14–3.21 g/cm^3	1.67	Nearly insoluble

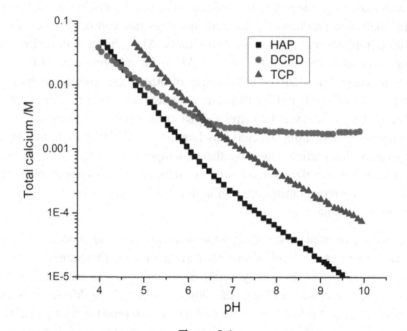

Figure 8.1

Solubility of selected calcium salts as a function of pH [5] as determined as a total amount of calcium released while regulating pH.

There seems to be much more comprehensive interest in the process of using particulates of CaHAP either as formulated fillers in grouts and cement pastes and also as starting materials in various deposition strategies to coat metallic implants for example. β phase tricalcium phosphate is found in a range of bone tissue-engineering applications and amorphous calcium phosphate is found as a time-release enamel deposition scheme being released from chewing gums [2–4]. It is all quite fascinating to consider the range of uses for these reactive and inert fillers and how they are ultimately deployed.

With the need for implants with higher strength and stiffness that can be fashioned without the long-term risks associated with metal ion release, larger ceramic monoliths have been produced using aluminum oxide and zirconium oxide in both orthopedics and dentistry. And with the compelling need to produce instrumentation that is compatible with MRI capability, there are efforts to produce clips, cutters, clamps, and other hardware that can be outfitted from ceramic components during continuous, MRI-guided surgeries. Here, the forms of these materials are covered, including their phase structure, their general processing strategy, and performance attributes.

8.3 Aluminum Oxide: Al_2O_3

Aluminum oxide (Al_2O_3), mined and refined into controlled particle size and composition, is commonly sintered to produce consolidated structures that can be polished and finished to yield ceramic implants and other related structures. Al_2O_3 has a high melting point (2072°C) and is found most commonly in its α-Al_2O_3 form, corundum. Al_2O_3 processed into biomaterial constructs usually still has traces of other metal oxides, including silica (0.1–0.2 wt%) and iron oxide (0.03 wt%). The complications with finding thermally stable molds and the inherent residual stresses that arise when melt processing are such that it is less common. Consolidating structures by heating very small particulates at high enough temperature that particles fuse together at temperatures much lower than the melting point as they lower their surface area (a surface energetics approach to reducing free energy). Sintering temperatures are still high (1000–1300°C) but much lower than 2000 + °C to melt alumina.

Corundum forms in a trigonal crystal structure with a corresponding crystal density of 2730 kg/m^3. Depending on the level of impurities in the mineral, there are a number of other crystal structures achieved but these are generally more rare. As was mentioned in Chapter 7, Metallic Biomaterials, in characterizing metal alloy structures, X-ray diffraction is the tool of choice to confirm crystal structure. There are milling steps to produce finer particles and purification steps to remove oxides of silicon, iron, and others also coprecipitated in the mined minerals. High temperature oxidation (called calcining) is performed to fully convert aluminum to its +3 oxidation steps to fully oxidize aluminum in the particulates. Finer particle sizes correspond purer mineral and ultimately lower sintering temperatures. So relatively pure forms of alumina can be produced and consolidated into larger structures to represent implants.

Even in the short time that implant materials have been considered, caution has been placed squarely on the very low fracture toughness of ceramics in general. This focus on preventing catastrophic fracture of devices implanted in recipients has impacted considerations about implant composition, processing installation, and design and there has been a significant learning curve. As device design, production and installation have been increasingly optimized, there is a growing sense that these devices are less susceptible to early and catastrophic failure.

From a structural perspective, sintering efficiency and conversion is highly linked with reducing flaw density in the consolidated forms. Producing hip stem components from finer grained alumina particles will yield more complete densification (fewer pores). The larger the residual pores in the structure, more likely that the load at fracture is reduced based Griffith's-based fracture mechanics principles mentioned in Chapter 3, Bones and Mineralized Tissues.

There is a similar interest in combining oxides in the alumina matrix to reinforce it and to blunt-crack propagation under load. The naming convention associated with oxide ceramics notes that high alumina ceramics are denoted with alumina fractions higher than 97% by weight. High purity alumina has an alumina concentration of at least 99.7% by weight.

In terms of coconstituents used in making sintered composite or two-phase structures, magnesium oxide (MgO) in high alumina ceramics is perceived to positively retard alumina grain growth during sintering and reduce the chances for intergranular fracture which is often weaker [6]. The alumina–magnesia phase diagram is shown in Fig. 8.2 [7]. The distinction between binary metal alloy phase diagrams and ceramic phase diagrams is that the boundaries are elements with metals and compounds with ceramics. The solid solubility

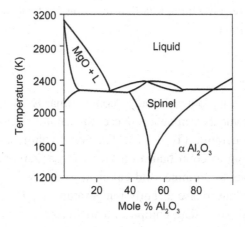

Figure 8.2
An example of the MgO–Al$_2$O$_3$ phase diagram where the components are compounds, not Redrawn from Kotka et al, US Patent 7045223.

of MgO in high purity alumina matrix composites is so low as to be sequestered at grain boundaries.

In the presence of other oxides such as zirconia in the 1%–2% range, sintering the alumina causes a phase transformation in the zirconia particulates from monoclinic to tetragonal. Again, the solid solubility of zirconia in alumina is very low and the zirconia is distributed adjacent to the alumina grains. If the metastable tetragonal phase or zirconia can be maintained upon cooling, when the structure is loaded, there is a stress-induced conversion of zirconia to the stable monoclinic phase absorbing energy in the process and also helping to blunt cracks that encounter the zirconia phase [8]. The success linked with raising the fracture toughness and ultimate strength of high alumina composites suggests that these are compositions are preferred to produce ceramic femoral balls and other bony implant devices derived from aluminum oxide.

There are a number of uses for Al_2O_3 beyond femoral ball construction for total hip arthroplasty. In orthopedics, alumina is used as a similar bearing surface in other total joint reconstructions. Alumina is also used in orthodontia as brackets that interface with archwires to apply lateral forces to the teeth in driving their migration. As it turns out, alumina can be produced as polycrystalline structures that appear white due to light scattering between grains as light propagates through it. There are also alumina brackets constructed from single crystal alumina (sapphire) that are machined to shape. The construction from a single crystal eliminates grain boundaries and creates an optically clear structure that can be also functional. Obviously, there are, cost, quality, and aesthetic drivers that motivate consumers of these devices to choose an option. Orthodontics is an area where the consumer has a direct bearing on the types of devices clinicians install as these are much more commonly marketed direct at the consumer similar to other areas in ophthalmology. The general idea though is that alumina is primarily considered for its potential as a hard tissue interface.

8.4 Zirconia: ZrO_2

Similar components have been produced from zirconia primarily focused also on femoral balls in modular total hip replacements. Zirconia is denser than alumina (5680 kg/m^3) and is another high melting temperature ceramic ($T_m = 2715°C$). For a volumetric replacement of tissue, the zirconia device is going to contribute to a larger mass. Zirconia is mined from ore, purified in similar schemes to alumina, and calcined to insure complete oxidation. It is found in its stable monoclinic phase at body temperature. Higher temperature processing required to sinter zirconia particulate compacts also causes solid-state phase transitions to both the cubic and tetragonal phases and the monoclinic. As a result, there can be some complicated phase structural evolution associated with zirconia and the presence of coalloying elements controlling the transformation rate. Probably the most common stabilizing additive is yttrium oxide (yttria) that is incorporated to aid in maintaining the tetragonal structure forming tetragonal zirconia polycrystals (TZP). It is possible to have only partially stabilized zirconia by adding insufficient amounts of stabilizer (usually 2%–3% on a molar basis) called metastable zirconia. With metastable zirconia, the presence of stress can cause partial transformation of tetragonal zirconia to monoclinic similar to what happens to zirconia when used as an additive with alumina. It is also possible that environmental factors could change the internal stress state more than is accommodated. The transformation can also strengthen the structure but if the response is too large, separate internal cracks can form catastrophically. The nuances of processing and structure are somewhat convoluted as there can be a gradient in zirconia metastability and loading is not always uniform or standard. There is a nice review of zirconia femoral ball development highlighting the mixed results as both the learning curve is ascended in producing these components and using them accordingly [9]. With these devices approved on an experimental basis only since 1985, it is safe to say that as more is understood about the link between composition, structure, and performance, better and more durable zirconia devices are likely to be achieved but the performance of the prior art is somewhat baked in relating to already installed implant devices that will have their own performance standard.

8.5 Porcelains

Probably the most common use of ceramics in biomaterials is in replacing dental superstructures, including crowns, bridges, and false teeth with dental porcelains. Porcelain is actually a multiphase ceramic structure formed from combinations of silicon dioxide and Al_2O_3. It is appropriate to present the SiO_2/Al_2O_3 phase diagram, shown in Fig. 8.3 and to

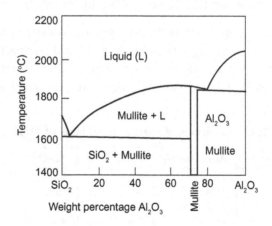

Figure 8.3
The SiO_2/Al_2O_3 phase diagram.

mention that based on the typical composition of the mixtures, most dental porcelains have compositions with SiO_2 content between 60% and 65% by weight and Al_2O_3 content between 7% and 15% [10], that places the composition within the two-phase (SiO_2 + mullite) region with nominally 10%–25% alumina in the mixture. Some fraction of the SiO_2 phase is crystalline in the form of crystabolite.

Porcelains are commonly sintered that requires adequate mixing of the two different particulates. Structural porcelains for producing crowns for grinding bite surfaces (molars) need better mixing of the disparate phases than porcelain veneers. The particulates are mixed in a gel-like slurry that holds the particles together before sintering and the gel can be poured or pressed into molds that are typically oversized relative to the final product. With the particulate coalescence comes shrinkage and the amount of shrinkage can be controlled to yield a correctly sized crown for installation.

With the two different particulates mixed together, there is a need to increase wetting between particles that is often done by adding acid fluxes that reduce the sintering temperatures required to activate the coalescence of the particulates. Fluxes for porcelain processing are often based on soda ash (Na_2O) or potash (K_2O). It is the delicate balance between formulation, sintering temperature, and shape that have led to optimized crown processing such that this is a generally routine operation conducted in dental fabrication laboratories. Typical formulated compositions of ceramic mixtures are shown in Table 8.2.

What is fascinating about replicating natural tooth structure is that our own teeth are not homogeneous. Teeth possess translucency gradient as one moves to the edges of the bite surfaces and this is most evident on the upper central incisors (your larger front teeth). In producing prosthetic teeth, one needs to control the level of tooth translucency which occurs by filling the perimeter of the tooth replicate with a gradient composition to allow for varying optical reflection and translucency along the prosthetic crown surface.

Correlating with sintering temperature is the strength, the density of the porcelain, and to some extent, the amount of shrinkage stress on the produced compact, particularly if it is sintered on a metallic base. There are different design requirements depending on where these porcelain structures are placed, and while there are occasional issues with individual

Table 8.2: Compositions of various porcelains of varying opacity

Form	SiO_2 (wt%)	Al_2O_3 (wt%)	K_2O (wt%)	Na_2O (wt%)	Balance/Other Oxides
I(t)	68.7	15.3	11	5	—
II(o)	58.4	15.1	6.1	15.6	4.8
III(t)	41.2	36.2	1	2.6	18
IV(t)	65.2	15.1	7.4	4.2	8.1
(t): translucent (o): opaque					

Source: From E.W. Phillips, R.W. Skinner, The Science of Dental Materials, WB Saunders, Philadelphia, PA, 1967 [11].

quality control, this area of structural ceramics has led to dental structures that are routinely made in exquisite detail and ever more complicated designs.

An excellent example of this interplay between the driving force for complete sintering and resulting properties is included in Table 8.3 and Fig. 8.4, respectively [12]. Raising the sintering temperature densifies the sintered compact, and with fewer pores contained in the structure, there is a corresponding rise in the Modulus of elasticity and compressive strength of the sintered element. As those pores are absorbed in the ceramic phase with particulate wetting, the result densifies as noted by the volumetric shrinkage.

8.6 Carbon

The notion of pyrolyzing, or energetically converting by plasma, organic matter and conveying the combustion by-products in the form of various solid phase carbonaceous constituents to a targeted surface encompasses aspects of chemical vapor deposition. Under precise process and compositional feed control, stable coatings can be deposited on substrates. Fluctuations in pyrolysis temperature, substrate temperature, and complexity can affect deposition thickness and composition. The rationale for coating surfaces of metallic implants that one can prevent potential corrosion reactions and blood coagulation responses when devices are installed in the vasculature (heart valves and stents). A schematic of the general system is presented in Fig. 8.5. A gas source within a functional chamber is directed toward a target surface. There are introduction ports into which organic reactants are fed into the chamber. The presence of either the plasma or the temperature of the feed gas is sufficiently high as to cause chemical reactions including combustion within the chamber. The feed stream velocity regulates the particulate velocity impinging the target

Table 8.3: The impact of sintering temperature on the resulting rise in both the Modulus of Elasticity, E, and compressive strength. The higher temperature increases the driving force for inter particle coalescence resulting in a larger resistance to deformation and increased strength [12].

Sintering T (K)	E, Gpa	Compressive Strength (Mpa)
1413	16.3	5.26
1433	26.2	6.8
1453	27.6	5.05
1473	36.3	7.66
1493	41.6	7.96
1513	44.1	9.06
1533	43.4	12.28
1553	46.1	12.84
1573	59.8	13.25
1593	67.3	13.43
1613	73.5	13.81

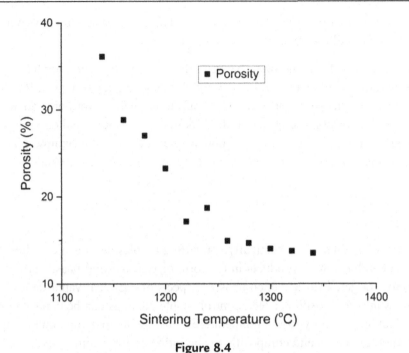

Figure 8.4
The effect of sintering temperature on resulting porosity in sintered hydroxyapatite, from [12]
1 standard deviation in porosity was approximately 1.5% by this determination.

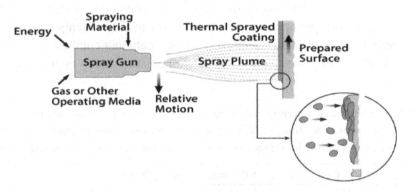

Figure 8.5
The scheme for directed particle deposition on a near net-shaped implant to enhance bone
growth.

surface and the particulate size regulates its inertial impact. Longer times correspond to
thicker coatings and typically, coating thicknesses are 1 μm or less in thickness.

The mechanics of deposition is essentially a directed spray of convective gases into which
organic products are combusted or precipitate in the directed stream. The coatings derived

from carbon have been used most extensively for cardiovascular valvular implant surfaces to retard platelet activation and other thromboembolic potential. The conditions are quite variable and it is possible to build structured carbon coatings that have long-range order as well as more glassy deposits.

8.7 Processing Schemes and Structures

The very high melting points of ceramics in general precludes their ability to be melt processed simply by pouring. Even liquid viscosities in the melt are much higher for ceramic liquids than for corresponding metals. It suggests that ceramics require other processing schemes than melt casting to produce preforms and other structures.

The most common way that structural ceramic monoliths are created is by sintering, which is a submelting coalescence of particles that has already been discussed on some general level. A schematic of the process is shown in Fig. 8.6. Mixtures of particles (gold) with liquid (black droplets) and liquid soluble polymer gluing agents (binders) are combined and

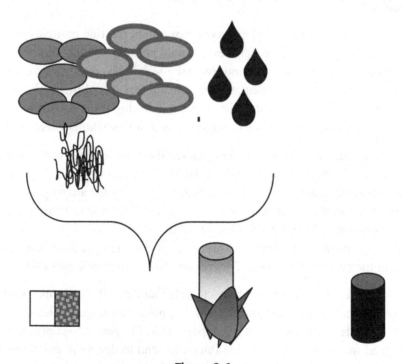

Figure 8.6

Schematic of firing process. Ceramic particles, liquid vehicle, and binder are mixed together and blended into slurries that can be compacted into a structure. Following the drying to liberate the vehicle, the solid compact can be raised above the decomposition temperature of the binder and trigger the fusion of particles in the compact.

mixed, dispensed into an appropriately shaped preform, and thermally processed to drive off the nonceramic components. The driving force for sintering is the reduced surface area of the sintered compact that leads to the understanding that an ensemble of smaller and finer particles will have a larger driving force for undergoing a submelting point fusion. One can actually calculate the surface energy of the ensemble as the surface energy of the particles summed up over the range of particle sizes. Comparing a single particle with a surface energy corresponding to the single radial surface exposed as opposed to a large ensemble of particles composing the same volume as the single particle, each with a dramatically smaller radius but with a much larger number of particles, clearly the ensemble is in a higher energy state and thermal processing will drive the ensemble to reduce the surface area exposed, all other attributes being the same. The reduction in the process temperatures compared to the melt for fine particle ceramic compacts is several hundred degrees. The lower the sintering temperature, the wider the choice of molding materials that can aid in processing and the lower the shrinkage strains produced in the compact during the cooling for the sintering procedures. In some instances, the shrinkage is so pervasive as to fracture compacts upon cooling without any intrinsic loading on the sintered product.

To sintering ceramics, one first needs to produce or obtain the fine particles of silica, alumina, calcium phosphate, etc. Sometimes, a single particle size and distribution is used, sometimes bimodal or multimodal distributions are used. For very high T_m ceramics in general, sintering requires finer particulate sizes ideally less than 1 μm in diameter. The smaller the diameter of the particulates, the larger the driving force for surface area reduction to occur and the more effective sintering is at lower temperature.

The particles are dispersed in a fluid medium called the vehicle (e.g., water or alcohol with other additives mixed subsequently mixed in). Binders are included which are essentially vehicle-soluble polymers added at small percentages allowing the shaping of more complex geometries and providing some minimum structural stability for transferring compacts to the furnace for sintering. Once the vehicle evaporates, the polymer remains acting as a kind of glue holding particulates together. To lower the sintering temperature more, often fluxes aid in oxidizing the particle surfaces and increasing the interparticle wettability.

The formulated mixtures are viscous fluids and gels that can fill molds appropriately. The evaporation of the vehicle dries the specimen to the point that it can be handled, stored, and later installed in the furnace to sinter the compact. Thin flat geometries dry very evenly and more complicated specimens with variable thickness tend to dry more unevenly. Once dried and stored, these pieces can be maintained indefinitely in what is called the green state or immediately directed to the sintering furnace.

Sintering follows a heating schedule shown schematically in Fig. 8.7, defined in part on prior successful experience in producing prototypes. Usually, there is a timed heating ramp that

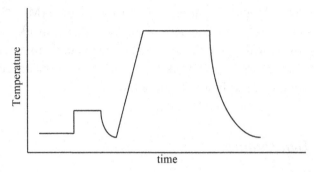

Figure 8.7
A typical heating schedule. The first heating is performed to drive off the vehicle and to retain the strength of the binder holding the compact together. The second heating is performed at high enough temperatures to burn off the decomposing binder and to sinter the particles in the compact together. Heating schemes are sophisticated to prevent the sealing of the outside boundaries of the compact that will doom the compact from reducing voids and preventing further densification of the compact.

drives off any residual vehicle, followed by an isothermal hold near the decomposition of the binder, usually 300–400°C. This stage is called binder burnout and the decomposition products outgas out of the structure leaving the low vapor pressure particles + any formulated fluxes. Following the binder burnout, the furnace is heated to high temperatures held for long times (10–12 hours at between typically 0.7 and 0.8 T_m based on the phase diagram for the formulated ceramic). That heated immersion results in sintering of the particulates, coupled with the loss of pore area within the volume of the compact and fewer particles exposed to free surfaces. From a physical standpoint, the particle compact is first reduced in density with the loss of the binder, followed by an increase in density as the pores are expelled from the interior of the sintered structure. The measured density with time is a quality assessment gauge as reference is made to the ratio of the measured density to that of the theoretical density of the crystals. Following the completion of the sintering cycle, the temperature is lowered usually in a controlled fashion to equilibrate the consolidated specimens at ambient temperature. There can be significant shrinkage of the structure upon cooling, with sufficient shrinkage strains to fracture the sintered specimens. Obviously, the heating schedules are optimized around strength, function, and replicating the desired shape of the compact. It is also worth noting that at least for dental composites, the molds that are constructed are often oversized so that the shrinkage can be accommodated as a tolerance in the design.

8.8 Mechanical and Physical Properties

There is a general trend between theoretical density and strength of ceramic particulate composites. As monoliths, published tables highlight general properties of consolidated ceramics, including that of Magnesia-partially stabilized Zirconia (Mg-PSZ) and tetragonal zirconia polycrystals (TZPs) [13]. The general message is that consolidated ceramics are denser than natural tissues, with strengths and moduli comparable to other metallic implant materials. For ceramics, the largest drawback from a mechanical perspective is their inherently low fracture toughness. Example properties for densified ceramics are shown in Table 8.4 [13].

8.9 Particulate Bioceramics

As, particulates, hydroxyapatite, other calcium phosphates and silica find larger use as fillers. From soluble calcium phosphates that are incorporated into growing bone structures to osteocondutive surfaces within injectable cements and scaffold structures for bone tissue engineering, to benign, drug-encapsulated hollow spheres and within other types of bioactive glasses, pastes, slurries, and cements.

In the most direct way, monoliths are unnecessary as particulates can be directly deposited into bone gaps in bone defect models. The quality of the healing can be resolved through in vivo testing and histology following sacrifice [14] Here, the size of particulates has ranged for various calcium phosphate particulates from 1 to 10 microns in diameter and the other particulates have been larger, typically hundreds of microns on average [3,15−17]. Smaller is likely better, but the main consideration is ability to be conveyed to the defect. Insoluble particulates are not likely to be altered as a result of interaction with adjacent cells but can provide surfaces that enhance the growth of bone mineral deposits from adjacent osteoblasts [18]. The presence of soluble particulates can obviously affect particle size as the particle dimensions changes and the soluble species can be harnessed by the cells [19,20].

Table 8.4: Example properties derived from consolidated alumina and zirconia ceramics used as monoliths

Property		Al_2O_3	Mg Phase-Stabilized ZrO_2	Tetragonal Zirconia Polycrystals, TZP
Chemical composition		99.9% Al_2O_3 + MgO	ZrO_2 + 8−10 mol% MgO	ZrO_2 + 3 mol% Y_2O_3
density	kg/m^3	>3970	5740−6000	>6000
porosity	%	<0.1	−	<0.1
Bending strength	MPa	>500	450−700	900−1200
Compressive strength	MPa	4100	2000	2000
Youngs Modulus	GPa	380	200	210
Thermal coefficient of expansion	μm/m-°K	8	7−10	11
Thermal conductivity	w/m-°K	30	2	2
Fracture toughness	MPa-m$^{0.5}$	4	7−15	7−10

Source: From C. Piconi, G. Maccauro, Zirconia as a biomaterial. Biomaterials 10 (1999) 1−25 [13].

There are some elements of alchemy and process control that still require optimization on subsequent bone formation. Certainly, the optimum particle size and distribution of various injectable particulates has not been fully evaluated and more work is needed, particularly related to mixed particle sizes and mixtures of different compositions [14]. The initial results suggest that the introduction of particulates can provide both source material and favorable surface features while enhancing bone formation.

8.10 Bioactive Ceramic Structures

The use of silica-based bioceramics that can be formulated with mixtures of SiO_2, CaO, Na_2O, and P_2O_5 forming glasses that have proven capable of forming interfacial bonds with living bone over periods of 1 month [21]. Detailed mechanisms of the reaction mechanism of these structures have been presented and include ion exchange and hydrolysis of the silica-rich layers of the glass surface. With time, there is dissolution and diffusion of Ca^{2+} and $PO4^{3-}$ ions that ultimately leads to the formation of an amorphous calcium phosphate structure on the surface [22]. Further interaction in the environment leads to added inorganic chemistry leading to direct bonding with the bone structure. The inclusion of so many compounds needed to work in concert within a wound site with variable pH suggests that there are likely narrow ranges of compositions that yield robust growth. There are ranges of glass composition that appear active in this response. As one evaluates more purified mixtures near the edges of the phase diagram, these structures appear more inert [21].

Schemes for producing consolidated forms of bioactive glass require precise thermal control as at higher temperature, there is a driving force to induce crystallization which would reduce overall solubility and a much larger driving force to actually sinter the particles increasing the density and making glass compacts much less porous, if not controlled [23]. Published processing schemes have produced porous structures from thermally processed particulates that have been partially sintered with porosities above 30% and pore diameters in the range of hundreds of micrometers [22].

Schemes to produce drug loaded bioactive glasses have been developed that require that the glass processing does not cause the drug to react or otherwise decompose. Research efforts have observed the efforts to incorporate primary growth factors into these structures as a way to enhance angiogenesis to the targeted bioactive glass implant location [24−26].

On the therapy front, similar sort of injection strategies can be undertaken, and the attributes of the benign ceramics are different. A range of silica-based dendrimers may be better described as mesoporous silica nanoparticles have also been produced on the range of 100 nm, generally much smaller in overall dimensions than for these particulate fillers discussed earlier. These porous glass bioceramics have a channel-like structure that can be loaded with a particular therapeutics and allow passive diffusion form the bioglass ceramic into the surrounding implant location with the notion that they are endocytosed carrying a drug along for the ride. The choice of therapy is rather widespread and can include fluorescing molecules like fluorescein, chemotherapeutics, growth factors, antibiotics like vancomycin, and combinations thereof [27]. For the hollow, permeable structures, the therapeutic payload has to be smaller than the pores in the ceramic and the timeline and threshold concentrations for dosing need to be well characterized. For the dendrimer-based superstructures, these are hybrid-type inorganic—organic structures and both the therapy and the organic building blocks are grafted onto the structure. Adequate chemical synthetic acumen is required to produce these structures and to also regulate dose and timeline for dosing [28]. Reactions that trigger the release of chemotherapeutic, growth factor, virus, or antibiotic usually is in the form of an enzyme reaction, pH change, or other activation process to fractionate the dendrimer structure. The ideal hybrid dendrimers are small enough to be cleared in the renal system.

The production of bioglass ceramic structures arise from several different strategies but the most common is to include in the particulate low melting fluxes and additives that lower the sintering temperature of the glass into the range that does not negatively affect their overall porosity allow for tissue ingrowth, a large challenge.

8.11 Relationship With Environment

Clearly, the functionality of these components either a monoliths or as particulates dispersed or added in bulk is key. The assessment of functionality for monoliths is tied to structural details, dimensional tolerances, strength, stiffness, ductility, pore structure, and flaw size and distribution. Functional assessment of particulates is much more complicated as no specific structural detail is key. For therapeutic release, both with in vitro and in vivo assays, cell and tissue assessment can be performed. Drug fluence is assessed and its impact of drug release on physiology or disease is often performed by other assays (mineral density, blood tests, urinalysis, imaging, biopsy, etc.)

8.12 Functional Usage

With consolidated ceramics being comparable to metals in terms of mechanical performance, it comes as no surprise to find ample research and clinical evaluations of ceramic biomaterials as hard tissue replacements. In orthopedics, bearing surfaces abound with consolidated alumina and zirconia devices. With the demand associated with degenerative joint diseases for implants for knees, hips and shoulders, there is plenty of demand for low-wear and low-friction replacement devices.

In dentistry, consolidated structures are commonly used in prosthodontics and general dentistry for crowns, bridges, and veneers. The goal in ceramic consolidation is to match the tint of the surrounding teeth. For structural uses for molars and bridges, dental porcelain is consolidated often on some sort of metallic base usually from gold or gold/nickel alloys. The key feature in material processing are that the sintering temperature has to be low enough to insure that the base does not melt.

Porous structures are useful in orthopedics as scaffolds into which surrounding bone infiltrates. Porous bioinert ceramics are very useful for spinal fusion surgery in which two disks are ultimately fused into one through the introduction of a porous scaffold plug between them. Bone infiltration using porous scaffold structures can be resolved in various bone gap presentations that can arise from cancer resection, particularly with oral cancers and with some needs in trauma care with regard to fracture fixation.

In particulate form, various bone augmentation procedures are performed by depositing particulates near surrounding bone stock in an attempt to activate more prolific bone growth near defects. Candidates for dental implants also sometimes have a need for larger bone stock to install the bone substructures safely without fracturing the mandible or maxilla. Particulate filling through an oral surgical intervention is one scheme for increasing bone thickness there.

8.13 Conclusion

Presented in Chapter 8, Ceramic Biomaterials, have been details regarding the structure and performance of ceramic biomaterials. Ceramics can form crystals like the metallic biomaterials discussed in Chapter 7, Metallic Biomaterials. They can also have sufficient defect structure to form less ordered glassy structures upon cooling. We have presented phase diagrams, formulations, and processing schemes to produce these as either consolidated monoliths, coatings, or as particulates, or fillers in other matrices such as degradable polymers discussed in Chapter 9, Polymeric Biomaterials and Chapter 11, Orthopedics.

It has been discussed that in consolidated forms, the structures produced for ceramics rival metals in terms of strength and stiffness. Ceramics tend to be more bioinert and that bodes well for cells adjacent to these surfaces and a key feature. These structures are also more fragile and susceptible to crack propagation, so the presence of flaws, pores, and their distribution is what is often a limiting factor for strength and durability.

We find many uses for ceramics particularly in hard tissue bone augmentation procedures and increasingly as inert coatings on more reactive metal structures. The primary performance gauge for bone infiltrating structures is the presence of continued mineralization and cell viability that is assessed by techniques discussed in Chapter 5 as well as by microscopy. We have presented other niche areas that might offer more promise for the future, particularly if advanced diagnostics and treatment will make use of higher magnetization in situ imaging techniques.

8.14 Problems

1. The apparent density of porous ceramic structures can be done using an Archimedes density measurement. By measuring the mass of an object both in air and in a submerged condition (e.g., water), the relative mass difference is a measure of the buoyancy of the structure being evaluated.

    In particular, if we measure a porous hydroxyapatite (theoretical crystal density, $\rho = 3126$ kg/m^3) form with a dry mass of 6 g and a separate mass of 3.6 g in a submerged aqueous condition (the density of water is 1000 kg/m^3 or 1 g/cm^3), determine both the *apparent measured density* of the specimen and the fractional porosity. The measured density of a material with zero porosity should be the theoretical crystal density, and that ratio of measured to theoretical density is unity. The pore volume or fractional porosity is 1 $-$ (measured density/theoretical crystal density). The relevant equation is shown below.

    $$\rho_{\text{meaured}} = \left(\frac{mass_{\text{dry}}}{mass_{\text{dry}} - mass_{\text{wet}}}\right)\rho_{\text{fluid}}$$

2. If the same sample was immersed in a different fluid medium (ethyl alcohol with a density of 789 kg/m^3), determine the submerged mass?

3. If we sintered this structure at a lower temperature, explain whether you would expect the wet mass in either medium be larger or smaller?

4. Given the planar pore structure produced in a porous hydroxyapatite-coated bioceramic described in the paper by Ben Nissan et al [1], estimate the average pore size and the 2-D planar porosity. Sophisticated determinations would use image analysis software but estimates are sufficient for here Fig. 8.8. The scale bar is 100 microns in length.

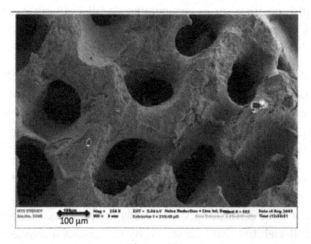

Figure 8.8

An example porous structure. *Reproduced with permission from Ben-Nassan et al. [1].*

5. What might be learned by CT as opposed to the 1-D radiographs shown in Fig. 8.1?

6. Is coral presented as osteoconductive or osteoinductive in this case?

7. If one made a Alumina/air composite using 350 GPa for the modulus of bulk Alumina, that followed a "rule of mixtures" behavior, ($E_{composite} = \Sigma v_i E_i$) where v is the volume fraction of each phase and E is the corresponding modulus of that phase, determine how much porosity is needed to match the stiffness of cortical bone.

8. Dental crowns, made from mixtures of silica and alumina called porcelains, are often sintered on gold alloy bases to simulate a normal-tooth superstructure (what is exposed). As shrinkage occurs with sintering, differential cooling strains can arise at the interface between the two materials. Explain why these types of crowns might be more susceptible to fracture.

9. Included in Fig. 8.3 is the phase diagram for alumina/silica. Based on the fact that sintering usually accomplished at $0.75 T_m$, where T is in °K, determine an appropriate sintering temperature for a 20 wt% alumina-composite porcelain mixture (the balance is silica)

10. Does Al_2O_3-SiO_2 exhibit eutectics as were discussed in Chapter 7, Metallic Biomaterials? (Fig. 8.3)

References

[1] B. Ben Nissan, A. Milev, R. Vago, Morphology of sol-gel derived nano-coated corraline hydroxyxpatite, Biomaterials 25 (2004) 4971–4975.

[2] M. Szpalski, R. Gunzburg, Applications of calcium phosphate-based cancellous bone void fillers in trauma surgery, Orthopedics 25 (5) (2002) S601–S609.

[3] S.V. Dorozhkin, Calcium orthophosphates, J Mater Sci 42 (4) (2007) 1061–1095.

[4] M. Di Stasio, M. Nazzaro, M.G. Volpe, Release kinetics of calcium and quercetin from chewing gum as a novel antiplaque and antimicrobial device., Curr Drug Deliv 10 (2013) 261–267.

[5] P.G. Koutsoukos, Current knowledge of calcium phosphate chemistry and in particular solid surface-water interactions, 2nd International Conference on the Recovery of Phosphorus from Sewage and Animal Wastes, Noordwijkerhout, Netherlands, 2001.

[6] F. Macchi, Alumina ceramics in joint prostheses, J Bone Joint Surg Am 87–88 (2015) 62–63.

[7] M. Kotka, J. Stone-Sundberg, J. Cooke, R. Ackerman, H. Ong, E. Corrigan, Spinel articles and methods for forming same (2006) U. S. Patent # 7045223.

[8] J. Wang, R. Stevens, Zirconia-toughened alumina ceramics, J Mater Sci 24 (1989) 3421–3440.

[9] I.C. Clarke, M. Manaka, D.D. Green, P. Williams, G. Pezzotti, Y.H. Kim, et al., Current status of zirconia used in total hip implants, J Bone Joint Surg Am 85 (Suppl 4) (2003) 73–84.

[10] C. Panzera, L.M. Kaiser, Dental porcelain composition, U. S. Patent # US5944884 A (1999) issued August 31, 1999.

[11] E.W. Phillips, R.W. Skinner, The science of dental materials, 6th Ed., WB Saunders, Philadephia, PA, 1967.

[12] O. Prokopiev, I. Sevostianov, Dependence on the mechanical properties of sintered hydroxyapatite on sintering temperature, Mater Sci Eng A Struct Mater 431 (2006) 218–227.

[13] C. Piconi, G. Maccauro, Zirconia as a biomaterial, Biomaterials 10 (1999) 1–25.

[14] H. Oonishi, L.L. Hench, J. Wilson, F. Sugihara, E. Tsuji, S. Kushitani, et al., Comparitive bone growth behavior in granules of bioceramic materials of various sizes, J Biomed Mater Res 44 (1999) 31−43.

[15] J.E. Barralet, L. Grover, T. Gaunt, A.J. Wright, I.R. Gibson, Preparation of macroporous calcium phosphate cement tissue engineering scaffold, Biomaterials 23 (15) (2002) 3063−3072.

[16] C.P.A.T. Klein, J.M.A. de Blieck-Hogemrst, J.G.C. Wolke, K. de Groot, Studies of the solubility of different calcium phosphate ceramic particles in vitro, Biomaterials 11 (7) (1990) 509−512.

[17] M.E. Saadalla, N. Ahad, I.R. Gibson, J.C. Shelton, Comparison between commercial calcium phosphate bone cements, Key Engineering Materials 218−220 (7) (2002) 331−334.

[18] J.O. Hollinger, An introduction to biomaterials, in: M.R. Neuman (Ed.), Biomedical Engineering series, CRC Press, Boca Raton, FL, 2012.

[19] E.D. Eanes, Amorphous calcium phosphate, Monogr Oral Sci 18 (2001) 130−147.

[20] M. Julien, I. Khairoun, R.Z. LeGeros, S. Delplace, P. Pilet, P. Weiss, et al., Physico-chemical-mechanical and in vitro biological properties of calcium phosphate cements with doped amorphous calcium phosphates, Biomaterials 28 (6) (2007) 956−965.

[21] D. Williams, Concise encyclopedia of medical and dental materials, Pergamon Press, Oxford, UK, 1990.

[22] M.N. Rahaman, D.E. Day, B.S. Bal, Q. Fu, S.B. Jung, L.F. Bonewald, et al., Bioactive glass in tissue engineering, Acta Biomater 7 (2011) 2355−2373.

[23] D. Bellucci, V. Cannillo, A. Sola, An overview of the effects of thermal processing on bioactive glasses, Sci Sinter 42 (2010) 307−320.

[24] R.M. Day, Bioactive glass stimulates the secretion of angiogenic growth factors and angiogenesis in vitro, Tissue Eng 11 (2005) 768−777.

[25] J.K. Leach, D. Kaigler, Z. Wang, P.H. Krebsbach, D.J. Mooney, Coating of VEGF-releasing scaffolds with bioactive glass for angiogenesis and bone regeneration, Biomaterials 27 (2006) 3249−3255.

[26] H. Keshaw, A. Forbes, R.M. Day, Release of angiogenic growth factors from cells encapsulated in alginate beads with bioactive glass, Biomaterials 26 (2005) 4171−4179.

[27] I.I. Slowing, L. Vivero-Escoto, C.W. Wu, V.S.Y. Lin, Mesoporous silica nanoparticles as controlled release drug delivery and gene transfection carriers, Adv Drug Deliv Rev 60 (2008) 1278−1288.

[28] M. Vallet-Regi, M. Colilla, B. Gonzalez, Medical applications of organic-inorganic hybrid materials within the field of silica-based bioceramics, Chem Soc Rev 40 (2011) 596−607.

CHAPTER 9

Polymeric Biomaterials

Learning Objectives

By reading this chapter the reader should be able to

- Understand the nomenclature relating to how polymers are classified, something of their chain length, purity, and regularity.
- Discern the distinctions between synthetic polymers that tend to have very simple repeat structures, and proteins that require more knowledge of the amino acid structure in defining how it organizes in 3-D.
- Understand the linkage between chain length and functional transport of molecules in the melt. This is commonly assessed by melt viscosity.
- Note that polymers, even under optimum conditions, are never completely crystalline. There is always an amorphous fraction.
- Understand that for all the discussion about phase behavior in metals and ceramics, the compositional differences in repeat structures, branches, and copolymeric elements tend to make phase behavior in polymers rather moot. We describe characteristics such as melt temperatures and crystal structures of phases present, but if every different chain length is considered a different molecule, phase behavior becomes mired in multicomponent systems.
- Recognize distinctions between different classes of polymers, and how they might be deployed. Polymers that are melt extrudable into fiber and or tube forms are most useful, and helps to explain the wide variety of polymeric sutures that are available.
- Polymers undergoing mechanical extension as occurs in drawing tend to strengthen the fiber direction and orient the fibers accordingly. Orientation is lost at higher temperatures when larger molecular mobility is apparent.
- Competently describe a few areas where polymers are used.
- Understand that as-produced properties of polymers only tells a part of the story. Biodegradable structures interact with body fluids and swell, undergo chain scission, and reduce mass, mechanical behavior, and molecular weight of the degrading polymer with suture time.

Biomaterials. DOI: http://dx.doi.org/10.1016/B978-0-12-809478-5.00009-2

9.1 Introduction

Many different polymeric structures can be synthesized as potential biomaterials. Any general representation of a polymer is a more like a chain or a linkage of repeating structures or units, which are called monomers. In terms of nomenclature, we think of the repeating chemistry as the repeat unit and the number of repeating links in each chain that is defined as the degree of polymerization, n. If the molar mass of the repeating unit is known, one can define the molecular mass of a mole of the same length chains as the molar mass of that polymer chain as the product of the number of links in the chain and the molecular mass of the repeat unit.

Conventional synthesis protocols in industrial production rarely produce polymers that have the same chain length but often a broad distribution; the chains are all long chains, but some are longer than others. We think of this distribution of chain lengths as a polydisperse mixture and as a result, there is a need to quantify the chain length and variance in terms statistical averages that are discussed in more detail in Chapter 5, Property Assessments of Tissues.

As an example, if we consider the structure of polypropylene, a common polyolefin polymer that is spun to produce sutures, the repeating structure is essentially the same as propylene, and it is actually synthesized from propylene as the monomer. In this instance the repeat structure has the structure of propylene, the molecular mass of propylene, and if the degree of polymerization of the chain is known (assume for this example 20,000 links), and the mass of a mole of polymer chains is the product of the molar mass of the monomer and the degree of polymerization, n, as shown in Eq. (9.1).

$$\text{Mw}_{\text{repeat unit}} {}^{*} n \, (\text{degree of polymerization}) = \text{Mw}_{\text{chain}} \tag{9.1}$$

Note there are many different repeat structures that can be polymerized and some common polymers along with their corresponding molar masses/repeat unit are shown in Table 9.1. It is the realm of synthetic organic chemistry to identify reaction sites on different monomers that can react that leads to repeatable, chain like structures. Polymers are classified by the mechanism used to polymerize the structure, the monomers from which they are derived, or the product molecule that is formed as a result of reaction among other things. Polymers can also be distinguished by molecular weight as that correlates with both lower processibility and higher melt viscosity.

In terms of polymerization mechanism, there are several typical schemes used to polymerize monomers. They are broadly classified as either a radical scheme where advancement occurs through the controlled reaction with formed radicals in the bulk, or as

Table 9.1: Molar masses of different polymeric repeat units

Monomer	Formula	Repeat Unit	Molar Mass of Repeat Unit
Ethylene	Polyethylene 	C_2H_4, saturated	28 g/mol
Propylene	Polypropylene 	C_3H_6 saturated	42 g/mol
PMMA	Poly Methyl Methacrylate 	$C_5H_8O_2$	100 g/mol
Polyethers: polyethylene oxide (PEO)/ propylene oxide (PPO)		Variable	Variable
Polyethylene terephthalate (PET), a polyester	Polyethylene Terephthalate (PET) 	$C_{10}H_8O_4$	192 g/mol

(*Continued*)

Table 9.1: (Continued)

Monomer	Formula		Repeat Unit	Molar Mass of Repeat Unit
Nylon 6,6, a polyamide	Nylon 6,6		$C_{12}H_2N_2O_2$	224.3 g/mol
Nylon 6	Nylon 6		$C_6H_{11}ON$	113.2 g mol

a condensation mechanism in which the business ends of each monomer form well-defined products such as an amide, an ester, or a urethane bond as a result of polymerization. Readers are highly encouraged to read related textbooks that have further details about specific polymers not covered here including Refs. [1–3]. Hollinger and Ratner are particularly useful as they mention specific host interactions and describe aspects of wound healing foreign body response, enzyme release, and other cellular aspects of wound healing linked with different polymer chemistries presented on the surfaces of implants.

9.1.1 Radical Polymerization

Radical polymerization, also known as addition polymerization, results from the formation of a stable radical which is the basis for each propagation step. Radical polymerization is effective in polymerizing a range of polyolefins, polystyrene, acrylates, and other vinyl polymers that contain unsaturated alkene chemistry. Radical chemistry requires a radical initiator that decomposes by exposure to heat, light, pH changes, or other chemistry to form radicals. Example initiators include peroxides such as benzoyl peroxide seen in Fig. 9.1, camphorquinone and azo-iso butyronitrile among others. The range of functionalities and the ability to use light in particular increases the allure that these types of chemistries can

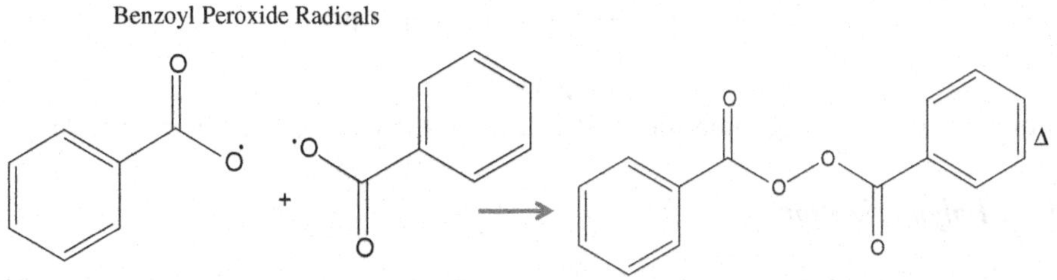

Benzoyl Peroxide Radicals

Figure 9.1
Benzoyl peroxide radical formation reaction, which can decompose through the O—O peroxide linkage into two radicals through heat or by chemical reaction to cleave it.

be used in vivo. Beyzoyl peroxide like other initiators has a O—O bond that cleaves with much less energy than the rest of the molecule and reliably can produce radicals.

Thinking in simple terms the initiator might be defined as I, cleaving into two radicals, R, as seen in Fig. 9.2.

Following the formation of the R* radicals from the controlled decomposition of a radical initiator, the formed radicals migrate in the solid or liquid state in an attempt to stabilize the radical into a covalent bond. For a simple alkene monomer, M, like propylene or methyl methacrylate (MMA), forming a stable bond with one end of the unsaturation leads to the radical propagating through the unsaturated bond and the formation of new radical of similar reactivity now attached to a slightly larger molecule, as shown in Fig. 9.3.

That propagation step recurs often and as polymer forms, there is phase transition from liquid to solid as a result of the many unsaturated reactions that result. Well-defined polymerization schemes are often terminated, but for in vivo polymerization, this is less of a consideration. In the end, many propagation steps ensue and polymer with large molecular weight often created very rapidly which is subsequently reprocessed into a useful shape/design. Nonetheless, there are many different monomers that can be polymerized by radical chemistry schemes. Polymers derived from unsaturated monomers that react with formed radicals are often named from the monomers from which they are derived. Thus while propylene is unsaturated, polypropylene (PP) is not. Some radical chemistry can be performed in vivo, while other radical polymers are produced off line and molded/crafted into shape afterwards.

$$I \quad \rightarrow \quad 2\ R^{*}$$

Figure 9.2
Radical initiation, the first step in radical polymerization.

$$R'^* + M \quad \rightarrow R'^* \text{ and so on and so on...}$$

Figure 9.3
Propagation steps consuming monomer and extending the chains that possess the radical ends.

9.1.2 Step Polymerization

Here the business end of each reactant is expected to add to a growing chain through well-defined reaction pathways to create high polymer. Examples of polymers produced by step or condensation polymerization include polyesters, polyamides, polyurethanes, and polyethers. In step polymerization, every reactant is as likely as the rest to undergo a reaction, there is no activated form like a radical to enhance polymerization in its adjacent vicinity it experiences through Brownian motion.

As an example, let us consider the polymerization of polyethylene terephthalate (PET), a common polyester used in making Dacron fabrics which are part of valvular graft constructions. Two reactants are required to produce PET, terephthalic acid, and ethylene glycol, both difunctional monomers, having either two acid functions or two ol functions at each end. It is well known that acids and ols typically react to form an ester linkage, with water being evolved as a small molecule as a product of the reaction. These two reactants form an ester bond and water. Conceptually this is shown in Figs. 9.4 and 9.5.

Each formation of an ester bond creates another small molecule, often water as a by-product, as is the case in polyester polymerization and many different step growth polymerization procedures yield a small molecule as a result.

If this reaction is performed at high temperature, the produced water tends to vaporize and condense on the top of the reaction vessel. Hence, it is named a condensation reaction. Under conditions of tight stoichiometric control, thousands of ester reactions can form leading the formation of thousands of molecules of water and the average chain linkage gets longer and longer. Under step polymerization, most of the molecules in solution are of similar chain length and increasing over time. Compare that to radical polymerization where most of the molecules are monomers and only a few reaction centers are active. This synthesis leads to a more bimodal molecular weight distribution that tilts toward a larger mass fraction of polymer over time. Polyesters, like other condensation polymers, usually contain atoms other carbon along the backbone, which is distinction with radical polymers that are usually all-carbon. Examples of the types of molecules required to produce various condensation reactions are included in Table 9.2.

Other polyester structures can be formed by altering the chemistry of the center segments maintaining the reactive end groups to still form the same condensation reaction. By substituting propylene glycol for ethylene glycol, ester reactions still form, but the repeat unit now contains propyl segments that repeat as opposed to the ethyl segment. Both are still polyesters but they might have different molecular mobilities and chain architecture.

If A represents a reactive end group like the acid function in terephthalic acid.

And B represents the reactive ol group in ethylene glycol, then terephthalic

acid looks like AFA and ethylene glycol looks like BGB.

IF A and B form water for example, then

AFA + BGB → AFGB + AB.

Figure 9.4

The end groups of the two difunctional monomers react to produce a larger molecule with new chemistry (FG) that represented the repeat structure of the growing polymer along with the formation of a small molecule (AB) which is water in the case of PET.

Table 9.2: Molecules used to produce various condensation reactions

Difunctional AFA Chemistry	Difunctional BGB Chemistry	Bond Formed	Small Molecule Produced
Terephthalic acid	Ethylene glycol	Ester, PET	Water
Terephthalic acid	Butylene glycol	Ester polybutylene glycol PBT	Water
Hexamethylene diamine	Adipic acid	Polyamide Nylon 6,6	Water
Decamethylene diamine	Adipic acid	Polyamide Nylon 10,6	Water
Hexamethylene diamine	Sebacoyl chloride	Polyamide Nylon 6,10	HCl
Hexamethylene diamine	Sebacic acid	Polyamide Nylon 6,10	Water
Methylene diisocyanate	Ethylene glycol	Urethane	None
Methylene diisocyanate	Butylene gycol	Urethane	None
Bisphenol A sodium salt	Phosgene	Polycarbonate of bisphenol A	NaCl

9.1.3 Copolymerization

There is no reason why only one is limited to a single monomer being polymerized (homopolymerization). Mixed feedstocks of unsaturated monomers for addition polymerization can lead to the inclusion of more than one monomer in a growing polymer chain. The production of a commercial product called low-density polyethylene (PE) is actually a copolymer of ethylene and longer chain length hexene for example that leads to the occasional inclusion of a branch in the other linear chain of a cluster of ethylene linkages. The branches tend to disrupt the energetics of crystallization and lead to the formation of a lower crystallinity polyolefin, and if the level of crystallinity is lower, so is the density of the bulk product since the crystals are more densely packed.

The extensive usage of pressure sensitive adhesives for diagnostic electrical sensors, adhesive tapes for IV fixturing and even commercial products such as nail polish are commonly produced from copolymers of ethyl hexyl acrylate (EHA) mixed with other acrylates and methacrylates like MMA or acrylic acid (AA). These polymers contain no crystallinity at all and depending on the MMA versus EHA content, one can tailor the glass transition temperature relative to body temperature. Copolymeric resins with larger EHA content have lower glass transition temperatures and are softer and more rubbery than resins with less EHA content, hence their use as elastic tapes and adhesives. Again, if both EHA and MMA polymerize by radical reduction of the unsaturation in these monomers, they are reacted in similar ways but have different side chains attached.

In comparing the copolymerization of condensation polymers such as polyamides and polyesters the only relevant chemistry is tied to the reactions occurring at the end groups. In other words the formation of PET is formed from the reaction of ethylene glycol and terephthalic acid, as shown in Fig. 9.5. Long-chain polyesters are produced under well-controlled conditions of high temperature and controlled humidity. As a result, medical devices produced from these feedstocks are packaged or processed into useful materials but the synthesis occurs off line.

While PET is made from the diacid and di-ol mentioned above, other polyesters can be formed from the reaction of other glycols with terephthalic acid and ethylene glycol with other acids. Thus it is possible to have chains in which some interior lengths between reactive end groups are different along the chain, even through ester reactions are still occurring during its condensation polymerization. This observation also leads to the conclusion that we need to be a lot more specific about condensation polymers given the wide breadth of molecules that could be reacted to form polyesters, polyamides, polyethers, and urethanes. One can produce both rigid or flexible amides, esters, and urethanes by controlling the length of flexible and rigid blocks between end groups, one can control the phase behavior of multiphasic structures that are still defined broadly as one class of ester, amide, or urethane, for example.

Also when considering the copolymerization of two different monomers or reactive end groups, there is the potential to form alternating copolymers or more randomly sequenced clusters of monomers. If there is a driving force for monomers to add to themselves, there is the potential to form block copolymers where large sequences of similarly added monomers propagate. The synthesis of block copolymers is very common in polyether

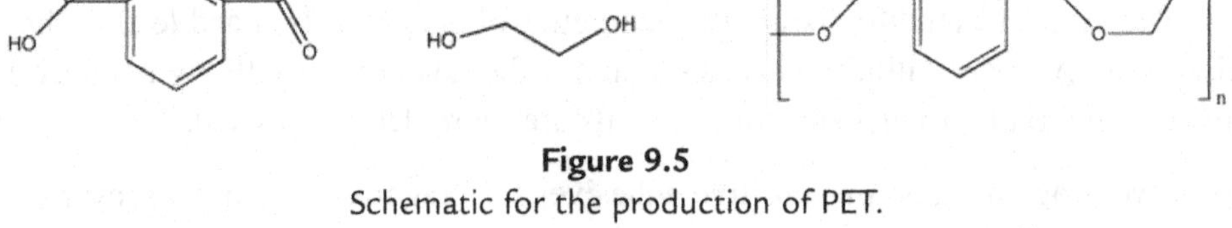

Figure 9.5
Schematic for the production of PET.

chemistry and there are many types of amphiphilic copolymers that are based on mixed ethers like PE oxide that is hydrophilic that is bound to PP oxide that is more hydrophobic which is generally very biocompatible. There are other block copolymers based on PEO and polycaprolactone (PCL). In these types of block copolymers, there is a need to define the general molecular weight the mass fractions of the block constituents, and lengths of the individual blocks. There can also be one link between blocks, as in a di-block copolymer, and there are also tri-blocks and with many more blocks linked to a structure, one can achieve what are noted as star polymers.

The ability to use different monomeric feedstocks has enabled the production of a wide variety of linear homopolymers that are covalently bonded along the backbone of each polymer chain. The ability to formulate combinations of feedstocks has led to a much richer capacity to build more controlled microstructures with individual chains and at the bulk level when groups of chains encounter one another.

There are other polymers that can be produced that have residual unsaturation contained within them including those based on butadiene, isobutylene, and silicones. All of these can subsequently link separate chains together in a crosslinked structure. There are instances when elastomers like isobutylenes and butadiene are interacting with biological structures, often as compliant coatings to soften haptic interfaces with skin and other biological tissues. The crosslinked structures are often more difficult to characterize as they as insoluble and chain architecture and network structure can vary, but it is worth noting that in addition to linear polymer structures, network polymers can also form. There is a tremendous level of collective interest in what is called thiol-ene or click chemistry that has the ability to harness reactions between thiol-based amino acids and other formulated thiols that are capable of reacting with unsaturated "ene" functions [4].

In summary, two primary synthetic methods have been presented that can produce a range of different polymers. Radical polymers often leverage C−C unsaturation and as a result, radical polymerization yields polymers that retain an all-carbon backbone. One common result of radical polymerization is that resins produced from this are less hydrolytically sensitive as water interacts more commonly with only the side chains of radical polymers and not the main chain. Condensation polymers typically retain features of the terminal chemistry of the reactants and as a result, more hydrolytically sensitive O and N are often found in the backbone. Copolymers of each synthetic type can be produced by judicious selection of either different unsaturated monomers or different chain sequences between end groups of monomers participating in condensation reactions. Linear, alternating, and block copolymer structures can be produced and crosslinked structures can be formed through further reaction with any residual unsaturation after polymer synthesis. Clearly there are many different structures that can form and the properties that are derived from what is produced are a direct result.

9.2 Phase Behavior of Polymers

If one was rigid in their interpretation of phase behavior of organic molecules, phase diagrams like those for metal alloys and ceramic mixtures could be produced for example between butane and docecane, a 20 chain hydrocarbon with the same repeat structure as butane but longer. Owing to the lack of control available through most synthetic radical and condensation polymerization schemes, there is already some potential problems in describing phase behavior of polymers of varying chain length. It is hard to identify objectively how many different constituents are mixed into a broad molecular weight distribution, let alone a mixture with two different homopolymer chains with different repeat structures.

But polymers clearly have phase behavior, some form crystals and have crystal structures. Crystalline polymers have identified melting points although there are so many defects in most polymers that they are generally considered semicrystalline at best. One could characterize the viscosity of molten mixtures that show a strong nonlinear positive correlation with increasing molecular weight. Increasing temperature above the melt temperature often reduces the melt viscosity and combinations of too high a temperature and too high a shear rate required for processing have the potential to degrade the polymer chain into smaller chain lengths.

9.3 Classes of Common Biomedical Polymers

9.3.1 Polyolefins

Polymers derived from gas and liquid-based hydrocarbons are commonly referred to as polyolefins and these resins have been used for decades tied to both fiber and suture production, many orthopedic bearing surfaces are derived from the ultrahigh molecular weight form of PE, gas permeation membranes, and hardware linked with clips, fixtures, trays, and packaging found in the operating and patient care rooms. Polyethylene, polypropylene, and polybutene are all considered polyolefin's.

9.3.1.1 Polyethylene

PE's most valuable use within medicine is in its ultrahigh molecular weight form, UHMWPE, used as bearing surfaces in total joint replacements, as noted in Fig. 9.6 where n ranges in the 1000s to 10,000s. These include the acetabular cup in total hips, the tibial tray in total knees, and there is a similar surface in the shoulder. PE has the same basic repeat structure as wax that is an oligomer but with PE, each chain is much longer or has a longer degree of polymerization. When chain extended to have molecular weights above 5 MDa, UHMWPE sufficient chain regularity to form crystals that melt in the range of 135–145°C. PE normally crystallizes in an orthorhombic crystal structure and has a density

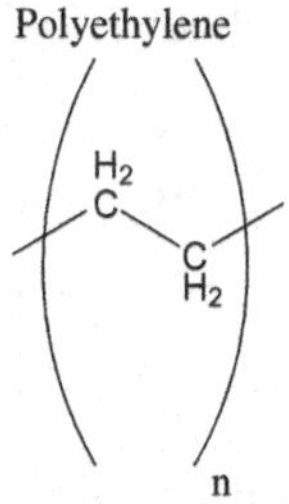

Polyethylene

Figure 9.6
Repeat structure for polyethylene.

that ranges between 0.86 g/ml for totally amorphous, molten PE to a theoretical density of 0.996 g/ml in a fully crystallized form, and in a processed form, typically 0.92–0.95 g/cm^3.

As the molecular weight of UHMWPE is so high, even in a molten state, UHMWPE is extremely viscous, so much so that it is virtually unprocessible by conventional melt extrusion techniques, and a process called ram extrusion is used to provide sufficient momentum to change the shape of UHMWPE into a useful near net shape form. UHMWPE is then typically machined to shape, polished, and dry sterilized after being packaged. More recently, UHMWPE has undergone heat treatment at elevated temperatures and below T_m to repopulate the surfaces with longer chains, not those cut as part of the machining process.

UHMWPE is softer than the metal and ceramic counter surfaces used in total joints which preferentially leads to wear and abrasion of particles, even of UHMWPE that are expelled into the joint cavities. The PE fragments that are ejected into the surrounding joint cavity are inert to surrounding cells, the PE fragments can encounter sentry cells that recruit monocytes and neutrophils in futile attempts to reduce these fragments. But with no solvent that can dissolve PE, there is little the foreign body response can affect in these particles and a process where the surrounding tissues deteriorate due to the immune function action. There is a time lag association with particle production and triggering osteolysis, and some joint replacements are loaded more than others, so they might be more prone to lead to pain responses earlier than others. So while PR is a great bearing surface, having a higher molecular weight increases the wear resistance but that benefit is offset by the fact that there is no known solvent and fragments that are collected are never effectively digested.

9.3.1.2 Polypropylene

The inclusion of an additional methyl group in the repeat structure of PE yields PP, another widespread commodity polymer that has found extensive usage in medical devices as well. The repeat structure of PP is shown in Fig. 9.7. PP is a polymorph but its preferred crystal structure is monoclinic, albeit with generally lower crystallinity than PE (0.90–0.91 g/cm^3), and it has a melting point of $\sim 165°C$, ($T_g = -15°C$). Owing to the smaller chain lengths in

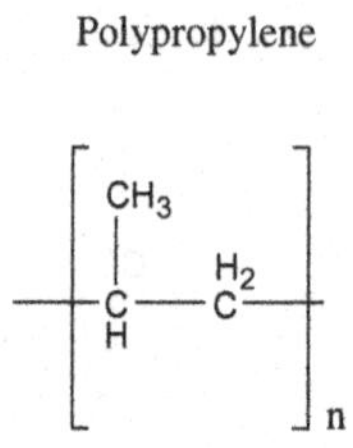

Polypropylene

Figure 9.7
Repeat structure of polypropylene.

PP relative to UHMWPE, PP is much more melt processable by conventional techniques like extrusion and injection molding.

The use of PP in general medicine has been most widespread as fibers and meshes tied to repairs within internal medicine. Polypropylene sutures are commonly produced by melt extrusion through fiber spinneret dies and the melt that is extruded through it is drawn through fiber spinning operations to induce large amounts of orientation designed to strengthen and stiffen the fiber relative to the bulk. The sutures are either single strand or braided structures and hooks/needles are attached as needed before packaging and sterilization. The impact of orienting these fibers leads to much lower levels of creep under load but also the potential that the fibers could be fractured during unusual loading events.

The drawing parameters and the size of the extrusion dies regulate the fiber diameter that is ultimately produced. Faster spinning speeds orient the fibers more, but that same fiber diameter could be achieved by lower orientation from a smaller diameter die. The amount of orientation has a big impact on properties and as-spun properties of sutures are very well characterized to insure their effective usage in a wide variety of suturing uses.

Further, ensembles of oriented fibers can be stitched together to form mesh-like structures that allow for tissue ingrowth within them making them ideal candidates for organ and tissue ruptures that might occur where there is a need to reinforce the natural tissue. Hernia repair commonly includes the installation of sterilized meshes that are stitched into and around the herniation in an attempt to stabilize the fascia and prevent further pain and anguish [5]. These types of meshes have been used for a number of years and the outcomes have been very successful.

There are many other uses for PP and other polyolefins in medicine, tied to packaging, trays, and other hardware found in various clinics and hospitals. If there is a comfort level is using these commodity polymers to create viable designs, then the only larger question is really tied to cost and budget and as opposed to the fact that only PP works, for example.

9.3.2 Beyond olefins: Acrylates

The capacity to perform in vivo polymerization has led to significant usage of acrylate and methacrylate chemistry for use in medicine. Acrylates are typically polymerized by addition schemes and can be formed in the presence of fillers that raise resin viscosity prepolymerization and also increase optical scattering in these noncrystalline, amorphous resins. Many acrylate-based monomers have been used and a table of common acrylates is shown in Table 9.2. Owing to the lack of stereoregularity during polymerization, acrylates are devoid of long-range order and form amorphous, often, transparent resins. Perhaps their widest use is as mix and set or photopolymerizable cements and adhesives. Here the focus is on four different acrylate chemistries that are highlighted in more detail. But the general message is other acrylate chemistry will have a similar scheme for polymerization and further characterization.

9.3.2.1 Methyl methacrylate

PMMA, shown in Fig. 9.8, is polymerized from MMA and is a widely used commercial grade resin that finds extensive use as plastic lenses, and lighter substitutes for silica-based window glass. MMA has been formulated into powder + liquid versions of bone cement that are commonly mixed and injected during the setting of some total joint prostheses. Bulk PMMA has a T_g of $\sim 105°C$, above which the resin is regulated by liquid behavior, and below which it is a glass.

PMMA that has been polymerized and shaped into molds have proven useful as ocular implants, contact lenses, and in filled conditions as tooth replicates. But these areas have been eclipsed by larger use of polymerized PMMA powder + liquid monomer bone cements used for fixturing prostheses. In two separate reservoirs, polymerized PMMA powder is comixed with an initiator that is stable under most storage conditions. The liquid fraction contains MMA monomer + an activating reactant that forms radicals for example from benzoyl peroxide and a stabilizer to maintain the monomer for appropriate shelf life. When

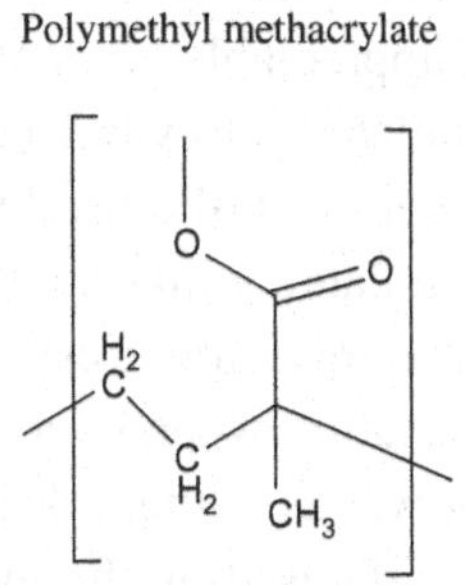

Polymethyl methacrylate

Figure 9.8
Repeat structure for polymethyl methacrylate.

the powder and liquid are mixed to yield a reactive dispersion or slurry the activator triggers radical initiation from the powder and the radicals propagate the radical addition reactions in the liquid phase. Polymerization occurs over less than 10 min and is exothermic hearing both the implant and the surrounding tissue. Temperature rises of as much as 10°C are common, but this clearly regulated by how many reactions are occurring at any one time and the thermal capacity of the components being installed. For procedures like kyphoplasty which will be discussed in Chapter 11, Orthopaedic Biomaterials and Strategies, there is no thermal sink and the heat is transferred to the surrounding tissues as it is injected. One is limited in terms of the total exotherm by the volume of what is injected and what fraction is monomer.

For injectable cements like bone cement, there are no specified rules on exactly when to inject, nor are there requirements about degassing the dispersion prior to injection. Injecting early has the benefit of a lower initial viscosity making it easier to inject but there is more monomer injected at this stage and permeation into the surrounding tissues may lead to a chemical necrosis. There is a need to manage both the thermal rise of the cement from polymerization and what chemical absorption there is into the tissue. Note that for metallic implants the implant is an effective heat sink and that tends to lower how high the temperature of the resin achieves during injection and setting.

Note that for knees and hips, both of these joints are normally under compression, so the stress state is less likely to cause joint separation. The cement requirements may be larger for shoulders where the joint is more often under tensile loading. Nonetheless the composition of typical cements are noted in Table 9.3 as are the general strength characteristics found in Table 9.4. It is noted that since these are mixed products, the presence of air bubbles and voids will impact the strength and density characteristics of these condensed structures.

9.3.2.2 BisGMA

For dental cements, photopolymerizable resins and sealants, the most common resin used is bis glycidyl acrylate, bis glycidyl methacrylate (BisGMA) is a very viscous liquid in its monomer form, and by dilution with appreciable amounts of other reactive comonomers, to lower viscosity BisGMA can be formulated into varnishes, brushable adhesives, and relatively viscous paste-like fillers. There is still a need to trigger the polymerization which for BisGMA has been commonly formulated with dimethyl para-toluidine and camphorquinone. The combination of camphorquinone (CQ) and N, N dimethyl para toluidine (DMPT) leads to radical formation when exposed to blue light typically in the range of 470 nm by these dental light wands. Other adhesive, sealant, and composite restorative systems have been developed based on the mixing of two-part, BisGMA resins. Activation ensues and rapid conversion occurs within minutes. Polymerization may be incomplete during 1−2 min of illumination and recognize that radical propagation could

Table 9.3: Composition of a typical bone cements used for fixturing total joint replacements

		B-Cement, Medical Contract Manufacturing, BV Nijmegen, NL [6]	Stryker Simplex B Bone Cement [7]
Solid phase components		40 g in a package	
Polymerized MMA	Inert filler	87.5%, w/w	15%, w/w
Styrene-MMA copolymer			75%, w/w
Barium sulfate	Inert radiopaque tracer	20%, w/w	10%, w/w
Benzoyl peroxide	Radical former	2.5%, adsorbed in powder	
Liquid components		16 g in an ampule	20 g in an ampule
Methyl methacrylate	Monomer	84.3%, v/v	
Butyl methacrylate	Monomer	13.1%, v/v	
N,N-Dimethyl para toluidine	Activator that cleaves benzoyl peroxide	0.6%, v/v	
Hydroquinone	Stabilizer to prevent polymerization during storage	Trace, ppm level	

Table 9.4: Properties of radiopaque bone cement [8]

Property	Average Value
Young's modulus (in compression	2.2 GPa
Tensile strength	28.9 MPa
Compressive strength	91.7 MPa
Density	1.1–1.2 g/cm^3
Water sorption	0.5% max
Shrinkage upon polymerization	∼3.5%

continue during dark phases following activation. The use of BisGMA is widespread throughout many dental clinics and the use of sealants has had a dramatic effect on reducing the number of cavity filling procedures due to dental caries. The use of sealants has also changed the dental practice from one of fixing defects to focusing on preventative oral health and has been a great success.

Photopolymerization has also been leveraged in other areas of medicine using other types of reactive acrylate resins such as polyhydroxyethyl methacrylate. Ingenious ways have been to take the same concepts developed by line of sight schemes used in dentistry to perform similar types of polymerizations elsewhere in vivo. A great example that shows the utility of reactive resin dispersion results from addressing abdominal adhesions. These conditions occur when segments of the intestinal track tend to fuse together. Aspects of muscular contracture tend to pull on segments of the intestinal track and can lead to blockages or adhesions requiring surgery to remove the blocking segments. Patients susceptible to one adhesion are likely to form more later and as a preventative, efforts have been made to disperse resins like hydroxyethyl methacrylate using an atomizer and trigger polymerization in a much wider field of view. The sealed areas are less likely to trigger these fusions and a better quality of life can be achieved free of subsequent adhesion surgeries. Here is an area where the concept of a reactive resin is not necessarily new, but where the understanding of the disease state and optimizing both chemistry and dispensing systems, huge potential exists in other areas of medicine untapped and without advanced tools.

9.3.3 Condensation polymers: Polyamides

It was discussed previously polyamides are condensation polymers formed from reactions between acids and amines, that yield the formation of an amide bond, not unlike how proteins are also formed. Nature can perform protein synthesis at ambient temperature while most synthetic polyamide production occurs at much higher temperatures. Discussed in more detail here are two different types of polyamides.

9.3.3.1 Nylon polyamide 6,6

Nylon 6,6 forms from the amides that are regularly produced from reactions between adipic acid and hexamethylene diamine, shown in Fig. 9.9. The 6,6 nomenclature highlights the number of methyl carbons interspersed between the carbonyls and between the amine functions. Nylon 6,6 is a semicrystalline polymorph but all of the crystals form triclinic structures with different unit cell dimensions and reasonable crystallinity is achieved in the

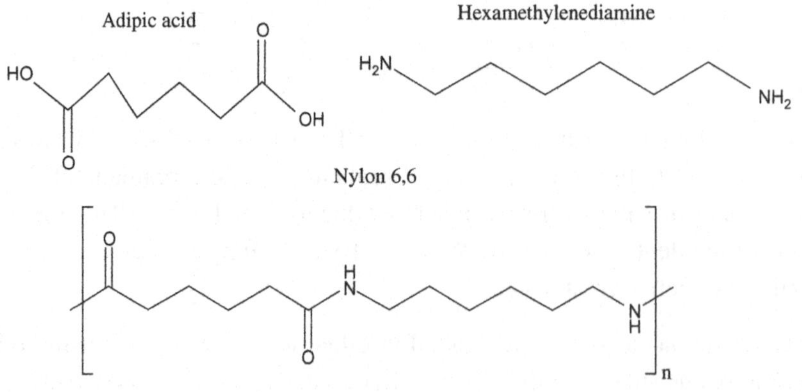

Figure 9.9
The Nylon 6,6 repeat structure and the difunctional components of adipic acid and hexamethylene diamine used to produce the chain extended polymer.

range of 30% of the volume. The density of nylon is typically about 1.1 g/cm^3 Nylon 6,6 melts at ∼250°C, and melt processing temperatures are typically about 25°C higher than that. Like other melt-processed polymers, Nylon 6,6 has been shaped and drawn into sutures, and stitched into other mesh-like products.

As part of the postprocessing sequences following drawing, sutures can also be solution-processed at room temperature through antibiotic treatment baths that can deposit chromic acid, a very effective antibiotic on the surface. These treatments can be integrated with spinning line and before take-up.

A distinction between polyamide biomaterials that are implanted and those from polyolefins for example is that polyamides are more hygroscopic, swell in the presence of water that tends to lower the strength and stiffness of the polyamide, and if implanted for a long enough period, will also be susceptible to enzymatic proteolysis, as the same bonds that are breaking down proteins will also break down these structures as well.

Engineering polymers such as Nylon 6,6 have also been formulated into melt-processed composites and foams. The base resin melt can be processed above 250°C, and if fillers and particulates can be formulated into the melt, composites can result. Using salt fillers the salts in the composites can be leached out to produce foams and scaffolds that can allow for later infiltration. But controlling the size and distribution of the fillers the pore size of the foam can regulated. And by adding inert insoluble fillers like calcium hydroxyapatite or even other more reactive or soluble particulates, the potential to consider polyamide-based degradable bone scaffolds is possible. The enzymatic degradation rates are rather low though for polyamides like Nylon 6,6.

9.3.3.2 Polyamide 6.10, others

By altering the aliphatic sequences using different monomers used in the formation of the amide bonds, one can alter the length of each repeat unit and chain flexibility. By choosing sebasic acid as opposed to adipic acid, one can form nylon polyamide 6,10 as opposed to 6,6. Both nylon forms have amide groups within the repeat structure, but are likely different in terms of their overall water sorption characteristics, T_g, and melting temperature.

9.3.3.3 Polycaprolactum, Nylon 6

Other polyamides can be synthesized by ring opening mechanisms as can form by the thermal decomposition of caprolactum to form nylon polyamide 6. The reaction is included in Fig. 9.10 and it is worth noting that sutures have also been produced from these structures and they are often copolymerized with nylon salts to produce Nylon copolymers of 6,6 and 6.

The properties of Nylon sutures are functions of the degree of orientation that is formed. A comparison of bulk nylon structures versus oriented sutures is included in Table 9.5.

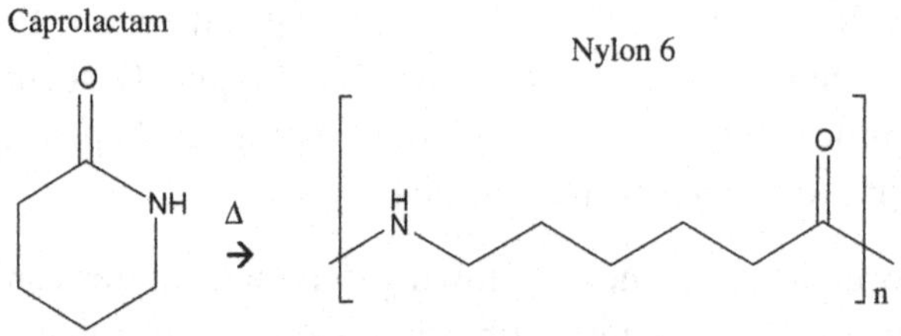

Caprolactam

Nylon 6

Figure 9.10
A ring opening synthesis is used to trigger the chain extension of caprolactum to form Nylon 6. Note that no small molecule is produced from the opening although this is also considered a condensation reaction.

Table 9.5: Bulk versus oriented nylon properties

	Nylon 6 Bulk	Nylon 66 Bulk	Nylon 6.10 Bulk	Nylon 6 & 66 Sutures, Range
Young's modulus (GPa)	2.1	2.8	1.8	1.8–4.5
Tensile strength (MPa)	83	76	55	460–710
Knot strength (MPa)				300–330
Elongation (%)	300	90	100	17–65

Data collected from J.B. Park and R.S. Lakes, Biomaterials, an Introduction, 2nd ed., Plenum, NY, 1992.

9.3.4 Condensation polymers: Polyesters

Similar condensation polymers can be achieved by end group reactions of acids and ols to form esters, and many of them linked together form a polyester. Polyester biomaterials have been very common used, and Dacron polyester, formed from PET has been polymerized and processed into sutures, fabrics used for suturing vascular grafts, heart valves. An excellent review is included in [9]. Smaller chain lengths have been duly noted to be degradable by hydrolysis facilitated by the presence of ester cleaving enzymes called esterases. And other bulk polyesters from polycarbonate have been the preferred material of choice for housings used in heart/lung bypass devices, for example. Here, we will discuss specific polymers, and note the biodegradable elements of these structures that have the capacity to more harmoniously interact with the healing body.

9.3.4.1 Polyethylene terephthalate

PET is the semicrystalline polymer formed from terephthalic acid and ethylene glycol, the repeat structure which is shown in Fig. 9.11.

It forms a relatively rigid structure with a T_g of approximately 70°C, a melting point of ~250°C, and crystallizes in a triclinic structure. The density of PET ranges from 1.33 g/cm^3 for the amorphous region to about 1.5 g/cm^3 for the crystal regions. The bulk density is somewhere in between. Like other melt processible polymers, extrusion, and drawing can

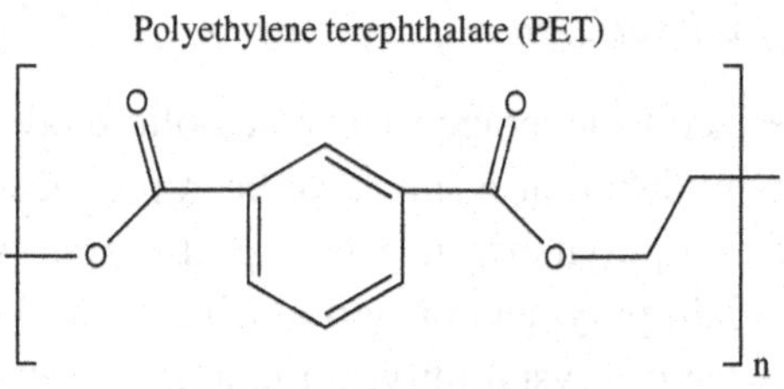

Polyethylene terephthalate (PET)

Figure 9.11
The repeat structure of polyethylene terephthalate.

produce sutures and fabric structures, and for vascular grafts, Dacron PET has been one of the two most common choices. The ability to stitch PET into the fabrics has led to their integration with other devices such as heart valves to include fabric superstructure around the device. These devices are of such high molecular weight as to not be readily biodegradable, but PET has some water absorption due to the ester bonds in the backbone and typically absorbs X% in the bulk structure. They were also fashioned into meshes for hernia repair but those based on PP performed better [10]. PET is clearly a tough and ductile polymer and much success has been achieved from sutures and other graft structures produced from engineered polyesters.

9.3.4.2 Polycarbonate

Alternative chemistry can be utilized to form polycarbonates, nominally produced from bisphenol A, whose repeat structure is shown in Fig. 9.12. Polycarbonate is commonly produced from the reaction of bisphenol A and phosgene to form a carbonate bond, which is similar to an ester bond. Polycarbonate is a more advanced engineering resin in part due to its larger level of ductility and toughness over other resins. Polycarbonate has not been used in large volume regulated implants, but reservoirs for heart/lung machine reservoirs are made from injection-molded polycarbonate.

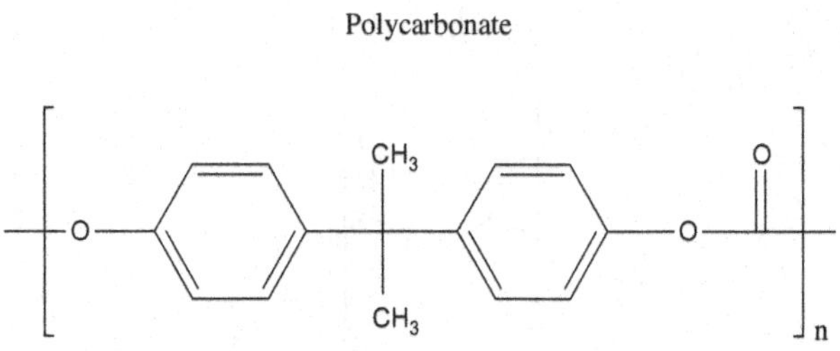

Polycarbonate

Figure 9.12
The repeat structure for the polycarbonate of bisphenol A.

9.3.4.3 Polylactic acid/polyglycolic acid/polycaprolactone

Other polyesters are synthesized to leverage their metabolic biodegradation into readily digestible fragments and many different resins have been produced from glycolic acid, lactic acid, and by ring opening polymerization of caprolactone. All of these forms can be made into low molecular weight polymers or into much longer chains. As homopolymers, each polyester has some degree of crystallinity; for example, polyglycolic acid (PGA), resulting from the polycondensation of glycolic acid, forms an orthorhombic unit cell, the repeat structure which is found in Fig. 9.13.

But when glycolic acid and other acids like lactic acid are mixed as comonomers, the polymerization of a copolymer tends to reduce the level of crystallinity and that has a dramatic effect on increasing the hydrolysis potential of these resins once installed. PGA copolymers of low molecular weights of ~ 3 kDa can be deployed as degradable sutures where only a few cleavage reactions are sufficient to reduce the strength of sutures made from PLA/PGA copolymers to ultimately fail within 10 days. The primary mechanism of chain fracture is hydrolysis of the ester linkages, which can be catalyzed in the presence of acids and bases and also in the presence of esterases. Much larger molecular weights of degradable polyesters can be fashioned into plates and screws for internal fixation that have deterioration rates more on the scale of years than days for low molecular weight PLGA sutures. If one can harness the ability of the body to heal itself over time, the potential to create biodegradable scaffolds and structures to stabilize fractures and other biomechanically weak regions and transfer the load back to the healing bone stock over time. The biochemical conversion forming glycolic and lactic acid from hydrolysis of PGA and PLA lowers the pH of the localized environment, enhancing the deterioration rate as it progresses but the lower pH can also interfere with natural biochemical processes linked with healing.

If biodegradable structures can be coformulated with a second monomer to regulate the crystallinity, and with the knowledge that lower crystallinity sutures have faster deterioration rates, it is also possible that these same resins could function successfully as

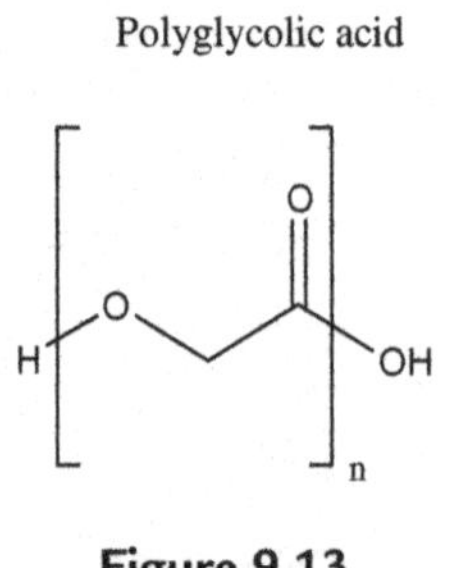

Polyglycolic acid

Figure 9.13
Repeat structure formed from polyglycolic acid.

regulated-dosing, drug delivery vehicles controlling the composition of these copolymers at higher molecular weight. Copolymerization is a strong influence on the resulting mechanical properties, based on the constituents used for copolymerization, as noted in Fig. 9.14 for PLA−PCL. PLA has significant crystallinity and that yields a relatively stiff bulk semicrystalline form with a modulus above 3 GPa. But copolymerization tends to disrupt the crystal forms and the presence of the more flexible PCL into the structure lowers the quasi-static modulus even more.

For PLA/PGA resins packaged with a drug for any controlled release therapy, the drug must be stable during elevated temperature processing, and not react with the resin reducing its effectiveness. Anything that alters the structure or reactivity of the drug as it is released with the surrounding environment is a potential risk factor complicating dosing relative to more normal IV or oral therapy. Oral dosing is also linked rapid metabolism often from gut acids and enzymes that are significantly reduced what is actually bioavailable to be absorbed into the bloodstream. Many different components could conceivably be packaged with these types of degrading structures including antibiotics, soluble minerals, chemotherapies, etc. Some examples of polyesters, both degradable and nondegradable structures is shown in Table 9.9, PLA and PCL data from [11] and included in Table 9.6.

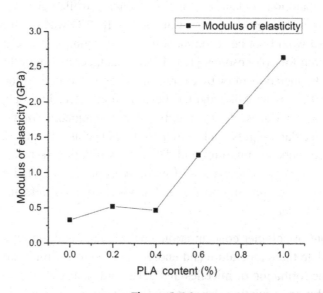

Figure 9.14
The influence of the PLA content on the modulus of elasticity of PGA copolymers. *From M.E. Broz, D.L. VanderHart, N.R. Washburn, Structure and mechanical properties of poly(d,l-lactic acid)/poly (e-caprolactone) blends, Biomaterials 24, 4181−4190.*

Table 9.6: Properties of different polyester materials. Note that the orientation and drawing of suture materials changes their properties from the bulk

	PET	PET Sutures	PLA	PCL
Young's modulus	3.1 GPa	1.2–6.5 GPa	2.65 GPa	0.33 GPa
Tensile strength	0.047 GPa	0.51–1.06 GPa	0.035 GPa	0.011 MPa
Knot strength		0.3–0.39 GPa		
Elongation	50–300%	8–42%	4%	32%
Density	1.37 g/cm^3		1.26 g/cm^3	

Data found in M.E. Broz, D.L. VanderHart and N.R. Washburn, Structure and mechanical properties of poly(d,l-lactic acid)/ poly(e-caprolactone) blends, Biomaterials 24 (2003) 4181–4190.

9.4 Polyethers

Soluble polyethers such as PEO and polypropylene oxide (PPO) and copolymers thereof constitute a completely separate area of injectable biomedical polymers that form soft structures and micelles. The ether segments of chain have significant molecular mobility readily increase the overall chain flexibility so even at high concentration, these materials are much more flexible than methacrylates or other vinyl polymers, for example.

The overall biocompatibility of PEO and PPO have been well demonstrated in the literature through animal studies for PEO molecular masses as high as 10 kDa [12]. Anybody who has encountered the need for colonoscopy will recognize the use of low molecular weight PEO as a bowel preparation, a clear, essentially bioinert, swollen gel that pushes everything else through leaving a clear pathway for colonoscopy. If PEO was not biocompatible, clinicians in internal would not be recommending our consumption of a gallon of fluid PEO gel during bowel prep for colonoscopy [13]. There is conjecture about the clearance of PEO and PPO, whether by metabolism or by excretion by inert transport to the urine. At high molecular weights, PEO is wax-like and has been used effective hydrophilic coatings on nonfouling biomaterial surfaces. PEO is highly soluble in aqueous solution even at relatively large molecular weights, and ultimately finds use as a biocompatible viscosity modifier in ranges of aqueous mixtures and dispersions found in skin care, creams, emollients, and salves. Block copolymers of more hydrophilic PEO and more hydrophobic PPO have actually more commonly been found as viscosity modifiers and thickeners in skin care creams and sunscreens.

The capacity to control polymer concentration, chain length, and the ratio of PPO to PEO allows one to regulate the temperature and energetics of self-assembly out of aqueous solution through the formation of micelles and gels. And as a result, there are schemes to harness self-assembly in regulating the precipitation of drug-included micelle structures where the additive is a ternary constituent affecting the driving force for copolymer solidification. Examples of how the coformulation of chemotherapies and growth factors with otherwise biocompatible copolymeric polyethers have been considered as injectable copolymer dosing and are described in more detail in Section 9.12.

9.5 Silicones

Other soft polymers with similar chain flexibility can be produced from precursors to form linear polydimethyl siloxane and other structures that can retain unsaturated bonds that can form crosslinks. Again, longer chain lengths correlate with higher resin viscosity, but like polyethers, silicones are very flexible and soft have larger molecular mobilities as materials above their glass transition temperature. The backbone structure of the Si—O silicone has a glass transition temperature at much lower temperatures than a normal all-carbon backbone found in additional polymers, for example. It is also an example of how the inherent silicone flexibility offers advantages in terms of insertion stresses and strains used in ophthalmology for flexible lenses, and in more flexible tubing. Key areas for use of silicones relates to ocular implants, vascular grafts, and as hydrophobic coatings and surfaces linked with wound care.

9.6 Natural Polymers

As was discussed in Chapter 2, Cell Expression: Proteins and Their Characterization, proteins found in connective tissues such as collagen, elastin, and keratin, hydrophilic protein hybrid structures such as polysaccharides, and other expressed specialized proteins such as insulin, HDL, and LDL lipoproteins and immunoglobulins found in the vasculature, all have polymeric structures, chain lengths on par with other polymers, and a similar long-chain molecular dynamics. The reader is encouraged to reread those sections in larger detail as there are large disparities in how synthetic polymers are produced and aspects of repeat structure and chain architecture and complexity. A comparison between nylon polyamides and proteins yields similar reactions formed from the combination of amine and acid end groups to yield amides, but nylon requires much higher temperatures, while protein synthesis occurs at body temperature, albeit slowly and under directed synthesis controlled by the ribosome. By increasing the number cells where primary protein synthesis is occurring, reasonable production rates can be achieved. There are other monographs that have more detail about these interesting structures, including Brekke et al. [14] and Rauh et al. [15]. It is also worth noting that polyamides like proteins are subject to hydrolysis in the presence of proteases and other enzymes that cleave amide bonds to form combinations of acids and amines. It is not a surprise to find the outcome of protein digestion is a lower pH as a result of the acids that are formed.

9.7 Other Polymers

There are many other polymer structures that could be mentioned in terms of their relationship to biomaterials, including latex rubber materials based on natural elastomers and polyisoprene, fluoropolymers, and other vinyl resins, their historical use, and current usage characteristics. Plasticized polyvinyl chloride had been used for years tied to transfusion bags for blood and other biologics, and the volume usage was enormous. Issues about the plasticizer extraction into the blood has led to the development of more common silicone tubing but the need for flexible and inert tubing remains for a variety of infusing systems. Similar trends to the resins presented already should be apparent. There are synthetic schemes for production, quality measures in terms of chain length, variability, functional attributes such as optical transparency, melt viscosity, and cellular activity and biocompatibility assessment using different assays. Rather than presenting this is a complete zoology of different resins and how they might be deployed, it seems more productive to pivot and look at groups of areas where resin deployment is rich and varied due to multiple materials competing to address similar clinical challenges. Let us focus simply on a few key ones up front as they often overlap.

9.8 Hydrogels, Scaffolds, and Other Degrading Structures

Key to a much wider array of biocompatible soft materials are those that are so hydrophilic as to appear as swollen networks similar to ground substance that are also water insoluble. Owing to the high sorptive capacity of these resins, they have proven very useful as tissue-engineering matrices, as drug delivery vehicles, and as fluid-based sealants. The variety of structures that can be formed is quite varied, as is the chemistry as to how these are ultimately harnessed into useful structures.

With tissue-engineered matrices the goal of the hydrogel is to provide a 3-D microenvironment that can successfully maintain cells that can proliferate without biochemical stresses that might arise from cytotoxic interactions with the matrix. Examples of resins that have been developed include those based on hydrophilic polysaccharides such as the salts of sodium alginate, a very hydrophilic resin that can crosslink in the presence of calcium as ion bridges. The precursors are biocompatible as is the calcium trigger. Clearly some aspects of mechanotransduction regulate cellular expression in cells contained in immobilization matrices of different network density. Copolymeric hydrogels have already been discussed relating to PEO–PPO-based systems and many other copolymeric hydrogels have been produced from hydrophilic segments such as PEO, and PCL being linked with segments like PLA and others. Natural polymers such as chitosan, hyaluronic acid, chondroitin sulfate, and dextrin have been similarly fashioned and there is a great section on these materials in Ref. [16]. The functional mechanical properties of copolymeric hydrogels are strongly dependent on the water content in the structure, and exquisite control is needed to produce reproducible results about mechanical behavior in these systems. Many measurements have been taken and typical moduli of elasticity are in the range of 1 MPa, similar to the mechanical behavior of natural tissues such as skin [17]. The ability to regulate the copolymer volume relative to the fluid in which its encased has the potential to produce even softer structures, as evidenced by hydrogel foams [18].

From a molecular design perspective, if polyester type structures are known to undergo biodegradation, the larger question is how to regulate the degradation response to match attributes of the healing profile. By altering how many degradable functional units are found along the backbone, understanding how the local pH of the microenvironment changes as a result of the wound healing cascade, and by controlling the molecular weight of the network structure, it is possible to design molecules that have a robust deterioration rate, without unnecessarily risking the patient to complications if a structure failed prematurely. Well-controlled studies exist as models to standardize how to perform these assessments. Included is data from a study performed by Metz et al. on both in vitro and in vivo degradation rates of 3-0 Maxon fibers ($D = \sim 250$ μm) implanted into a rabbit peritoneal cavity, with the notion to evaluate a suture fracture strength after different incubation times [19].

9.9 Polymeric Sutures

The need to close wounds is of concern to everyone involved in surgery, from the ER to transplants, to internal medicine, plastic surgery, and many other clinical subdisciplines. The practice linked to binding tissues together is a key learned skill among practitioners. There are many factors that are involved in the successful resolution of a wound site, whether part of a trauma or a scheduled procedure. If the focus is on suturing, the tissues involved in the wound closure (including their size, structure, and strength), the relative sterility of the environment, the presence of body fluids in and around the wound site, and the relative mobility of the wound are all factors to be considered by the clinician involved in closing it. The choice of wound closure is ultimately made by the clinician based on both the type of wound and their preferences and experience from prior outcomes.

For thousands of years, many sutures were made in attempts to bind wounds together and these have come from a range of natural materials [20] such as horse hair, hide, cellulose, linen, and catgut among many others leading up through the 1940s. Industrial development and production led to much larger availability of many new types of resins that could be adapted into potential suture materials. That listed included PP, nylon, and polyesters both as single fibers and as braided structures. Their performance was gauged relative to catgut which was established as a standard practice in wound closure even with issues of immunological response over time.

Clinical wound management evolved as did the practice of wound closure. It was seen that nylon and polyester sutures swelled and softened in wet environments as they absorbed body fluids in the wound site. Sutures could still perform their function holding separated tissues in close proximity and as tissue strength of the wound resolved, these were commonly cut and extracted from the tissue ends if used for skin binding. Clinical wound management also evolved as knots were perfected and the number of suturing sites was optimized for the type of wound site, whether fascia, skin, blood vessels, etc.

In the 1970s, new resins and suture materials were developed and produced with the notion that the degradation rate could match in some way the residual strength evolution of the wound, thereby transferring a larger fraction of the strength across the interface back to the native tissue without undesirable tissue reactions that result from the metabolism of the degrading structure.

Synthetic absorbable sutures based on low molecular weight, polyglycolic acid (Dexon, Davis, and Geck Corp) and polyglycolic-co-lactic acid (VIcryl, Ethicon J&J) were developed in the 1970s and have led to significant research and development on new types of low molecular weight polymers that could harness the needs of a biodegradable suture better than what was commercially available. A separate overriding development in the United States was the Medical Device Act of 1976 that led to a much higher threshold of testing and evaluation for new types of sutures invented afterwards. Suffice to say that there are many different choices available for clinicians engaged in wound closure.

Sutures are produced primarily by melt processing through an extruder and pushed through an extrusion die called a spinneret and drawn by spinning wheels that orient the fibers and can induce further crystal formation in these semicrystalline fibers. The optimization of drawing temperatures, line tension, and the die dimensions all tend to affect the overall dimensions of what can be produced. Typically to make small diameter fibers, it is operationally easier to have large hole diameter in the die and apply more tension on the crystallizing fiber than to have a smaller diameter hole from in the die. The fiber diameter decreases due to a Poisson's contraction. The larger the compressive force in the die region of the extruder, the more the fiber expands once it is liberated from the compression in the die. Orienting the chain lengths in the direction of draw strengthens the stiffens the suture but leaves it with less ductility and it is more prone to fracture.

Stronger/stiffer fibers can be made by drawing them. Fluctuations in the line tension and instabilities that can affect the mass flow rate in extrusion-based feeding systems and a somewhat variable diameter along the spool even though the conditions are designed to yield an average fiber diameter. As a result, fibers are classified in terms of an acceptable range of fiber diameters and classifications exist for different resins under the assumption that their properties are similar for similar draw extensions which would lead to similar fiber diameters.

There are extremely comprehensive books dedicated to sutures, the nuances of suturing, knots, environment, and binding location [21]. The goal is simply to present characteristics and properties of different common fiber types, with some comment about where they have been used (Tables 9.7–9.9).

The exposure of these hydrolytically sensitive and sorptive polymers structures creates changes in density and water content, mechanical behavior, and later as hydrolysis occurs, further changes in molecular weight, pH, and other structural changes. Efforts to track the mechanical losses that accompany hydrolytic deterioration are shown for a PCL–PLA copolymer that was dissolved in a 50% water solution prior to initiating a polymerization with traces of an acrylic monomer to bind the segments together [23]. As the samples were exposed to a fresh DI water solution, further swelling and hydrolysis occurs as noted by the lower modulus when tested over time under quasi-static loading conditions, which is shown in Fig. 9.15. The kinetic model for deterioration appears to follow an exponential decay with a single time constant [23].

Similar data exist for sutures evaluated under either in vivo or in vitro conditioning to compare the deterioration rates. Included here is data published showing the deterioration of 3.0 Maxon (PGA-trimethylene carbonate) fibers implanted in the peritoneum of rabbits and tested after controlled implantation periods, as shown in Fig. 9.16 [18]. In this instance, force data are shown, but that could be easily transferred into strength data.

9.10 Drug Delivery: Hydrophilic and Amphiphilic Polymers as Vehicles

Probably the largest area in terms of impact where the confluence of polymers as regulating media in medicine has evolved has been in controlled release drug delivery systems both as oral therapy and also as injectables. There are a number of relatively simple natural polymers such as carboxymethyl cellulose, alginates, and those based on xanthum gum that can be mixed with various drug components, and the release characteristics are such as to bypass the bulk of drug metabolism that often arises in the enzyme destruction occurring in the organs tied to digestion including the stomach, liver, and kidneys. By reducing what normally ingested in oral therapy by pills that rapidly dissolve, one can actually package smaller doses in the drug and allow for a more efficient metabolic uptake in the intestinal track following drug cammoflauging in digestive track. Analgesics have been by far the most common repackaged drugs which have led to new intellectual property in these gel-based systems. The dissolution and/or permeation of the drug from the gels is more tortuous and a more sustained release pattern can be achieved by packaging hydrophilic drugs in more amphiphilic molecules.

There are several reasons why repackaging of drugs within controlled release vehicles may actually lead to a more effective dosing. One is that it is possible that toxicities that might accumulate from the rapid rise in metabolites from each drug has the potential to stress the cells in the digestive track leading to inflammation in the form if hepatitis and renal

Table 9.7: Summary of different suture materials including their form

Nonabsorbable	Sutures		Crystal	Supplier
Classification	Tradename	Physical framework	Structure	
PET polyester	Ethibond	Braided multifilament, coated	Triclinic	Ethicon
PET polyester	Mersilene	Braided multifilament bare	Triclinic	Ethicon
PET polyester	Ethiflex	Braided multifilament coated with PTFE	Triclinic	Ethicom
PET polyester	Dacron	Braided multifilament bare	Triclinic	Covidien
PET polyester	TiCron	Braided multifilament coated w/ silicone resin	Triclinic	Covidien
PET polyester	Surgidac	Monofilament or braided multifilament	Triclinic	Covidien
PET polyester	Tevdek	Braided multifilament coated with PTFE	Triclinic	Teleflex
PET polyester	Polydek	Braided multifilament with PTFE	Triclinic	Teleflex
PBT-copolymer polyester	Novafil	Monofilament	Triclinic	Covidien
Polyamide (PA) 6 &66	Ethilon	Monofilament	Triclinic	Ethicon
PA 66	Nurolon	Braided multifilament coated	Triclinic	Ethicon
PA 66 & 6	Surgilon	Braided multifilament coated with silicone	Triclinic	Covidien
PA 66 & 6	Dermalon	Monofilament, no coating	Triclinic	Covidien
PA 66 & 6	Sutron	Monofilament	Triclinic	Ergon sutramed
PA 66 & PA 6	Supramid	Core (PA 66) + sheath (PA 6)	Triclinic	B Braun
Polypropylene	Prolene	Monofilament	Monoclinic	Ethicon
Polypropylene	Surgilene	Monofilament	Monoclinic	Covidien
Linen		Twisted	?	Unilene
Silk	Silk	Braided multifilament	?	CP Medical
Silk	Silk	Braided multifilament		Teleflex
Silk	SofSilk	Braided multifilament		Covidien
Absorbable	Sutures	Synthetic		
Polyglycolic acid (PGA, also polyglycolide)	Dexon S	Braided multifilament, bare	Orthorhombic	Covidien
PGA	Dexon Plus	Braided multifilament, with surfactant coating	Orthorhombic	Covidien
PGA	Dexon II	Core (PGA) with PCL–PGA sheath	Orthorhombic	Covidien
Polyglycolic acid–polylactic acid (PGA–PLA) (90/10) or PLGA	Vicryl	Braided monofilament	Disrupted orthorhombic	Ethicon
Polydioxanone (PDO or PDS)	PDS	Monofilament	Orthorhombic [22]	Ethicon

(Continued)

Table 9.7: (Continued)

Nonabsorbable	Sutures		Crystal	Supplier
PGA-polytrimethylene carbonate Catgut	Maxon Catgut, surgical gut	Monofilament Twisted strands	? Plain and chromic acid treated	Covidien Multiple suppliers

Adapted from C.C. Chu, J.A. von Fraunhofer, H.P. Greisler, Wound Closure Biomaterials, CRC Press, Boca Raton, FL, 1997 with updates based on corporate changes.

Table 9.8: Summary from the US Pharmacopoeia and the European Pharmacopoeia relating to suture dimension classifications

USP Nonsynthetic Absorbables	USP Nonabsorbable and Synthetic Absorbables	EP Absorbables and Nonabsorbables	Suture Diameter Minimum (μm)	Suture Diameter Maximum (μm)
	11/0	0.1	10	19
	10/0	0.2	20	29
	9/0	0.3	30	39
	8/0	0.4	40	49
8/0	7/0	0.5	50	69
7/0	6/0	0.7	70	99
6/0	5/0	1	100	140
5/0	4/0	1.5	150	190
4/0	3/0	2	200	240
3/0	2/0	2.5	250	290
2/0	0	3	300	390
0	1	4	400	490
1	2	5	500	590
2	3	6	600	690
3	4	7	700	790
4	5	8	800	890
5	6	9	900	990
6	7	10	1000	1090

Adapted from C.C. Chu, J.A. von Fraunhofer, H.P. Greisler, Wound Closure Biomaterials, CRC Press, Boca Raton, FL, 1997.

disease. It is also possible that there is a reason to level out the dosage to a more consistent level which might be achieved by more controlled release systems. Finally, one has the potential to regulate potential side effects, for example, with chemotherapeutics if the drug component can be packaged in such a way as to regulate its efficacy.

There have been a number of systems that have been considered to package different therapeutics that really suggests future research potential more than anything else. As examples, amphiphilic copolymers based on PEO—PPO—PEO have been packaged with a number of different therapeutic components to gauge improvements in patient outcome, efficacy in drug release, and correlating structural details of the drug in copolymer with its overall bioavailability.

Table 9.9: Table of defined properties defined by the suture dimensions of some specific biodegradable sutures as produced

Suture Type	Diameter	Naming Designation	Quasi-static Modulus of Elasticity	Tensile Strength	Yield Strain
Dexon		2/0	7.58 GPa	830 MPa	22.2%
Polydioxanone PDS	0.585 mm	2	2.31	500	
PDS	0.498	1	2.19	520	
PDS	0.432	0	2.22	495	
PDS	0.345	2/0	2.32	505	
PDS	0.294	3/0	2.30	520	
PDS	0.221	4/0	2.44	570	
PDS	0.174	5/0	2.30	535	
PDS	0.112	6/0	2.20	620	
PDS	0.01	7/0	2.43	--	

Note that fiber strengths are designated typically units of g/denier, but with the conversion factor of stress units as 1 g/denier correlates with 0.137 MPa.

Adapted from C.C. Chu, J.A. von Fraunhofer, H.P. Greisler, Wound Closure Biomaterials, CRC Press, Boca Raton, FL, 1997.

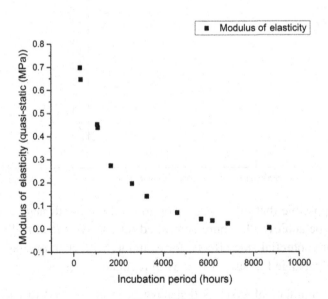

Figure 9.15

The reduction of modulus for a PEG-PLA copolymer incubated in fresh DI water following polymerization. Note that the hydrolysis yields an exponential deterioration rate. *Graph reproduced from A. T. Metters, K. S. Anseth, and C. N. Bowman, Fundamental studies of a novel, biodegradable PEG-b-PLA hydrogel, Polymer 41 (2000) 3993–4004.*

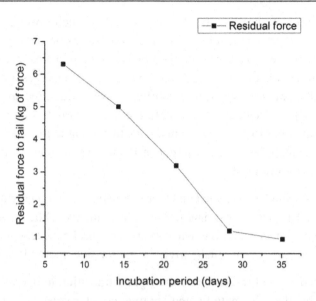

Figure 9.16

Force required for fracture of Polydioxanone/PGA (Maxon) fibers implanted and incubated in a live animal over a period of days. Note a similar deterioration in strength. *Graph reproduced from S. A. Metz, N. Chegini, and B. J. Masterson, In vivo and in vitro degradation of monofilament absorbable sutures PDS and Maxon, Biomaterials 11 (1990) 41–45.*

One particular PEO–PPO–PEO copolymer, synthesized commercially as a tri-block system in which each block has a molecular weight of about 4 kDa, is known commercially as Pluronic F127 and Poloxamer 407. Copolymers of PEO and PPO have been mixed with many different model therapeutics in an attempt to link the structure of what forms at ambient temperature and body temperature, including analgesics [24], antibiotics [25], steroidal inflammatories [26,27], chemotherapeutics including methotrexate [28], cisplatin [29,30], carboplatin [31], and paclitaxel [32,33]. Nishiyama goes through an extensive review highlighting the wealth of details on different copolymers and structures that have been attempted [34]. One can imagine the wealth of potential permutations making it very difficult to somehow an optimum functional drug delivery system a priori. It is still in the research, development, and demonstration phase to identify the hydrophilicity of various candidate drugs worth packaging, an optimum structure that is both biocompatible and allows for controlled release. Some gels are based on erosion and consumption of the biodegradable elements in the vehicle while others as simply a passive delivery system regulating the release rate without creating new surfaces, for example.

9.11 Conclusions

A comprehensive effort in Chapter 9 has looked at the structure and properties of conventional homopolymers, copolymers, and other hydrophilic structures. Polymers due their lower melting temperatures can be melt processed at much lower temperatures than other material classes. Polymers can be processed into fibrous products such as sutures, films, reactive fluids in the monomer state, and biodegradable plates and screws. The bottom line is that protocols exist to gauge the compositional changes and the chemical structural changes that can arise when hydrophilic network structures are ultimately used as temporary fixation, sutures, and devices all with the notion of deterioration. Polymers without such profound deterioration mechanisms or those that tend to degrade into byproducts that can sometimes trigger a larger inflammatory response tend to be removed before longer term exposure exists.

Similar exposure tests could be conducted on other polymers and vinyl polymers and polyolefins tend to be so hydrophobic as to be invariant when installed in vivo. Other systems, particularly forming heterochain polymers with more than carbon in the backbone tend to absorb water, but many instances, it is not enough to actually trigger bond scission, more like a swelling process.

Obviously bulk polymers and resins above their glass transition temperature are much more compliant and flexible than the metallic and ceramic counterparts. The ability to match more closely tissue mechanics will go a long way in producing better overall outcomes.

A wide variety of possibilities exist for in vivo processing is possible. The wide range of photochemistry can be applied to perform photochemistry so long as there is line of sight and photopolymerization is quite a common tool for causing bond formation to occur in vivo. It is also possible to rely on passive self-assembly in solutions and to use the solubility of amphiphilic copolymers as a tool where solutions can be injected and upon subtle heating from in vivo metabolism, that can be enough to trigger the formation of gels. It is possible to envision a wide variety of therapeutic deliveries that could be harnessed by controlling the compositions and locations where deposition occurs and by understanding how additives influence the phase structure of the self-assembling micelle or gel structure.

9.12 Problems

1. You have a chain with a repeat structure representative of MMA. There are 1000 links in that chain, calculate the molecular weight.
2. Look up the structures of polyhydroxyethyl methacrylate (PHEMA) and polylactic acid (PLA), and explain why one polymer is more susceptible to bulk hydrolysis than the other.
3. If the amorphous regions of a semicrystalline polyester are more apt to absorb water, explain how the degree of crystallinity affects the degradation rate of PGA, for example.
4. You are tasked with suture selection for a vascular grafting on an average cardiovascular patient only to find out that same suture is selected for a patient is hypertensive. Explain the possible mechanical responses of the suture to the overload condition. Hint, there are three possibilities.

5. Draw a dynamic gravimetric analysis curve (mass vs. time) for two different polymers, one, a polyolefin produced by radical polymerization, and a polyester, when exposed to a hot and humid environment capable of some hydrolysis. Compare the two behaviors of the polymers and explain why one might actually have some mass gain initially?

6. For the dynamic modulus curve shown as a function of time for the PLA−PCL composite in Fig. 9.15, determine the time constant linked with exponential decay of the modulus with biodegradation.

References

[1] B.D. Ratner, Biomaterials Science: An Introduction to Materials in Medicine, Elsevier/Academic Press, Amsterdam, 2013.

[2] W.M. Saltzman, Tissue Engineering, Principles for the Design of Replacement Organs and Tissues, Oxford University Press, New York, 2004.

[3] J.O. Hollinger, M.R. Neuman (Eds.), An Introduction to Biomaterials. Biomedical Engineering Series, CRC Press, Boca Raton, FL, 2012.

[4] C.E. Hoyle, C.N. Bowman, Thiol-ene click chemistry, Angew. Chem. 49 (2010) 1540−1573.

[5] J.P. Arnaud, J.J. Tuech, P. Pessaux, Y. Hadchity, Surgical treatment of postoperative incisional hernias by intraperitoneal insertion of dacron mesh and an aponeurotic graft—a report on 250 cases, Arch. Surg. 134 (1999) 1260−1262.

[6] G. Lewis, L.H. Koole, C.S.J. van Hooy-Corstjens, Influence of powder-to-liquid monomer ratio on properties of an injectable iodine-containing acrylic bone cement for vertebroplasty and balloon kyphoplasty, J. Biomed. Mater. Res. B-Appl. Biomater. 91 (2009) 537−544.

[7] Stryker. *Simplex P Bone Cement: Unique Formula and Manufacturing.* 2016; Available from: http://www.stryker.com/en-us/products/Orthopaedics/BoneCementSubstitutes/005885.

[8] S.S. Haas, G.M. Brauer, G. Dickson, A characterization of PMMA bone cement, J. Bone Joint Surg. 57 (3) (1975) 380−391.

[9] D.D. Jamiolkowski, E.J. Doemier, The poly (alpha-esters), in: J.O. Hollinger (Ed.), Introduction to Biomaterials, CRC Press, Boca Raton, FL, 2012.

[10] G.E. Leber, J.L. Garb, A.I. Alexander, W.P. Reed, Long-term complications associated with prosthetic repair of incisional hernias, Arch. Surg. 133 (1998) 378−382.

[11] M.E. Broz, D.L. VanderHart, N.R. Washburn, Structure and mechanical properties of poly(d,l-lactic acid)/poly(e-caprolactone) blends, Biomaterials 24 (2003) 4181−4190.

[12] C. Fruijiter-Pollath, Safety assessment of polytethylene glycols PEGs and their derivatives used is cosmetic products, Toxicology 214 (2005) 1−38.

[13] M. Arora, P.I. Okolo, Use of powder PEG-3350 as a sole bowel preparation, clinical case series of 245 patients, Gastroenterol. Hepatol. 4 (2008) 489−492.

[14] J.H. Brekke, G.E. Rutkowski, K. Thacker, Hyaluronan, in: J.O. Hollinger (Ed.), Introduction to Biomaterials, CRC Press, Boca Raton, FL, 2012.

[15] F. Rauh, M. Dornish, R. Street, A.R. Shrivats, Complex polysaccharides: chitosan and alginate, in: J.O. Hollinger (Ed.), Introduction to Biomaterials, CRC Press, Boca Raton, FL, 2012.

[16] C.M. Agrawal, J.L. Ong, M.R. Appleford, G. Mani, Introduction to Biomaterials, Cambridge University Press, Cambridge, UK, 2014.

[17] S.J. Bryant, K.S. Anseth, Hydrogel properties inlfuence ECM production by chondrocytes photoencapsulated in polyethylene glycol hydrogels, J. Biomed. Mater. Res. 59 (2002) 63−72.

[18] K. Park, H. Park, Super absorbant hydrogel foams, 1998, US 5750585, issued May 12th 1998.

[19] S.A. Metz, N. Chegini, B.J. Masterson, In vivo and vitro degradation of monofilament absorbable sutures PDS and Maxon, Biomaterials 11 (1990) 41−45.

[20] T.M. Muffly, A.P. Tizzano, M.D. Walters, The history and evolution of sutures in pelvic surgery, J. R. Soc. Med. 104 (2011) 107–112.

[21] C.C. Chu, J.A. von Fraunhofer, H.P. Greisler, Wound Closure Biomaterials, CRC Press, Boca Raton, FL, 1997.

[22] M. Jaidann, Etude de L'orientation et la Structure Cristalline Du Polydioxanone, Ph.D Dissertation, Departement de Chemie, Université Laval, Laval, QC Canada, 2008.

[23] A.T. Metters, K.S. Anseth, C.N. Bowman, Fundamental studies of a novel, biodegradable PEG-b-PLA hydrogel, Polymer 41 (2000) 3993–4004.

[24] B. Foster, T. Cosgrove, B. Hammouda, Pluronic Triblock copolymer systems and their interactions with Ibuprofen, Langmuir 25 (2009) 6760–6766.

[25] M.L. Veryries, G. Couarraze, S. Geiger, F. Agnely, L. Massias, B. Kunzli, et al., Controlled release of vancomycin from poloxamer 407 gels, Int. J. Pharmaceut. 192 (1999) 183–193.

[26] C. Nagant, P.B. Savage, J.P. Dehaye, Effect of pluronic acid F-127 on the toxicity towards eukaryotic cells of CSA-13, a catonic sterioid analogue of antimicrobial peptides, J. Appl. Microbiol. 112 (2012) 1173–1182.

[27] P.K. Sharma, S.K. Bhatia, Effect of anti-inflammatories on Pluronic F127: micellar assembly, gelation, and partitioning, Int. J. Pharmaceut. 278 (2004) 361–377.

[28] J. Pluta, B. Karolewicz, In vitro studies of the properties of thermosensitve systems prepared on Pluronic F-127 as vehicles for methotrexate for delivery to solid tumors, Polim. Med. 36 (2006) 37–53.

[29] A. Silvani, P. Gavianni, E.A. Lamperti, M. Eoli, C. Falcone, F. DiMeco, et al., Cisplatinum and BCNU chemotherapy in primary glioblastoma patients, J. Neurooncol. 94 (2009) 57–62.

[30] A. Sonada, N. Nitta, S. Ohta, A. Nitta-Seko, S. Morikawa, Y. Tabata, et al., Controlled release and antitumor effect of pluronic F127 mixed with cisplatin in a rabbit model, Carciovasc. Intervent. Radiol. 33 (2010) 135–142.

[31] A.A. Exner, T.M. Krupka, K. Seherrer, J.M. Teets, Enhancement of carboplatin toxicity by Pluronic block copolymers, J. Contolled Release 106 (2005) 188–197.

[32] W. Zhang, Y. Shi, Y. Chen, J. Ye, X. Sha, X. Fang, Multiunctional pluronic P123/F127 mixed polymeric micelles loaded with paclitaxel for the treatment of multidrug resistant tumors, Biomaterials 32 (2011) 2894–2906.

[33] W. Zhang, Y. Shi, Y. Chen, J. Hao, X. Sha, X. Fang, The potential of Pluronic polymeric micelles encapsulated both paclitaxel for the treatment of melanoma using subcutaneous and pulmonary metastatic mice models, Biomaterials 32 (2011) 5934–5944.

[34] N. Nishiyama, K. Kataoka, Current state, achievements, and future prospects of polymeric micelles as nanocarriers for drug and gene delivery, Pharmacol. Ther. 112 (2006) 630–648.

Nanomaterials and Phase Contrast Imaging Agents

Learning Objectives

The reader should come away from this chapter with

- a larger view of ensembles of nanomaterials that, while not consolidated structures, have functional attributes that aid in resolving enhanced phase contrast
- an understanding of what derives phase contrast using X-rays, MRI, and positron emission tomography (PET) scanning
- an understanding that live imaging has a more stringent set of constraints for nanomaterial usage than in assays for biopsy
- examples of how radiology is linked with treatment efforts
- the ability to couple nanomaterials with minimally invasive catheter designs adds to opportunities to treat/manage cerebrovascular conditions that in the past were considered inoperable.

10.1 Introduction

Most biomaterials textbooks that comment on nanomaterials consider primarily either scaffold structures or mineralization as key examples. Bone and the mineralized isolates as carbonated apatites forming in an organized collagen matrix [1], for example, have broad X-ray diffraction patterns in part due to the both the number of defects in the growing mineral phase and to the nanoscale structure that contribute to less coherent scattering [2]. The broadening is sufficiently large as to make an absolute structural determination of the crystal structure of minerals in bone challenging [3]. There are countless studies to point out that there are many human and mammal interactions with nanoparticles exist, many from a toxicological standpoint, and there appear to be distinctions between stable nanoparticles that interact with human hosts and nanoparticles that are metabolized from soluble and digestible proteins for example [4]. Yes, the discussion and extensive use of mineralization from either a tissue engineering realm or innately related to growth and development in vivo to frame the discussion of nanomaterials skews the value and critical need for injected nanomaterials in advanced diagnosis and radiology.

Biomaterials. DOI: http://dx.doi.org/10.1016/B978-0-12-809478-5.00010-9

The confluence of the separate and distinct revolutions in both nanomaterials synthesis and characterization and advanced computing has led to new paradigms in cellular, tissue, and clinical diagnostics. Within the United States, this new thinking moved the National Institutes of Health in the late 1990s and early 2000s to create a roadmap for advanced medical research. The outcomes from the roadmap pointed to elements suggesting that technical advances in science and engineering that are likely to have profound the way medicine is practiced in terms of earlier diagnosis of disease. As an example of scope and scale, the US Centers for Disease Control (CDC) has published recent statistics about the increasing rate of scheduled diagnostic imaging which shows a dramatic uptick in the usage of diagnostic imaging technology which is being fueled by better diagnostic imaging phase contrast enhancement schemes. The results are shown in Fig. 10.1 [5]. The comparisons

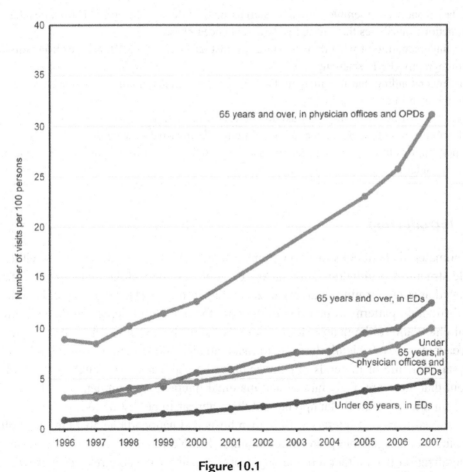

Figure 10.1

Data from the US Centers for Disease Control (USCDC) to represent the number of doctors visits per 100 people on an annualized basis. The same groups of people are being diagnosed more often in 2007 than in 1997.

drawn are between older and younger patients and those visiting the emergency department (ED) as opposed to an outpatient department or facility (OPD). If one broadens their perspective beyond live, diagnostic imaging to consider fluorescence-based assays, the scope is dramatically larger from a research and biopsy perspective. With this in mind, it is still important to consider where and how these advances might have their largest effect as injectable nanomaterials [6].

One cannot predict which diagnostic discoveries have the largest impact on improving health but it is safe to say that identifying actionable disease states earlier in their course has the potential to transform manageable diseases into cures and makes the interventions less traumatic and invasive. As a result, there will be a larger emphasis on earlier diagnosis which relies on low-dose radiographic tools and other imaging techniques like MRI, ultrasound, and PET scanning that are thought to be benign. It is a huge investment when one considers the number of procedures being performed and the overall cost of that relative to the overall gross domestic product. Healthcare expenses range on the order of 15%−20% of the entire $1 Trillion GDP and diagnostics are a large fraction of that overall expense. In this chapter, we will present phase contrast agents that are compatible with various diagnostic methodologies both commonly used today and those that are expanding in terms of clinical use. For a number of years already, enhanced diagnostics has been practiced in both X-ray transmission and MRI. These are reviewed here and references are pointed to metabolic phase contrast agents used, for example, in PET, a powerful emerging imaging modality and hybrid systems that operate both in terms of diagnostics and potential therapy.

Based on size alone, nanomaterials can be widely dispersed within tissues and within fluid pathways. Their size also enhances their permeability and based on renal clearance, smaller nanomaterials are more likely to be cleared to the excretory system allowing their temporary residence for enhanced diagnostic imaging in live systems, assuming they are benign, but that is not the only consideration [7]. If the constraint of introducing these into live animals are applied, there is still tremendous potential for nanomaterials to be used as probes within cell and tissue culture, as is already being done with fluorescence-based assays and considering the separate use of quantum dots [7−9]. Overall, the ability to reliably and controllably synthesize and distribute nanomaterials has large impact now and what is interesting is that there is always an appetite for newer, better, and more tolerable phase contrast fluids to enhance disease diagnosis in living systems.

10.2 X-ray Diagnostics and Phase Contrast Agents

The use of X-ray diagnostics has been a staple of radiology clinics and emergency rooms worldwide. The facile and widely used X-ray transmission tools allows X-ray to be a preferred tool to assess micro and more comprehensive skeletal fractures, bone density, to direct orthopedists and general surgeons in the repair of damaged and diseased bone stock.

X-ray diagnostics has helped direct strategies to install a range of skeletal implants and to help direct repair strategies for both internal and external fixation. A large reason for the emphasis on skeletal and dental structures is the effective gradient between the concentration of X-ray scatterers within bone and dental tissues relative to soft tissues. The mineral precipitates are much more effective scatterers and the gradient in scattering with bone density is a key reason that bone density varies inversely with the transmitted intensity to the detector.

X-ray imaging technology originally used X-ray diagnostic films that were cumbersome to manage, susceptible to print and image quality including deteriorations in image quality from scratches in the film with successive viewings, and generally large doses were used to image the film. With advances in higher sensitivity X-ray films, the dose required for analysis was lowered making each imaging experience safer. The films still required large storage facilities for image libraries and image management was a problem that has been generally solved through digital archiving so rather than brick and mortar space requirements, there are now gigabit data storage requirements and beyond. The ability to move the source and detectors relative to the object allowed for the rapid expansion of computer tomography which dramatically improved the imaging modality to generate 3D renderings of 2D images, but the dose required for CT is much larger per imaging event.

Smaller, more focused devices are commonly used in dental offices for imaging of tooth structures, pointing to areas of enamel demineralization, indicated by darker regions in teeth, where X-rays are more effectively transmitted. The films produced are smaller but storage of the films was still required.

With advances in digital capture and digital signal processing, the ability to directly collect X-ray transmission radiographic attributes electronically, replicate the imaging from the films for display, and store them in much denser electronic data storage facilities. This alternative storage format has allowed the hospitals to repurpose large amounts of space in radiology clinics for other things.

The use for radiology tied simply to fractures, bone density assessments, and other assessments in hard tissues would suggest that investing in technology probably pays off eventually. But there has been as much interest in considering the use of radiology in other areas of the hospital. There has been a tremendous amount of interest in mammography to perform early diagnosis of breast cancer passing low-energy X-rays through compressed breast tissues. The results have been quite good at identifying inhomogenieties in breast tissue, some of which arise from breast tumors and some from microcalcifications that also scatter X-rays more efficiently than the surrounding tissue leasing to false positives. Many other uses of X-rays in diagnosing disease within soft tissue have also been realized with phase contrast agents.

10.2.1 GI Blockage Assessments

For a number of years in internal medicine, obstructions in the digestive track have effectively been identified using gastrointestinal dispersions and slurries that contain X-ray phase contrast agents. The ideal advanced phase contrast agent for X-ray diagnostics is an insoluble and benign metal salt with high scattering centers. Various Ba-based and I-based salts have been produced with very low solubility in vivo [10,11]. The salts can be ingested or injected and conveyed through the digestive track. Upon encountering an obstruction, fluid slurry movement stops and the location of the obstruction can be identified by X-ray. Obstructions and stenosis (radial restrictions) in the esophagus [12], the small [13], and large intestine [14], shown in Fig. 10.2, can be all resolved by adding these slurries accordingly. It is also possible to identify organ leakage, for example, from the margins of the stomach (or spleen or appendix) or other digestive organ since the phase contrast agents do not dissolve or permeate through the digestive track.

In terms of formal design requirements for these radiocontrast agents, ideally these are highly insoluble salts in vivo. They can be milled into particles (smaller is not necessarily

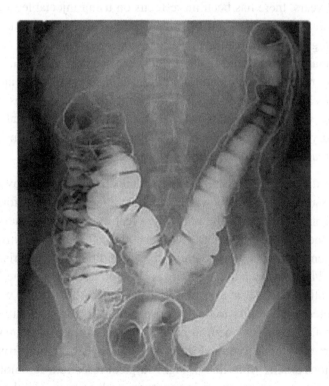

Figure 10.2
Lower GI determination by X-ray imaging using barium sulfate as a phase contrast medium. File provided through the Creative Commons Share Alike 30 unported license.

better, but small enough (µm sized) to be both injectable, homogeneously distributed within a fluid slurry, and not interacting in any direct way with the biological tissues the particles encounter. Barium sulfate ($BaSO_4$) is highly insoluble and the Ba^{2+} has a very large nucleus, making it a much more effective scattering center than even mineral deposits within bone. As a result, highly concentrated slurries are not required to achieve appropriate positional details from subsequent X-ray diagnostics. To resolve where a specific blockage or stenosis is located, it is a matter of following the transport of the radiocontrast agent through the digestive track and identifying locations of stenosis and blockage. The phase contrast introduction can be performed by oral ingestion of the slurry for the upper digestive gastro-intestinal (GI) diagnosis and by enema for the lower intestinal track. Ideally, the scatters should be readily available and inexpensive, both characteristics of Ba-based and I-based salts. Future development could address how patient ingestion could be a more tolerable experience.

10.2.2 Cardiovascular Phase Contrast Angiography

Within the last 20 years, there has been more focus on using injectable radiocontrast agents in interventional neuroradiology. Abnormalities in neurovascular flow can cause a range of symptoms, including vertigo, thrush, hypoxia, and arise from ischemias, from naturally forming vascular malformations and fistulae, and arteriovenous malformations. The defects can be observed by normal X-ray imaging but the use of phase contrast angiography, where radiocontrast agents are directly injected into the neurovasculature to observe flow patterns creates a much more detailed roadmap for intervention. Typical abnormalities that can be noted include aneurysm and angiography can be linked with other imaging modalities, examples of which are shown in Figs. 10.3 and 10.4 below [15].

Following detailed diagnosis, interventional procedures to redirect neurovascular flow, reduce arterial pressure on aneurysms walls, or block defective and malformed blood transport pathways are considered. The impressive feature with these interventional procedures is that most are executed intravascularly through minimally invasive catheterization schemes reducing the potential for morbidities directly arising resection and the recovery time. Phase contrast angiography is done on a nearly routine basis now and it is done on an outpatient basis. It is awesome to consider that for people with profound cerebrovascular defects, the ability to be diagnosed and resolved without requiring a craniotomy is a profound improvement in patient care, performed at dramatically lower cost when one considers the months required in recovery and rehabilitation from craniotomy and functional morbidities arising from line of sight surgical resection. It is not possible to eliminate the need for craniotomy in crisis situations such as trauma and energency room (ER)-type presentations but craniotomy can be rendered a rarer outcome through larger use of minimally invasive angiography.

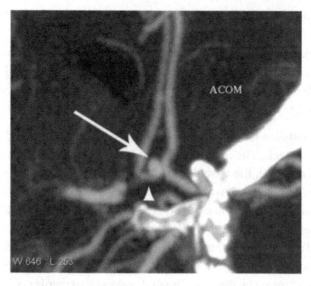

Figure 10.3

Iodine-based X-ray phase contrast in angiography showing a berry aneurysm, with the long arrow. *Reproduced with the permission of JA Hirsch, Massachusetts General Hospital Radiology Rounds, 2008: 6:1.*

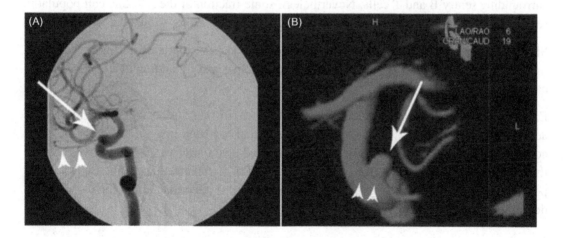

Figure 10.4

Iodine-based X-ray phase contrast agent for X-ray angiography, again (A) identified by the long arrow in the phase contrast image and (B) the volume rendered image. *Reproduced with Permission from JA Hirsch, Massachusetts General Hospital Radiology Rounds, 2008: 6:1.*

With all of the fanfare associated with catheter-based angiography for diagnosing cerebrovascular abnormalities, it is worth noting that there is still a palpable complication rate somewhere between 0% and 1% that arises simply from diagnostic imaging defined as neurological deficit following the procedure [16,17]. Complications include ischemic stroke, hemorrhagic stroke, and other patient-related intolerances associated with the radiocontrast agent. The severity of the complication can range from essentially no long-term morbidities to sudden death. The takeaway is that diagnostic procedures are becoming more routine and with that, clinical experience with deploying catheters and radiocontrast agents has improved patient outcomes from diagnosis. It is conceivable that other, better diagnostic injectables could reduce patient intolerances more effectively and improve patient outcomes further.

The design requirements for radiopaque phase contrast agents are quite different than for those for the digestive track. The ideal neurovascular radiocontrast agent are soluble, possess a very short residence time in the vasculature, can be readily cleared through the renal system without damaging it, not activate platelets, and provide a strong radiopaque signal locally where injected. Both lipid-based iodo oils and aqueous-based iodo ionic salts compounds have been developed as radiocontrast agents. As lipid-based iodo compounds are less soluble in blood and their residence time in the bloodstream is longer, they are used less frequently than aqueous-based agents. With aqueous injectables, there are both ionic and nonionic based iodine aromatics that have been developed, examples of which are shown in Figs. 10.5 and 10.6. The salt-based systems possess a higher osmolaiity and seem to have a larger interaction with the patient population triggering allergen immunoglobulin responses. The non-ionics cannot dissociate, and their higher stability reduces the interaction with the surrounding sentry B and T cells. Nevertheless, some fraction of the immune cell population senses the injection. The most common iodo-based injectables are shown below.

Substitutions to these molecules have been made to make these injectables more neutral in pH to reduce vasodilation potential from acidic injection and by adding calcium to reduce cardiac toxicity.

Exquisite maps of the soft tissue conveyance of these slurries can be achieved with these additives, as shown in Fig. 10.7, (A) an aneurysm that has been imaged using phase contrast fluid injections first before embolization and again afterwards (B) clearly showing the isolation of the aneurysm from the vasculature. Phase enhanced angiography is a powerful imaging modality, even more so when localized injections allow for a determination of localized blood flow.

Figures 10.5 and 10.6
Examples of iodine-based salts used as radiopaque phase contrast enhancement agents.

When injected, radiologists actively monitor the patient for any adverse complications, those that range from mild to severe and shown below in Table 10.1. Vascular clearance is commonly achieved through the kidneys, and patients are screened for poor filtration capacity [glomerular filtration rate (GFR) <30 mL/min] and excluded from phase contrast

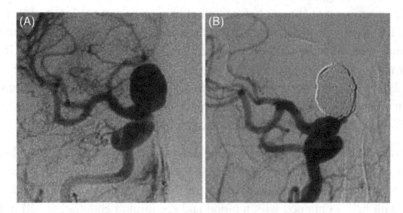

Figures 10.7

A and B Angiography results using an x-ray phase contrast fluid before (A) and after (B) embolization in isolating the aneurysm from the vasculature. Continued darkness in the embolized region indicates incomplete isolation with continued risk of rupture without further isolation. *Reproduced with permission from the Society for Neurointerventional Surgery (SNIS), through www.brainaneurysm.com.*

Table 10.1: Side-effects of x-ray phase contrast injection in the vasculature linked with angiography: The first list includes mild reactions, followed by moderate and more severe. Summarized in a range of patient education blogs linked with phase contrast angiography, one example is https://www.radiologyinfo.org/en/info.cfm?pg=safety-contrast#safety-side-effects

Nausea, vomiting	Altered taste	Sweats
Cough	Itching	Rash, hives
Warmth (heat)	Pallor	Nasal stuffiness
Headache	Flushing	Swelling: eyes, face
Dizziness	Chills	Anxiety
Shaking		
Moderate symptoms include:		
Tachycardia/bradycardia	Hypotension	Bronchospasm, wheezing
Hypertension	Dyspnea	Laryngeal edema
Pronounced cutaneous reaction	Pulmonary edema	
More severe symptoms include:		
Laryngeal edema (severe or progressive)	Profound hypotension	Unresponsiveness
Clinically manifest arrhymias	Convulsions	Cardiopulmonary arrest

Replicated from T. Clifford, K. Daley. Medical Imaging/Interventional Radiology, A Competency Based Orientation and Credentialing Program for the Registered Nurse in the Perianesthesia Setting, *American Society of Perianesthesia Nurses, ASPAN 2009.*

imaging to avoid kidney failure in these patients. It is also known that the phase contrast agents are toxic to the renal cells, so reimaging is considered very carefully.

Angiography is extremely powerful to identify anomalies in cerebrovascular flow patterns and also gauge the success of the interventional strategies in neurosurgery. Pictured below are phase contrast angiograms of iodo-injected regions of one particular blood vessel that shows a rather prominent aneurysm before and after a coiling procedure to fill the aneurysm and remove vascular pressure from the aneurysm wall. The darker fluid-filled regions are indicators of more scattering of the phase contrast media and show in the first a large sacular aneurysm. The second picture shows local blood flow in the same region after the embolization within the aneurysm. The lack of the phase contrast agents found within the aneurysm when they are injected into the bloodstream suggests that the vascular pressure isn't not directly pressurizing the aneurysm wall after embolization.

So radiocontrast fluids co-locate with blood in the vasculature and allow for relatively easy identification of vascular anomalies. The larger question about these fluids relates to their inherent safety. The longer the residence time for these injectables, the more likely they will interact with cells contained within blood and the intimal endothelial cell lining.

10.3 MRI Phase Contrast Agents

Similar types of angiographic imaging can be done using MRI, with the same notion of injectable phase contrast agents to provide more effective image contrast. The basis for magnetic resonance imaging relies on the fact that all proteins, biofluids, polysaccharides, and the like contain hydrogen as part of the structure. There are whole courses dedicated specifically to radiology and MRI specifically but for the sake of the effort here, it is fair to note that there is both a lot of hardware and signal processing required to produce images similar to the X-ray images described earlier. The MRI unit generally contains a large, fixed magnet called the bore that operates conventionally at between 0.5 and about 2 Tesla of magnetic field strength [18]. Newer systems in development have field strengths of as high as 7 Tesla [19]. These are enormous wound magnets and the mechanical requirements needed to improve functionality include using superconductor wires to lower the resistance of the system, cooled by liquid helium. The magnet aligns the spin states of the hydrogen atoms in proteins, bone blood, inserted into the tube, human, animal, or otherwise either toward the head or the feet. The opposing spins cancel generally each other out but there a small fraction of spins that remain as unmatched pairs. Coils that transmit radiofrequency pulses are positioned and energized such that they cause the unmatched spins to absorb the resonance energy required to switch their spin orientation [19]. As the pulse is turned off, the unmatched spins revert to their prior state and emit the resonance energy. The speed by which these revert back (a relaxation time) is an indication of the chemical environment from which the resonances occur and the intensity of the signal is a function of the concentration of unmatched spins [19]. Phase contrast fluids are not in their own right required, but in terms of higher quality imaging, it is paramount to increase the signal strength over hydrogen that can be achieved by using nuclear sensitive phase contrast fluids.

MRI-based phase contrast agents are also nanomaterials, derived from metal chelates that have significant MRI resonances. The two most common metals used in MRI phase contrast are those based on chelates of gadolinium and manganese.

Similar diagnostics evaluations can be done to X-ray based angiography using these metal chelates, injected as an IV fluid push. The local environment flooded with the MRI diagnostic contrast agent immediately has a much more responsive MRI phase contrast signal than the surrounding blood into which it is injected. The net result is that one can generate a more detailed flow map of which vessels feed others, which are interconnected, and these can be compared with normal cerebrovascular maps. When abnormalities exist, the goal is to identify whether identified symptoms are linked with the nuances of the flow pattern and to resolve whether intervening can either minimize the risk of a subsequent rupture or blockage or mitigate symptoms that can often be quite debilitating. As you can imagine, a lot of both expense and time goes into properly diagnosing these individuals who can present with headaches, vertigo, and in some instances, brain bleeds or in other instances no symptoms at all. Getting a detailed map allows a more informed strategy to decide whether one can intervene to obtain a meaningful outcome that has the potential to improve a patient's health.

Gadolinium and, to a lesser extent, manganese can be reacted to form either organometallic ionic salts or nonionic chelates that are hydrophilic, soluble within the bloodstream, and contribute a strong paramagnetic species to raise the sensitivity of the tissues into which these fluids and dispersions are injected. Example structures that have been synthesized include a range of cage-like organic molecules such as those included in Fig. 10.8 [20]. The most common organic cage molecule for MRI phase contrast is diethylene triamine pentaacetic acid (DTPA). In these molecules, the paramagnetic transition metal (Gd^{3+} or Mn^{3+}) is situated in the middle of the cage and shares electrons to stabilize the structure. Both ionic salts (charged) and nonionic organometallic structures have been produced.

Based on the molecular structure of these example organometallic cages, the typical size of these molecules is on the order of $1-2$ nm in diameter, small enough to be cleared within the renal system with pore dimensions likely 10 times bigger. The competitive interest in developing new phase contrast agents is linked with improving phase contrast sensitivity, increasing tolerance in vivo, increasing its clearance capacity, and shortening its residence time overall. Improved resolution is linked with lowering the concentration of what is ultimately injected. There are patient sensations to the injections of these contrast agents as well, but the sorts of anaphylactoid responses generated with iodo-based X-ray phase

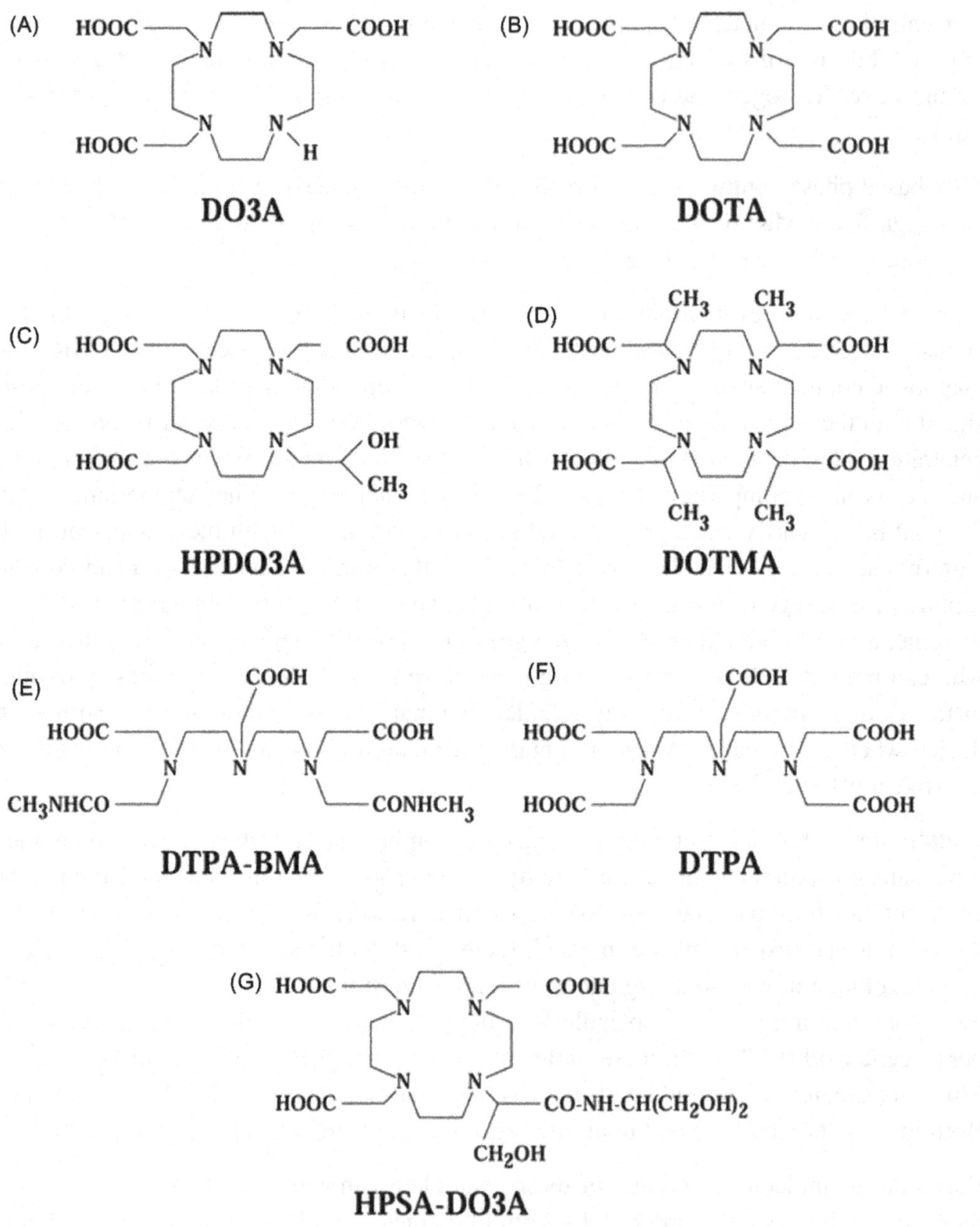

(A) DO3A

(B) DOTA

(C) HPDO3A

(D) DOTMA

(E) DTPA-BMA

(F) DTPA

(G) HPSA-DO3A

Figure 10.8
Example compounds that have been synthesized that have enhanced MRI signaling and could be injected as a phase contrast fluid during in situ MRI.

contrast agents are not as common. The larger concerns associated with MRI phase contrast agents are the residence time for these to interact with blood cells, and the clearance that is ideally rapid once injected. The capacity to probe benignly within the cerebrovasculature by MRI phase contrast agent injection allows incredible detail to identify the margins associated with tumors, growths, and other abnormalities. In Fig. 10.9, MRI images with and without phase contrast show the margins of a meningeal tumor that has grown within the skull [21]. Obviously with 3D imaging, slicing above and below this layered image would provide a scale for the sphericity of this particular tumor and point to treatment strategies that could include resection, embolization, therapeutic stereotactic radiation procedures, and chemotherapy.

For patients undergoing MRI radiography, significant attention is given to their renal health as older patients with lower GFRs tend to retain the phase contrast agent at higher levels for longer times. It is generally known that with the onset of middle age, there is a continued reduction in GFR that can accelerate with further aging [22,23]. The awareness that older patients are getting more frequent diagnostic imaging has raised the risk that renal complications can arise for older patients and patients with less renal clearance capacity undergoing phase contrast MRI. The complications have led to increased screening procedures to lower the potential that phase contrast radiography clogs the nephrons in the kidneys. The condition where these nanomaterials are incapable of being cleared and reduce the effective GFR is called nephrogenic systemic fibrosis (NSF) and is linked with partial or total kidney failure following diagnostic imaging [24]. The ability to augment clearance

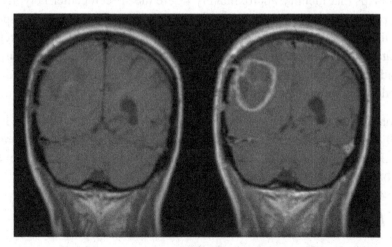

Figure 10.9
Brain mapping using phase contrast enhanced MRI to image a separated meningeal tumor which is far easier to identify than with conventional MRI without phase contrast (left). *Reproduced with permission from Gary Liney.*

by compulsory hemodialysis has the allure of reducing the complication rate associated with patients not screened out for NSF.

The ideal nanoparticle for enhanced MRI phase contrast radiography is much smaller than the pores in the nephron, paramagnetic, stable in vivo, not triggering platelet activation nor triggering a T-cell or B-cell response, has a short vascular residence time, and ideally recaptured in isolated waste treatment operations in the radiology clinic following diagnostic imaging. The fact that there are still complications arising from currently used phase contrast agents accounts for the continued drive to produce a more tolerable forms of benign phase contrast agents whose residence in vivo is short and uneventful.

From an imaging perspective, we know of phase contrast agents that can passively interact within the bloodstream, within the digestive track, and be used to provide shape and scale to tumor masses contained within subsets of the patient population. Both MRI and X-ray phase contrast can resolve differences in structure, composition, density, and comparisons can be made to assess each abnormality encountered.

Using active communication systems, we can command volunteers to observe images, listen to music, to voice, and other aural cues, sense odors, and interrogate changes in the MRI signaling in the brain when exposed to these cues, a functional response sense in situ by time resolved functional or fMRI. By comparing control images from activated images, one can resolve differences in the relaxation times associated with the magnetization of the tissues in the brain arising from cues. One can observe where these sensory signals are processed based on comparing the control image from the activated image. There are generic brain maps that identify approximately where the speech center is typically situated, but there are patients with profound alterations in brain function that develop speech centers elsewhere in the affected brain. The ability to resolve where these high-value regions of the brain are located is quite important for patients who are candidates for neurosurgery and the like. The relatively value of a brain region is defined in terms of eloquence and some areas are considered much more valuable than others.

It is not as common to subject these volunteers to phase contrast imaging as it is inherently more risky. But neurologists are increasingly able to understand cerebral responses in the context of fMRI mapping. What is missing is a mapping scheme to resolve metabolism which is the basis behind PET scanning.

10.4 PET Imaging

The signal detection for PET scanning is similar to what we use for X-ray radiography, in the sense that transmitted light is captured and partitioned relative to high transmission and low transmission regions as part of the process of processing the signal. What is different in PET scanning is the source. PET scanning uses a range of radioactive tracer molecules as ingested soluble salts that can mimic saline or glucose, allowing the tracers to be metabolized. Radioactive β emitters are produced from a variety of isotopes that can undergo nuclear decay as one proton is transformed into a neutron and there is a need to shed the positive charge. The emission yields positrons, electrons with a positive charge, that subsequently react with electrons to undergo an annihilation reaction that result in the production of gamma rays. ^{22}Na is one potential radioactive isotope having a relatively long half-life of 2.6 years. The nuclear decay emission is noted below.

$$^{22}Na \rightarrow {}^{22}Ne + 1e^+$$

The half-life corresponds to the rate of decay; a long half-life suggests a relatively sluggish decay rate. As positrons are produced (emitted) by the nuclear transformation, they interact with electrons yielding a light ray

$$1e^- + 1e^- \rightarrow h\nu(511\ eV)$$

As Na$^+$ ions in a radioactive saline solution are conveyed and sequestered, their localization is linked to where the annihilation reactions occur yielding emitted light. The only issue with using Na$^+$ isotopes that the intensity of the PET signal might be small if the emission is sluggish. A higher concentration of the positron source in saline to generate a larger signal. The other latent problem is that positron emission will continue until sufficiently decayed, whether sequestered in vivo or excreted. This conundrum has triggered more interest in considering other isotopes that might be more effective. Radioactive ^{18}F in fluorooxy glucose is one such isotope, which decays to oxygen with β emission half-life of 110 minutes. Using this compound suggests that complete decay of the introduced species should be nearly extinguished within 4−5 half-lives, less than a day during an outpatient procedure. Other light element isotopes such as ^{11}carbon, ^{13}nitrogen, and ^{15}oxygen can all be packaged into organics that can also be similarly metabolized and conveyed although some of these isotopes are increasingly rare and there is a cost consideration for the lack of availability.

A table of half-lives for and relative abundance for several candidate b sources is shown in Table 10.2.

Table 10.2: Half-lives of likely positron sources

Isotope	Injectable Compound	Half-life	Potential Usage
^{22}Na	NaCl	2.60 years	Metabolic gauge
^{18}F	NaF	110 minutes	Bone
^{52}Fe	Iron salts	8.3 hrs	Hemoglobin
^{124}I	I salts	4.3 days	Metabolic

From Brookhaven National Laboratory [25].

The intrinsic value of PET scanning is that metabolic activity can be linked between the ingestion of the radiotracer and the subsequent identification of annihilation reactions sensed by photodetectors usually in a CT-type configuration. If the radioactive source can be traced simply by identifying where the later illumination events originate once annihilation commences, clinical radiologists can resolve the activity of tumors and how much angiogenesis has occurred in raising the perfusion of the tumor mass relative to the surrounding tissues. It is also possible to colocate hot spots of perfusion that can be linked to other radiologic features. An example is listed in the figures below. The schematic for PET scanning is similar to other CT-type measurements, in that after ingestion or injection of the radioactive beta emitter, the patient is installed in a circumferential analysis chamber to detect radiation produced by positron annihilation and decay. Fig. 10.10 shows a typical slice showing the gradient in positron emission in different gross organs based on the body image which can be dynamic and remapped with time.

The strongest value is the ability to link hot spots in PET scanning with other organ specific tissues. Fig. 10.11 shows an X-ray CT image on the left and a corresponding PET image on the right for a human subject and it is clear that the photons are concentrated in the spleen, bowel, and kidney. The patient was subsequently diagnosed with a spleen tumor.

With all of the uses of nanomaterials in phase contrast enhancement tied to radiology, the largest concern is resolving how to clear these materials quickly and efficiently. We can consider a mass balance here, with the input being syringe injection usually by catheters that are colocated upstream from important features worth investigating more comprehensively. The pathways for conveyance, if injected into the cerebrovasculature, for

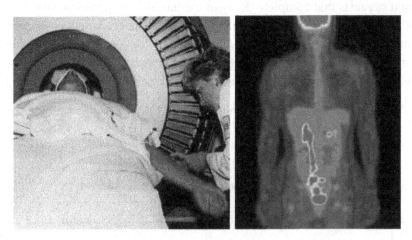

Figure 10.10
The PET scanner used at Boca Radiology Group, Boca Raton FL and examples of high emission regions (red in online version; grey in print version), suggesting high metabolism of ^{22}Na [26]. *With permission from the BocaRadiology Group.*

example would include an axial transport mechanism that over time will mix with the rest of the blood and dilute the particles to a nominal concentration. With continued perfusion and homogenization, the driving force for radial transport is reduced, but it does not preclude that some of the nanomaterials are taken up into the surrounding tissues while being recirculated.

Nanomaterials circulating in blood are conveyed to the renal artery and into the kidneys, where there is a separate larger driving force in the nephron for radial transport as the pore sizes in the kidney vasculature allow for small molecules, ions, and smaller metabolized proteins to be passed into the urine; see Fig. 10.12. The phase contrast agents are ideally small enough to be conveyed in a similar fashion. With patients with compromised renal function, they are commonly dialyzed immediately after imaging to remove the liability of continued recirculation of the phase contrast agents. The ability to alter the filtration capacity using different dialyzer constructions offers control to allow for more rapid

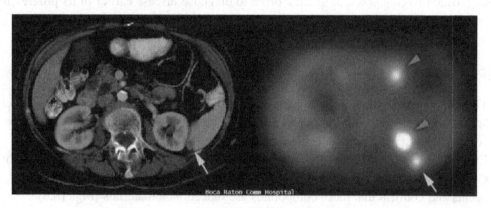

Figure 10.11
A rendering by both MRI (left) and PET in an abdominal slice. Note the hot spots with the arrows in both the spleen, bowel and kidney [26], again permission from the BocaRadiology Group.

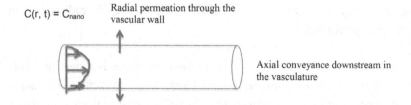

Figure 10.12
Schematic showing axial blood flow with radial extraction of phase contrast fluid and other metabolites within renal tissues.

clearance of the phase contrast agents after injection. With any circulating foreign species, the larger concern would be platelet activation triggering a potential clot.

10.5 Conclusion

The goal is not to make radiologists out of biomedical engineers who are interested in materials development. It is also important to note that the strong association with tissue engineering and nanomaterials is ultimately what leads to a larger compelling need for more effective diagnosis. The right type of functionally relevant nanomaterials is exactly what is needed. It has been shown here that injectable phase contrast fluids really are nanomaterials capable of normal clearance within the renal system allowing for their temporary residence to enhance imaging without further exposing the patient to complications. Different imaging modalities have been discussed yielding different attributes required for the different injectables. The future for further materials development for diagnostic imaging is bright and the drive to diagnose disease earlier in its progression only reinforces the need for better and more benign diagnostic strategies.

10.6 Problems

1. There might be compelling reasons to keep the MRI phase contrast patients in the clinic area in the hours after their procedure for both observation and to reclaim the phase contrast agent. What potential issues are there for both?
2. Explain why are insoluble salts preferable for X-ray CT phase contrast enhancement?
3. Compare intermolecular bonding dimensions for representative MRI phase contrast agents and confirm that these compounds are indeed nanomaterials (Fig. 10.8).
4. If fluoroxyglucose is added as 10 mL of a 10 micromolar solution, define the number of moles of molecules capable of continued radioactive decay after 11 hours if the half-life associated with the βemission is 110 minutes.
5. Draw how the number of radioactive molecules as a function of time, assuming that same half-life of 110 minutes. Assume a basis in terms of the number of initial molecules and show the data as a ratio of R/R0, the number of radioactive molecules relative to the initial fraction.

    $$\frac{\text{Log } (R/R0)}{\text{time}}$$

6. You are supporting a clinical radiology operation and there is a need to probe bowel obstruction. Explain what technique is most likely to be conventionally deployed?
7. One might expect high rates of metabolism linked with high perfusion organs such as the lungs, brain, or kidneys. Is PET scanning useful in diagnosing lung cancers or is perfusion so high in the normal lung that it is not possible to distinguish tumor from it?
8. Explain how might asymmetry in a cylindrical organ be detected with X-ray CT?

9. Cadmium-based quantum dots (QDs) are clearly nanomaterials that have very useful diagnostic capacity as well. Can you address whether there any reasons for shy these types of particles have found challenges in being adopted in normal radiological diagnostics?

References

[1] Y.Y. Hu, A. Rawal, K. Schmidt-Rohr, Strongly bound citrate stabilizes the apatite nanocrystals in bone, Proc Natl Acad Sci U S A 107 (2010) 22425–22429.

[2] M.J. Olszata, X. Cheng, S.S. Jae, R. Kumar, Y.U. Kim, M.J. Kaufman, et al., Bone structure and formation: A new perspective, Mater Sci Eng R 58 (2007) 77–116.

[3] S. Weiner, H.D. Wagner, The material bone: structure-mechanical function relations, Ann Rev Mater Sci 28 (1998) 271–298.

[4] C. Buzea, I.I. Pacheco, K. Robbie, Nanomaterials and nanoparticles: Sources and toxicity, Biointerphases 2 (2007). p. MR17-MR71

[5] USCDC, U.S. Health, 2009, Editor. 2010, US Department of Health and Human Services: Washington DC.

[6] F. Cellesi, N. Tirreli, Injectable Nanotechnology, in: B. Vernon (Ed.), Injectable biomaterials, Woodhead Publishing, Oxford, 2011.

[7] H.S. Choi, W. Liu, P. Misra, E. Tanaka, J.P. Zimmer, B.I. Ipe, et al., Renal clearance of nanoparticles, Nature Biotechnol 25 (2007) 1165–1170.

[8] A.M. Smith, S. Dave, S. Nie, L. True, X. Gao, Multicolor quantum dots for molecular diagnostics of cancer, Expert Rev Mol Diagn 6 (2006) 231–244.

[9] M. Longmire, P.L. Choyke, H. Kobayashi, Clearance properties of nano-size particles and molecules as imaging agents: considerations and caveats, Nanomedicine 3 (2008) 703–717.

[10] A.S. Ericksen, M.J. Krasna, B.A. Mast, J.L. Nosher, R.E. Brolin, Use of gastrointestinal contrast studies in obstruction of the small and large bowel, Dis Colon Rectum 33 (1990) 56–64.

[11] A. Momose, T. Takeda, Y. Itai, K. Hirano, Phase-contrast X-ray computed tomography for observing biological soft tissues, Nature Med 2 (1996) 473–475.

[12] J. Zhang, D. Tian, R. Lin, G. Zhou, G. Peng, M. Su, Phase-contrast X-ray CT Imaging of Esophagus and Esophageal Carcinoma, Sci Rep 4 (2014) 5332.

[13] D.J. Nolan, Barium examination of the small intestine, Gut 22 (1981) 682–694.

[14] I. Beggs, B.M. Thomas, Diagnosis of carcinoma of the colon by barium enema, Clin Radiol 34 (1983) 423–425.

[15] Miller, J.C., Cerebral Aneurysms. Radiology Rounds, A Newsletter for Referring Physicians from the MGH Department of Radiology, Cambirdge, MA 2008. 6.

[16] J.E. Heiserman, B.L. Dean, J.A. Hodak, R.A. Flom, C.R. Bird, B.P. Drayer, et al., Neurologic complications of cerebral angiography, Am J Neuroradiol 15 (1994) 1401–1407.

[17] R.A. Willinsky, S.M. Taylor, K. terBrugge, R.I. Farb, G. Tomlinson, W. Montanera, Neurologic Complications of Cerebral Angiography: Prospective Analysis of 2,899 Procedures and Review of the Literature, Radiology 227 (2003) 522–528.

[18] P. Armstrong, M.L. Wastie, Diagnostic imaging, 3rd ed., Blackwell Scientific, London, 1992.

[19] S.A. Kane, Introduction to Physics in Modern Medicine, 2nd ed., CRC Press, Boca Raton, FL, 2009.

[20] E. Girard, M. Stelter, J. Vicat, R. Kahn, A new class of lanthanide complexes to obtain high-phasing-power heavy-atom derivatives for macromolecular crystallography, Acta Crystallogr D. Biological crystallography online 59 (2003) 1914–1922.

[21] Liney, G.P. Magnetic resonance imaging. 2014; Available from: http://www2.hull.ac.uk/science/mri/whatismri.aspx.

[22] R.J. Glassock, The aging kidney: More pieces to the puzzle, Mayo Clinic Proceedings 86 (2011) 271–272.

[23] R.J. Glassock, C. Winearls, Ageing and the glomerular filtration rate: truths and consequences, Trans Am Clin Climatol Assoc 120 (2009) 419–428.

[24] R. Kawewlai, H. Abdujudeh, Nephrogenic systemic fibrosis, Am J Roentgenol 199 (2012) W17–W23.

[25] *Positron emitter table.* [cited 2015]; Available from: http://www.bnl.gov/medical/RCIBI/Sub-links/PositronEmitterTable.asp.

[26] *Boca Radiology Group (BRG).* 2014; Available from: http://bocaradiology.com/pet.html.

CHAPTER 11

Orthopedics

Learning Objectives

In terms of learning objectives, the reader should be able to:

- Recognize how fractured bones are stabilized by internal and external methods, comparing and contrasting healing rates and acceptance.
- Recognize the types of hardware, including rods plates, screws, pins, and integrated assemblies for both fixation and articulation.
- Identify schemes for joint stabilization for tendon and ligament reconstructions.
- Recognize how tissue engineered scaffold structures can be considered in terms of bone gaps and fusions.
- Compare and contrast allograft transplants versus synthetic and hybrid reconstructions identifying outcomes, risk factors, and other attributes.

11.1 Introduction

Bone and cartilage deterioration is commonly a function of both osteoarthritis and osteoporosis, diseases that can lead to cartilage deterioration, poor articulation (stick-slip frictional locking of the joint as opposed to smooth joint movement), and often pain and numbness, which are often the motivations for an office visit. It is important to understand something of the etiology and the epidemiology of fracture fixation and degenerative joint disease, and interventional strategies for both fracture fixation and joint disease as well. Comments are also included about materials discussed in Chapter 7, Metallic Biomaterials, Chapter 8, Metallic Biomaterials, and Chapter 9, Polymeric Biomaterials, relating to bone stabilization and joint replacement. Repair strategies for tendons and ligaments that are fast with the rise in terms of the number of procedures occurring. And finally, dental structures, which have common overlaps to orthopedics, as mandibular fractures are often an outcome of trauma, and the temporomandibular joint (TMJ) is another joint that also degenerates.

Biomaterials. DOI: http://dx.doi.org/10.1016/B978-0-12-809478-5.00011-0

11.2 Trauma-Induced Fracture and Repair Strategies

We have been stabilizing fractured bone segments for a long time. Resolved commonly by X-ray diagnostics, fractures are classified in terms of where they occur and the morphology of the fracture. Coupled with a determination of the general health, local vascular supply and age of the patient, strategies for initiating a bone reunion are initiated. Resetting fracture surfaces is essentially based on extending fractured segments sufficiently to realign the bone as one continuous bone and then immobilizing the fragments to maintain their local proximity. Immobilization by plaster and composite resin casting has been performed for many years, and while it is effective, there is often patient discomfort associated with hygiene, clothing, and with being able to access the skin, etc. (itchiness). Inflatable jacket systems after resetting allow for better hygiene and patient comfort but the removal and reinstallation of the jacket can sometimes be linked with misalignment if not sufficiently taut during bone reunion. So simple fractures, particularly in a healthy population, are adequately dealt using the immobilization schemes as identified above.

More complicated and energetic traumas can lead to more comprehensive fractures. For these more damaging and comprehensive fractures, internal reduction fracture fixation can be performed that requires an open surgery to install bone plates adjacent to the fracture site. The materials used are linked primarily with metals in Chapter 7, Metallic Biomaterials, and polymers and composites discussed in Chapter 9, Polymeric Biomaterials. Depending on where the fracture occurs and the relative amount of bone stock to work with, fixation is achieved through what is defined as external reduction, which doesn't require open surgery, but the minimally invasive installation of pins to colocate the fractured bone fragments together. The pins are extended often radially from the fracture site through the skin and connect that to a surrounding superstructure, a process called external fracture fixation with an external fixator. The details of these devices and a comparison/contrast assessment of the outcomes from using these devices and procedures are included.

What is evident is that not all trauma events lead to comprehensive bone fractures, there are traumatic events that can fracture ligaments (connective tissues from bone to bone) and tendons (connective tissues from bone to muscle) that are probably most commonly experienced in sports medicine. Various types of mechanical insults and jumping exercises can rupture tendons and ligaments and because of our inability to understand how to regrow a tendon or a ligament, often bone grafts are required to reattach these connective segments. Repetitive injuries such as shin splints and other bone bruising events can lead to bone microfractures, which are often resolved with rest and limited loading. It is also possible that trauma can be the initial trigger for later joint degeneration associated with hip contusions which are commonly poorly vascularized relative to other areas of bone and often lead to a condition of avascular necrosis, often of unknown origin.

11.2.1 Etiology and Epidemiology of Fracture

The causes for orthopedic intervention of fracture change with age and have changed with time as well. The segment most at risk for bone fractures is the elderly. De Laet et al. show, in Fig. 3.1, the relative fracture incidence as a function of both age and bone mineral density (in units of g/cm^2), and clearly show that for the same bone density, older patients are more at risk of fracture [1]. Gait instability, the ease of steady locomotion, instabilities, and slower neuromuscular firing response are noted with age, making seniors more likely candidates for a fall-induced trauma. Coupled with seniors having unstable mooring, their bone density also drops precipitously. Evidence shown in Fig. 11.1 suggests that the same insult on an older, more brittle bone is more fracture-prone. So not only are seniors more likely to fall, the fall is more likely to result in a fracture.

Traumas happen at all ages. The most likely scenario for a fracture-induced fall is the extension of limbs in bracing for the fall. People can be conditioned how to fall without extending an arm but children generally haven't mastered that around the jungle gym for example. Younger patients are flooded with growth factors during recovery and often resolve with the common casting strategies and simple resetting of the bones. They do not require more involved bone fracture fixation strategies unless the bones migrate too far apart or the fractured bone is fragmented.

Fractures also result from other traumas induced by any of a range of impact-based collisions. Fractures are more evident in populations already suffering from another disease, those undergoing chemotherapy, and those exposed to bone cancers. And there are different

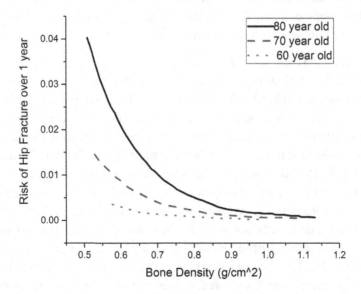

Figure 11.1
Incidence of bone fracture with fracture age as a function of femoral neck bone density. Redrawn from [1]

fracture modes that create specific crack morphologies and lead to a specific fixation strategy to stabilize it.

Fractures that are diagnosed requiring more comprehensive stabilization or in a patient population that might be more difficult to heal use both internal and external fixation schemes. The so-called internal reduction fracture fixation requires a surgery to install a bone plate or other fixturing device. Bone plates have a series of design features including the dimensions, the density and placement of holes to allow for bone screws to be threaded through the plate, and chamfers to more closely seat the screws in place. Depending on the geometry and length of the fracture, fixation can be done by single compression plate, or double fracture fixation plates where plates are installed on either side of a comprehensive fracture. In mandibular and skull fractures, there are bone plates that are curved as opposed to straight. There are a number of choices produced from medical grade orthopedic metals.

11.2.2 Materials of Choice in Fracture Fixation

High strength and high modulus plates from stainless steel and titanium are commonly produced, with the goal of intervention transferring the load to the bone plate near the bone fracture. Surgeons often choose where to place screws and now many attachments were made to create a stabilized fracture site based on the type of fracture presented, so often some holes are not used. Screw hole locations are often offset (not lined up in a row) to insure that all of the screws don't trigger axial crack coalescence in the plated cortical bone after fixation. It is common to avoid installing screws in and around the actual fracture site to reduce ion release from the screws that can interact with the growing osteoclasts demineralizing the fractured bone region and the remineralizing osteoblasts. A gap of at least 2−3 cm immediately around the fractured bone region devoid of attachments is typical.

Titanium ($E = \sim 100$ GPa) and steel ($E = \sim 220$ GPa) are often over-engineered relative to the load capacity of the residual healing bone stock, so the plates can be much smaller than the bone to which they are affixed. The repair should obviously not fail during healing, hence the motivation for a larger plate. A smaller cross-sectional area plate can sustain more than the normal body loads encountered during healing without yielding or fracturing. Healing can sometimes be retarded, as the healing bone is less likely to be mechanically stressed with the plate absorbing most of the load. Rods and plates are typically forged below the melting point of the metal to generate elongated grains in its extended direction. Forging can be accomplished in some metals at room temperature (cold working) and heating prior forging is defined as hot working. The plastic deformation imparted by forging raises the yield strength of the metal that is shaped. As a result, forging strengthens the plate in bending [2]. Holes are produced after forging, and some are chamfered to allow for better seating of screws with lower profile once fixtured. An example installation in stabilizing a wrist fracture is shown in Fig. 11.2 [3].

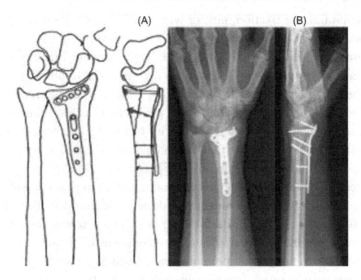

Figure 11.2
Volar fracture fixation plate used for wrist fracture coupled with parallel and perpendicular X-ray imaging of fixated fracture. The schematic is shown in (A) and the corresponding radiography images are found in (B). *Reproduced courtesy of D.L. Helfet, Hospital for Special Surgery. Available from: <http://www.hss.edu/orthopedic-trauma-case46-wrist-fractures.asp>, 2014.*

The use of biodegradable resins and composite plates such as those made from poly hydroxyl acids is increasingly common for internal reduction fracture fixation. The difference between using poly L-lactic acid (PLLA) ($E = \sim 10$ GPa) compared to steel or titanium requires larger PLLA plates to insure load stability. The payoff for using PLLA is that the molecular weight, crystallinity, and ultimately the mass of the plate can be controlled such that the hydrolysis rate weakens the structure and transfers more load capacity to the recovering bone segment over time. The hydrolysis rate for these higher molecular weight polyesters ($M_w = 50-100$ kDa) is in the order of months to several years, depending on the local pH and the degree of crystallinity. More crystalline structures tend to be more resistant to hydrolysis. The appropriate design of the degradation rate is slow enough so as to prevent premature loading of the recovering bone segment.

All of these open reductions risk infections from airborne bacteria present during surgery, and commonly, antibiotics are part of the recovery regiment to eliminate the potential for osteomyelitis that is difficult to eradicate if regions deep within bone are infected. Following fracture, it is surgeon's choice whether to remove the fixation plate and screws or not. There is no direct value in performing another surgery, and the extraction site can again become infected from the open removal. The liability risk of leaving the device installed without removal could lead to longer term ionic release which has been related to some types of subsequent osteosarcoma tumors [2] in veterinary uses. In the end, it is patient and doctor deciding together on removing these types of devices following recovery.

For closed reduction fracture fixation, pins or wires are installed externally to relocate fragments of bone segments together similar to Freeland [4]. The pins, again produced from steels and titanium, are positioned to compress the bone segments together temporarily, usually after reduction, coupled with generally some type of immobilizer to reduce motion and to prevent these fragments from drifting apart. This type of closed reduction fracture fixation is ideal for bones that are chipped, small phalangeal fractures, and fragmented bones. The goal of the pinning procedures is much like that for the bone plates, success is based on colocating fragments together and a combination of pins and a bone plate fixation are shown in Fig. 11.3 following Kamath et al. [5]. The benefits of pinning are that no open surgery is required, and one can use the installation direction to generate sufficient compressive force to drive fragments together. External reduction has the potential for infection as the skin barrier is broken in installing pins. The potential for airborne and skin infections to occur where the pins are located is evident. The clinician is clearly involved in identifying the state of recovery upon presentation, as well as infection risk, and when sufficient fusion has occurred such that the pins can be retracted allowing skin to heal where the pins were placed. External reduction fracture fixators are always removed after a period of weeks to months, depending on the rate of new bone formation at the margins.

A hybrid fracture fixation strategy uses externally installed pins that propagate through the bone stock as with closed reduction pinning, and are interconnected (usually screwed) through a superstructure called an external fixator. Cylindrical external fixators are commonly performed as an alternative to stabilizing lower leg bone fractures. The pins traverse the connective tissue and require screw connections or other hardware to link to an external scaffold. Excellent bone growth has been observed using this type of scaffold stabilizer [6]. There is subtly more micromotion of the fusing bone segments, which is

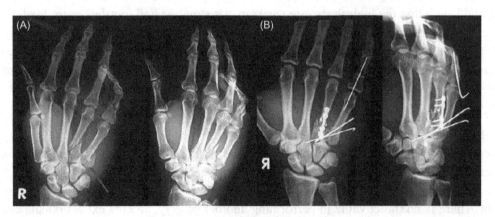

Figure 11.3
Combination reduction using wire pins to bind the proximal end of a fractured ring finger and a small bone plate. Presented are two preoperative views (A) with a more refined view and (B) two postoperative views showing both the pins and plate installed following [5]. *Reproduced with permission from J.B. Kamath, Harshvardhan, D.M. Nalk, A. Bansal, Current concepts in managing fractures of metacarpal and phalangess, Indian J. Plastic Surg., 44, (2011) 203–211.*

thought to stimulate new bone growth, compared to more rigid open reduction. Later in the recovery phase, the scaffold can be deconstructed in stages based on the amount of new bone synthesis. With several pins oriented at different entering angles to one another, cylindrical fixtures external to the connective tissue can be screwed into the pins.

11.2.3 Tendon and Ligament Repair

The damage to joint stability doesn't have to be directly related to bone fracture. Tendons and ligaments, specialized tissue linkages between differing bone and muscle segments, can also fail during trauma, depending on the loading mechanics. These types of injuries make up a large segment of athletic injuries and training efforts are directed at equipping athletes with more effective protective gear and exercise programs to strengthen muscles, tendons, and ligaments. Due to the increasing prevalence of sports medicine, efforts are also being made for high performers to reconstruct damaged joints either through synthetics or by transplants to make the repaired joints more stable. In front of the gliding knee joint, the patella (kneecap) is bound by two patellar tendons to hold this bone in place to insulate the joint from frontal impact damage. Behind the patella, three ligaments stabilize the knee, the anterior, medial, and posterior cruciate ligaments. The patellar tendon also helps to stabilize bone stability in the knee. Helmet impacts orthogonal to the normal bending direction of the knee can rupture any of these stretched ligaments. Ligaments can also fail just by an unusual planting of the knee. Anterior cruciate ligament (ACL) type injuries are fast on the rise, especially with female athletes. A recent review showed that the rate of ACL injury among female collegiate athletes is much higher than that for men, in some instances as high as $2 \times$ or $3 \times$ [7], as shown in Fig. 11.4. There are either differences in how female

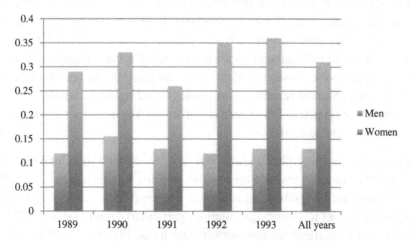

Figure 11.4
Data on ACL injury rate linked with collegiate athletes participating in soccer [7]. The rate data is normalized per 1000 athlete exposures (games/events). The rate statistics for other ligament injuries are invariant, as shown in Table 11.1 [7].

Table 11.1: Comparison study of gender versus incidence of several common diagnosed knee injuries among athletes

Column 1	Men's Soccer	Athlete Exposures (626,223) athlete events	Women's Soccer	Athlete Exposures (308,748) athlete events
Injured structure	#	Rate /1000 exposures	#	Rate /1000 exposures
Collateral ligament	319	0.51	192	0.62
Torn cartilage (meniscus)	119	0.19	105	0.34
Patella or patellar tendon	130	0.21	92	0.31
Anterior cruciate ligament	81	0.13	97	0.31
Posterior cruciate ligament	22	0.04	12	0.04

From E. Arendt, R. Dick, Knee injuries among men and women in collegiate basketball and soccer, Am. J. Sports Med. 23 (1995) 694–701.

athletes plant to pivot or change direction or the actual strength of the female ACL that makes it more susceptible to fracture and tearing.

Partial tears can be reunited arthroscopically, using nonbiodegradable sutures or bone screws for attachment, and following the recovery period, efforts are made to slowly test the repaired ligament along with strengthening the rest of the surrounding ligaments stabilizing the knee. Recovery is typically from several weeks to several months.

Complete tears typically require bone implants. Autografting can be done fractionating the middle third of the patellar tendon with the cut bone segments to which it is attached similar to Fig. 11.5. This graft is called a bone–patellar tendon–bone (BPTB) graft. This plug is fed through the failed ligament location and then the bone fragment is attached or screwed into the upper bone, as seen in Fig. 11.6. Stretching of the tendon after the bone fusion creates a biomechanical response in the autografted ligament similar to the original ACL with much larger joint stability. There are other graft possibilities for the ACL but the BPTB is the most straightforward.

There are demonstrations of synthetic grafts that have functioned in animal studies and human trials, but the standard practice for restabilizing the ligament-free joint is through either an ACL transplant allograft or an autograft. The inadequate fatigue resistance of synthetic ligaments has let to their fragmentation, particularly with Goretex PTFE grafts that tend to also embed particulates into surrounding tissue [9]. Any synthetic graft will likely require a bone attachment scheme and there are adequate options for the fixturing

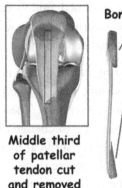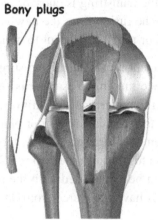

Bony plugs

Middle third of patellar tendon cut and removed

©MMG 2000

Figure 11.5

Fractionation of the patellar tendon as a autograft donor site for ACL reconstruction. *Reproduced with permission from the E-orthopod web site: http://eorthopod.com/patellar-tendon-graft-reconstruction-of-the-acl/*

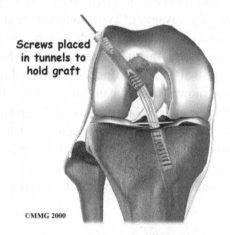

Screws placed in tunnels to hold graft

©MMG 2000

Figure 11.6

Reconstruction site showing the installation of the BPTB repair. *Reproduced with permission from the E-orthopod website: http://eorthopod.com/patellar-tendon-graft-reconstruction-of-the-acl/*

though allograft and autografts. The larger problem or synthetics is matching the force−displacement characteristics both initially and after many cycles of knee use for example.

Other donor sites for ACL reconstruction include the hamstring tendon graft which is increasingly more common. Grafts from the hamstring and the patella are successful and, if there is a preference, the hamstring is chosen, sectioned, and threaded into the adjacent bone region where the bone fusion fixes the newly formed ligament in place. Bone screws can also be used to bind or pin the ligament to an adjacent bone.

Of course, much of ligament repair is elective surgery. ACLs are not crucial for casual jogging, and even distance running. Yes there is some knee instability and perhaps slightly more pain, but it is not critical for an average runner. There are other sports such as tennis and basketball that require more foot planting to change direction, and these sorts of functional movements for elite athletes require surgical reconstruction if they fail and the athlete wants to return to their sport. Of course there is no guarantee that full range of mobility can be established with the same functional performance after grafting, but elite athletes have recovered from ACL surgery to have complete careers after that.

11.2.4 Spine Stabilization

Osteoporosis is a more profound regulator of quality of life as it relates to degenerative joint disease within the spine. The ravages of systematic vertebral compression fractures have been noted observing aged osteoporotic individuals who are stooped over in response to accumulating multiple compression fractures over time. That loss of bone mineral density and the corresponding strength and stiffness of the vertebral segments can lead to a primary compression fracture, shown schematically in Fig. 11.7. The effect of one vertebral fracture usually leads to a change in the biomechanics of the spinal loading and an amplification of the stress on the adjacent vertebral segments, which are likely to fail in due time, and the whole process progresses relentlessly. Coupled with the fractures are chronic pain, compromised movement capacity and difficulty in executing work schedules, decreased lung capacity, and depression among other things [10].

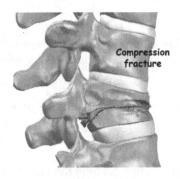

Figure 11.7
Example of a primary vertebral compression fracture. *Reproduced with permission from Getty Images.*

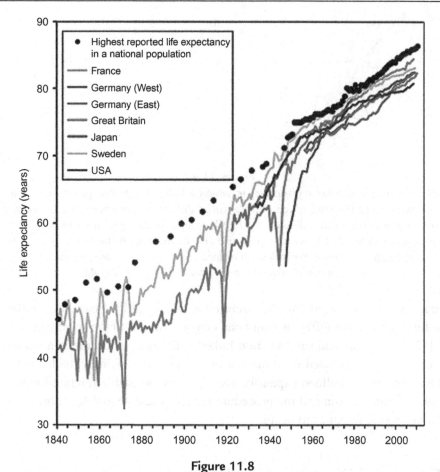

Figure 11.8

Female life expectancy in developed countries: 1840—2009. Source: *Highest reported life expectancy for the years 1840—2000 from online supplementary material to Oeppen J, Vaupel J. W. Broken limits to life expectancy, Science 296 (2002) 1029—1031. All other datapoints from the Human Mortality Database (http://www.mortality.org) provided by Roland Rau (University of Rostock). The figure is redrawn from a published image. Additional discussion can be found in K. Christensen, G. Doblhammer, R. Rau, J.W. Vaupel, Aging populations: the challenges ahead, The Lancet; 374(9696) (2009) 1196—1208.*

Nominally, 10% of the population in the United States is likely ostoporetic and that average lifespan is an increasing attribute as the number of septuagenarians, octogenarians, and those of the super-aged rise relative to a more modest birthrate [11,12], as observed in Fig. 11.8.

Efforts to stabilize the fulcrum compressing viable disks leading to unnatural sagittal spine curvature or kyphosis have advanced using inflatable balloon procedures to reestablish a more normal biomechanical dimension to the spine. The intervention called kyphoplasty is a minimally invasive catheter deployment procedure not that different than balloon

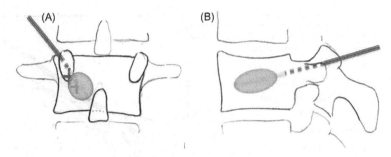

Figure 11.9

An example of a transpedicular kyphoplasty in which a balloon catheter (*green*, light gray in print version) is inserted into the void space of a fractured disk after reorienting the vertebral segment for a more normal orientation, followed by the filling of that cavity with bone cement (*red* tube, dark gray in print version). (A) A front view and (B) a side view of the spine. *From Y. Robinson, C.E. Heyde, P. Forsth, C. Olerud, Kyphoplasty in osteoporotic vertebralncompression fractures—guidelines and technical considerations, J. Orthop. Surg. 6 (2011) 43.*

angioplasty. The catheter is fed into the fractured vertebrae and the balloon is inflated with a reactive fluid not terribly different than bone cement, similar to the schematic shown in Fig. 11.9 [13]. The filling and solidification linked with injection occurs in a matter of minutes and the resin is isolated from the rest of the fracture region by the balloon [10,14]. The lift generated by the balloon expansion results in a more stable fractured region, and there is reduced chronic pain and the procedure reduces the potential for subsequent adjacent compression fractures to occur.

11.3 Trauma and Disease in Articulating Joints

More common with aging tissues is the development of pain and poor articulation of joints that can commonly be inflamed through overexertion, exercise, and everyday usage. Interestingly, traumas and contusions for example in the hip can lead to poor recovery and form vascular necroses where the femoral ball is insufficiently vascularized to affect a proper recovery. There are other avascular necroses, deteriorations of unknown origins that can also form necroses requiring replacement. Those affected by autoimmune disorders such as rheumatoid arthritis [15,16] and lupus [17] can also have larger inflammatory responses in joints and cartilage leading to cartilage deterioration. There is also open conjecture about whether runners [18] and weightlifters [19] can also have cartilage deterioration induced by the overuse and physical activity. These diseases can be managed to some extent by analgesic therapy, by minimizing activities that increase pain and further deterioration, etc. But often there is a latent need to replace inflamed joints to resolve chronic conditions and return patients to a more complete life.

11.3.1 The Epidemiology and Etiology of Joint Disease

There are four general common traits that can lead to degenerative joint disease. They include age (usually above age 45), gender (females generally are more susceptible), ergonomic overuse and repetitive injury, and obesity [20]. There is conjecture about whether it is possible to be a runner and never suffer the consequences of worn and torn cartilage, eventually [21]. The biomechanics of walking and running suggest that the heavier the center of mass is, the more compressive force there is on the knees, hips, and ankles and likely the larger chance of degeneration. An interesting comparison study is summarized in Table 11.2. If degenerative joint disease was only a function of body mass, one would expect the lowest joints under the most compressive load to cause pain first, but the ankle is so well designed, even with only a minimal amount of bone stock, knees and hips fail due to cartilage erosion long before the average ankle does [22]. The main takeaway relating to joint pain is that with the demographics of an aging population, skeletal and movement disorders are common with the most common experience being osteoarthritis. Arthritis, in general, is managed by analgesic therapy, rest to allow for healing, exercises, and physical therapy and controlled, weight-bearing exercise to rebuild muscles that can stabilize bone and retain bone density. In some instances, acute issues of arthritis can resolve, but degenerative arthritis is a progressive condition that often requires schemes to recontour or replace articulating surfaces to operate more smoothly and with less pain.

Table 11.2: Indication of osteoarthritis risk comparing runners and walkers and their self-reporting for both OA and Hip replacement

	Runners		Walkers	
	Men	Women	Men	Women
N (#)	46,819	27,933	3122	11,503
Incidence of osteoarthriris	1141	863	74	621
Incidence of hip replacement needs	208	51	36	78
Age (years)	46.1($\pm$10.7)	39.9($\pm$10.4)	61.5($\pm$11.2)	52.5($\pm$12)
Smokers (%)	1.33	1.65	3.4	3.6
BMI (kg/m^2)	23.9($\pm$2.5)	21.4($\pm$2.4)	26.6($\pm$4)	25.3($\pm$5)
Exercise energy expended (MET-hour/day)				
Walking			2.2	1.7
Running	5.44	4.98		
Years running or walking (AVG)	13.2	9.8	11.3	8.3
Marathons (#/last 5 years) (AVG)	1.95	1.15		
10 km performance (m/s) (AVG)	3.9	3.4		

From P.T. Williams, Effects of running and walking on osteoarthritis and hip replacement risk, Med. Sci. Sports Exerc. 45 (2013) 1292–1297.

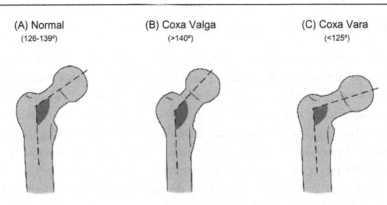

(A) Normal
(126-139°)

(B) Coxa Valga
(>140°)

(C) Coxa Vara
(<125°)

Figure 11.10
Examples of angular attributes of hip joints relating to the formation of Coxa Vera defects [26,27]. (A) A normal neck shaft angle, (B) a coxa valga angle, and (C) a coxa vara femoral anatomy.

There are instances where cartilage deterioration occurs much earlier in life. Hip malformities in which the femoral ball is more perpendicular to the compressive load direction occur in a small segment of the population [23]. Actually, what is more interesting is that the femoral neck angle at birth is normally 150°, and during development of the pelvis and with children becoming more ambulatory, there is a larger compressive load on the femoral ball causing it to tilt and lessen the angle [24]. Normal development leads to a femur to femoral ball angle approaching a nominal fixed angle of 125−135 degrees although this is widely variable among people of the same age. There are subsets of patients with more compliant bone that creates a defect called a Coxa Vara defect [25], as shown in Fig. 11.10. Due to differences in pelvic width between females and males, the angle in females is more slightly more perpendicular with a lower angle, one small reason why women are normally shorter but there is a wide variance among groups of individual ages, etc. Beyond puberty, there are fewer changes. Subsets of kids have what is defined as childhood inflammatory arthritis that tends to create both pain and cartilage erosion [28]. Early hip implants are recommended for patients with profound misalignment and Coxa Vara defects to reestablish a more normal biomechanical loading and to address the lingering pain [26]. Hip replacement for adolescents and young adults in their 20s is rarer compared to osteotomy [29], but it can be recommended if the native joint is sufficiently damaged [30].

It seems worth considering what else leads people to clinics with evidence of joint deterioration. There can be singular traumas that are correlated to some instances of later necrosis [31]. Gout can precipitate of uric acid within joints leading to three body wear during articulation [32], while alcoholism [33] and anabolic steroid use seem to have negative effects on maintaining functional chondrocytes within cartilage [33,34].

Perfusion-related diseases such as sickle cell anemia also tend to have negative effects on chondrocyte viability [33]. And separately, autoimmune triggers like lupus [33] can concentrate inflammatory responses within joints which also reduce chondrocyte viability. The takeaway is that the symptoms (cartilage deterioration, pain, and functional articulation) can be improved by joint replacement, but not necessarily by addressing the primary cause of the deterioration.

11.4 Joint Types

There are a range of different types of joints found human and veterinary medicine. They include saddle, hinge, ball and socket, gliding, and pivot type joints. Here we will present the typical joints that undergo these articulations and the types of diseases that manifest challenges to smooth articulation. Examples of such are included in Fig. 11.11.

11.4.1 Hinge Joints

The most common joints include the knee and elbow as noted in Fig. 11.11. Both joints are essentially trays, with the knee formed by the tibia and fibula onto which the distal end of the femur rotates as with a hinge, called the tibial tray. Separating the distal end of the femur from the tibial tray is growth of cartilage on the bony ends with a segment of cartilage interspaced in the joint called the meniscus. The cartilage is composed of type II collagen that is both tough and highly swollen with synovial fluid contained in the capsule. Articulation is through these internal rotations as would occur with a hinge. A separate lubrication mechanism arises with the squeezing of the cartilage that produces a liquid film that allows for even easier articulation.

Any malformities and tilt of the tray will overload the meniscus resulting in localized wear and also partial and complete tears with a range of morphologies. With a *valgus* knee, profound alterations in the load angle overstress the knee [35] that is commonly resolved, in part, by total joint replacement (TJR). Overuse events can cause vascular bruising and lead to either vascular (VN) or avascular (AVN) necrosis in which the bone stock is more poorly vascularized as it heals. Arthritis can also lead to a physical deterioration in the thickness of the cartilage on the articulating surfaces. And of course, extra mass from high BMI raises cartilage compressive force. In a large segment of the active and exercising population, cartilage tears can be observed but oftentimes, the presence of the tear is not necessarily linked with pain symptoms which is often more related to bone bruising and microfractures that can lead to fluid leakage within the bone stock. If cartilage damage is complete, bone on bone loading is more common and linked with acute pains and poorer joint articulation.

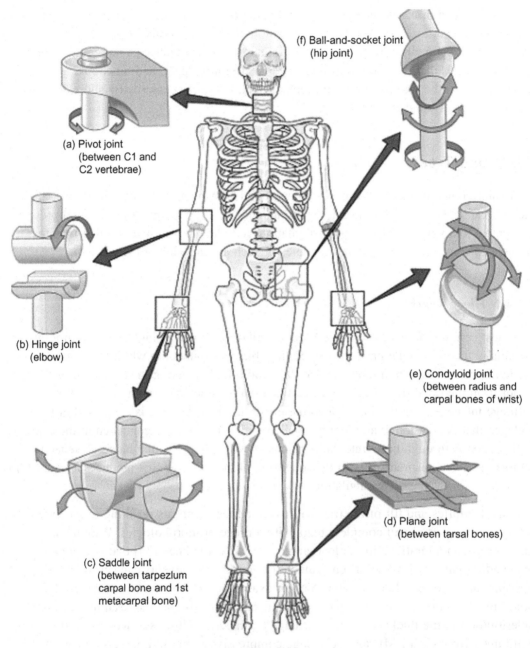

Figure 11.11
Schematic of different types of joints and articulation modes. *Published with permission from C Molnar and J Gair, Concepts of Biology, 1st Canadian Edition, BC Open textbooks, Download this book for free at http://open.bccampus.ca*

It is also thought that within reason, motions of the ankle and wrist can also be described as hinge joints, but that does not fully accommodate the multi-axial range of motion. Both the wrist and the ankle have a primary hinge opening motion, but clearly one can move the wrist and ankle in more than one degree of motion. Humans would have less robust fine motor skills and ballet would not exist if the wrist or ankle had only a single directionality.

11.4.2 Ball and Socket Joints

Ball and socket joints, found in both the shoulder and hip joint, are freely rotating joints. In the hip, the proximal end of the femur includes a femoral ball, and it fits into the socket identified as the acetabulum, contained within the pelvis. A similar joint construction is observed in the shoulder, but the hip is loaded in compression and the shoulder is loaded in tension from gravitational force on the extending arm. Cartilage is found on both articulating joint surfaces, and similar to the response with knees, the deterioration of cartilage can have biochemical origins such as what is found with arthritis. The femoral ball is susceptible to poor vascularity and this tissue is an early marker to observe both vascular and avascular necrosis in susceptible populations. Ultimately, people visit their doctors due to the joint pain that can require both a management and a mitigation plan.

Total shoulder surgery replacement is becoming more commonplace, perhaps in response to so many repetitive injuries associated with throwing and racket sports. Torn rotator cuffs in elite pitchers are ligament tears that can lead to an instability in the shoulder joint and the ball sagging from its optimum placement in the shoulder socket. In some instances, a rotator cuff arthropathy can develop from poor articulation that can necessitate the replacement of the joint. Similar arthritis and avascular necrosis can also cause cartilage deterioration. It is worth noting that in terms of the number of interventional procedures to repair the shoulder, there is more growth potential here than in other joints where there is a saturation in terms of existing and substantially equivalent devices.

11.4.3 Pivot/Rotary Joints

Pivot joints or rotary joints are found within the spine, as noted in Fig. 11.12. The angular motion of one vertebral segment relative to another as one bends forward from the waist compresses the anterior cartilage between disks and exerts a tensile force the posterior side. The motion is considered as a bending with a fulcrum in the center region of the spine where the spinal column is placed. Separate pivots can arise in patients suffering from scoliosis where there are observed nonlinearities in the vertebral alignment of the spine, and in vertebral compression fractures of the aged. Pain (either acute stabbing responses or a chronic low grade ache and numbness are the key observables here) and efforts are made to minimize symptoms and reestablish a more normal articulation. The numbness can arise

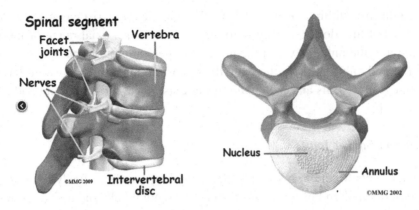

Figure 11.12

(A) Spinal cross-section showing vertebral segments linked through intervertebral disc joints, the spinal column with its nerve connections is shown as are facet joints attaching the vertebral to the spinal column. (B) Top view showing the intervertebral disc contains both a nucleus and an annular regions with different structures. *Reproduced with permission from E-orthopod website: http://eorthopod.com/thoracic-spine-anatomy/*

from herniation of the cartilage that bulge from the spine under load. The displacement can apply pressure to either the spinal column or neurons associated with communication and signaling within the spine. Repair strategies have considered both the removal of herniated cartilage followed by either vertebral fusion surgery, the installation of intervertebral cartilage segments to replace the herniation, and other internal fixation schemes to stabilize the spine otherwise.

11.4.4 Gliding/Saddle Joints

Other joints that are defined as gliding joints are linked with small bones in the hand and foot. The metatarsals and metacarpals are essentially bones that can slide across one another in articulating. In these instances, the bones create a shear force on the cartilage (Fig. 11.13).

Further extending in the hand and foot regions, there are saddle joints, where the presence of two bones that are situated in a saddle helps to orient and direct toes and fingers to all be directed into similar directions.

For those afflicted with carpel tunnel syndrome, autoimmune disorders such as Lupus and Raynaud's syndrome, often, the metacarpal joints are affected most acutely. Efforts to improve the ergonomics of mass production have proven insufficient so far in eliminating work-related accumulated damage patterns that can arise from repetitive motion injuries. Interventional strategies have led to individual surgeries to remove and isolate damaged

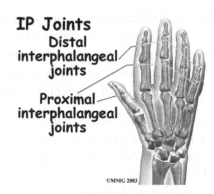

IP Joints

Distal interphalangeal joints

Proximal interphalangeal joints

©MMG 2003

Figure 11.13
Many of the joints in the hands are defined as saddle joints, including both the intraphalangeal (IP) joints and the metacarpal joints. Saddle joints tend to be drawn back into the saddle at equilibrium raising their stability. *Reproduced with permission from E-orthopod website: http://eorthopod. com/hand-anatomy/*

cartilage, but for systemic diseases, a drug-based or corticosteroid-based regimen to address inflammation and analgesic responses seem to be both more common and more likely leading to successful outcomes.

11.5 The Mechanics of Joint Replacement

There are many hardware requirements for performing joint replacement. In addition to the actual hardware that is installed, there are tools for cutting, resurfacing, in and aligning the joint for appropriate loading and gait. Some joints such as the hip are modular in design allowing the surgeon to choose specific hardware (ball diameter relative to cup diameter) to control gait and motion after recovery. This means that for a hip implant, often there is a selection process to identify an optimum series of components that are mated together. It is possible to have a stem produced from titanium, a cobalt-chromium, aluminum oxide or zirconium oxide ball, and a polyethylene bearing surface as the acetabular cup, all as one integrated assembly of different material constituents.

All of these components are made as discussed earlier. The high modulus metal or ceramic components for the knee, hip, or shoulder are cast or sintered appropriately, and often separately shaped. The polymeric bearing components are ram extruded into preforms and shaped by machining. If the implants are to be cemented into place, the bone cement is supplied as two parts, powder + monomer mixture, which is mixed, degassed, and conveyed into a dispenser following homogenization. All monolithic components are polished, packaged, and dry sterilized by gamma irradiation to an identified regulatory threshold dose. Any other surgical instrumentation and alignment tools are also packaged and sterilized. Quality control parameters assessed include hardness assessments, phase structure, dimensional tolerance, and roughness determinations for coupons also produced for destructive testing during manufacturing. The completed and sterilized packages are delivered to the surgeons in the operating room and deployed accordingly. The following tutorial walks one through the process of installing a replacement knee.

Upon surgically opening up the synovial capsule housing the failing knee joint, the surgeon can cut the bone stock to match the counter-surfaces to match the appropriate hardware. Starting with the distal end of the femur, vibratory bone saws are used to cut the bone to match the femoral implant contours. For this particular element, a hole is also created in the femur to accommodate the protrusion opposite the bearing surface. A similar slicing and hole construction is made in proximal end of the tibia to accommodate the tibial implant.

Knee implants are often cementless constructions while hip implants can often be fixtured using surgical bone cements, methacrylate-based grouts that polymerize in vivo following an ex vivo mixing and transfer to an injector device.

The tibial tray is designed with tabs on the top surface to allow the installation and fixturing of a polymeric bearing surface. For polymer–metal articulating knees, the most common synthetic bearing surface is produced from ultrahigh molecular weight polyethylene, UHMWPE. The chain length of UHMWPE that corresponds to molecular weights (as high as 5 MDa) is such that when formed into bearing surface materials, the UHMWPE is wear resistant to the sliding motions of the femoral knee component on the tibial tray. The bearing spacers are usually machined into an appropriate space to match the dimensions of the tray, and using an impactor (hammer), the spacer is lodged under the tabs of the tibial tray.

It is worth pointing out several features of the current state of the art in joint replacements and a regulated industry. First, there are a number of industrial companies that are producing nearly equivalent components in terms of form and function at least for hips, shoulders, and knees. In terms of modern devices, the general form and shape of hip devices do not deviate from those patented in the mid-20th century [36,37]. From those original patents whose protections have run out, there are new, subtly different designs that have been presented to the USPTO along with system level patents that couple the implant with other features including alignment systems [38,39], minimally invasive surgery tools [40], robotic surgery tools [40], and the sum of the device plus the system is packaged as the invention. From a regulatory standpoint, a wildly different design would require more qualification testing from the FDA in the general population. So implant designers are careful not to deviate from general understanding of what a hip, knee, or shoulder implant should represent.

New materials going into a new design warrant patent protection, as noted by the use of ceramic on metal [41], ceramic on polymer, ceramic on ceramic [42], and metal on metal [41] implants have been patented and tested under clinical trials and laboratory trial studies. A nice review shows the breadth of recent patent activity [43]. But the landscape is unusual in that in a highly regulated environment, there has been less movement toward generic devices as patents run their course as is so common with drug patents moving to generics with more regularity.

11.6 The Tribology of Joint Replacements: Impact on Joint Lifetime

The articulation of TJR components is essentially a test in friction and wear. Smoother surfaces are less prone to wear, and the presence of fluids at the interface can also lower both friction and wear rates. On the continuum of performance spectrum, the use of a softer, more compliant, and more forgiving bearing surfaces will likely lead to the softer component having excessive wear. The use of UHMWPE is certainly more wear resistant than polyethylenes of lower molecular weight but polyethylene wear rates using UHMWPE are reported to be between 0.1 and 0.5 mm/year on different substrates [44–46]. In addition the hygroscopic nature of cartilage is not conserved in hydrophobic polyethylene, thus, TJR with PE is a dry lubrication mechanism of articulation. On the other end of the performance spectrum are wear resistant materials such as the metal on metal joint constructions, but these have led to a condition called metallosis, in which the few metal particulates abraded during articulation are subsequently oxidized and embedded in surrounding tissues [47].

Polyethylene is a low friction polymeric surface, and higher molecular weight resins retard wear compared to a lower one [48]. The repeated sliding back and forth under load still creates a local abrasion that removes material from the softer side (the polymer in this case) usually in the form of microparticulates. The smaller the particles, the larger that are produced under the same erosion rate conditions. A more polished finish on the metal side of the implant can reduce the wear by smoothing edges that could cut into the softer bearing surface. But wear is an obvious outcome that requires consideration and design.

Functional wear is measured clinically by tracking the erosion of the bearing thickness over time after installation using diagnostic X-ray imaging. The polymer insert for both knees and hips ranges in thickness between 6 and 10 mm. Erosion rates are usually higher in the first year, and an average wear rate depending on the user is 0.05–0.3 mm/year [49]. It is easy to consider that with polymer wear rates on the order of 0.1 mm/year with micron-sized particles, and with the identified surface areas of implants undergoing erosion, billions of particles are ultimately expelled and they have to go somewhere. The wear particles derived from hydrophobic PE are also not biodegradable, nor do not melt nor swell under body exposure conditions. But with all implants that undergo wear and abrasion, the long-term concern is the upregulation or awakening of the immune system that targets these particles surrounding the implant location for digestion. The attempted digestion usually resorbs some of the surrounding tissues housing the implant leading to implant loosening, pain, and a condition called osteolysis.

Obviously, different patients have different devices, different body masses, are of different ages, and use their implanted devices in different ways. This could explain the wide variance in functional wear rate. Of course, wear is not sensed directly by the implant recipient, it is the interaction of the immune system with the wear debris that dictates a sensory response. There have been efforts associated with retrieval studies where implants have been removed and revised or presented at autopsy to gauge overall performance but these are only single measurements. Cumulative wear is resolved as a volumetric accumulation with years of implantation and comparisons are shown in Fig. 11.14.

The comparison to laboratory data is crucial to make larger predictions linking optimum material and process conditions to the lowest wear rates. Wear tests can be conducted on rotational pin on disk wear machines, and functional hip and knee simulators have also created to replicate similar mechanics associated with functional joints that have been loaded [53]. The benefits for doing simulated tests are that not only can deviations in wear rate with time be measured, but one can also observe the attributes of the wear debris produced.

The mechanics of a pin on disk sliding wear unit are relatively simple and allow for separate determinations of both stress and wear rate, but it is the analysis that is less clear. Turntables can freely rotate a plate of known roughness to replicate one side of a sliding joint. When a pin is placed on the rotating plate, the rotational speed of the plate is reduced

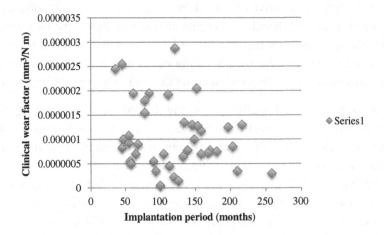

Figure 11.14

Data replotted from both Jasty et al. and Sychertz et al. and compiled by Eflick [50−52]. Note how few datapoints are at long time.

due to the frictional loss of momentum, and the product of the rotational speed and time yields a sliding distance. The normal force relative to the contact area of the pin on the rotating table gives an applied stress. The dependent variable, the mass wear rate, is taken by gravimetric determinations over time, or by resolving a thickness reduction and multiplying by the area of the sample, volumetric determination of lost sample volume can be determined. The slope of the mass or volume loss per unit time or per unit length corresponds to a mass wear rate. Applying a higher force will correlate with a higher wear rate. Performing similar tests immersed in a fluid in a different humidity will increase lubrication and lessen the amount of wear debris collected. And since the mechanics of sliding friction lead to frictional heating, the speed of the rotation and prior residues on the track might also influence the observed wear rate.

Wear can be reduced by altering the processing sequences that form the articulating surfaces. The bearing surface of UHMWPE is often machined to shape it and polished accordingly. The counter-surface is also polished to reduce roughness. Alternative process strategies to reduce wear might include near net shape forming of the polymer component to reduce the chance of reducing the molecular weight on the surface. Other schemes to harden the polymer component include ion implantation and chemical crosslinking. These components also undergo irradiation sterilization, which can alter the polymer structure. There ought to be a more informed discussion about how large of a dose is really needed to sterilize components, particularly as manufacturing operations are cleaner.

The production of wear debris and its negative consequences are exacerbated by the fact that a large number of small wear particles (micrometer sized and below) are ultimately produced. After enough of them are resident in the surrounding tissues, depending on the virility of the immune system of the host, they are sensed by resident sentry cells that recruit an inflammatory response to digest polyethylene particulate residues. The response of the recruited monocytes and polymorphonuclear cells is to lower pH and to digest and deconstruct the surrounding bone stock in a failed attempt to digest the polyethylene particles that are essentially inert. The resulting osteolysis can trigger a profound loosening of the implant in the surrounding bone tissue. The manifestation of symptoms is likely some instability and pain associated with more motion of the fixtured bone implants in the bone stock and usually results in a new implant called a revision device.

Two competing pressures are increasing the required design lifetime of various installed orthopedic implants. One is that there is an incremental increase in the lifetime of the general population. Implants were originally designed with the idea that the implant would outlive the patient and have proven functional for periods between 15 and 20 years, as indicated in Table 11.3. With more suppliers with generally equivalent device designs, that lifetime hasn't changed, although there have been some device designs that have failed prematurely leading to early revisions. If there is no change in when people are implanted

Table 11.3: Representative datasets from different research studies showing the age range, years post-follow-up and percentage revisions an indication of a device failure and a need to intervene [15, 30, 54−65]

Study	Ref. #	# of hips (Patients)	Mean age (years)	Range	Mean years follow up	Cemented THA (%)	# revised (%)
Bilsel et al.	[55]	37 (23)	22.3	17−30	11.3	62	3 (8)
Chandler et al.	[58]	33 (29)	23	14−29	5.6	100	7 (21.2)
Chmeli et al.	[59]	66 (39)	19.9	(11−29)	15.1	100	35 (53)
Dorr et al.	[56]	81 (69)	30	14−45	9.2	100	29 (33)
Dorr et al.	[57]	49 (35)	31.1	16−45	16.2	100	33 (67)
Halley and Charnley	[65]	49 (27)	26	NA	9.5	100	7 (14)
Kitsoulis et al.		20 (10)	15.8	13−24	9.2	100	10 (50)
Lachiewicz et al.	[64]	62 (34)	26	14−49	6	100	2 (3.2)
Learmonth et al.	[63]	14 (7)	16	12.−22	8.5	100	none
Maric and Haynes	[15]	17 (17)	18	14−20	9.3	76	1 (5.8)
Ruddlesdin et al.	[61]	75 (42)	14.6	11.−17	5.4	100	1 (1.3)
Sochart and Porter	[60]	83 (55)	24.9	17−29	20	100	44 (53)
Torchia et al.	[30]	63 (50)	17	11.−19	12.6	100	27 (43)
Witt et al.	[62]	96 (54)	16.7	11.3−26.6	11.5	100	24 (25)

and the lifetime of the devices hasn't been increased, there is an increasing chance that one implant lifetime isn't enough and a so-called revision surgery might be required. Also, by implanting in younger patients, the lifetime could be affected if younger patients are more active and create more excessive wear patterns for their implanted devices, or are healthier candidates for surgery and have actually better outcomes.

Obviously for other joint constructions, there are similar integrated assemblies that are combined to represent each joint. There are some subtleties relating to local biocompatibility of the so-called cemented and friction fitted joint reconstructions. Those joints retrofitted using a bone cement grout to fixture the joint require a larger cavity to be created to allow for the introduction of the cement before the setting of the component. The process of injecting the joint with bone cement has the potential to expose the living interface to both a potential chemical necrosis arising from monomer diffusion into the surrounding tissue if the cement is mixed and immediately injected, and a thermal necrosis resulting from the exotherm of the bone cement polymerizing in vivo adjacent to the living interface. Both of these potential necroses can lead to some fraction of atrophy and the clinician is the last processer controlling at what stage of advancement injection commences. Countermeasures to address concerns about necrosis suggesting waiting for the initial installation to reduce the amount of monomer injected, cooling the components before installation to increase their capacity for heat absorption, etc. They all have their drawbacks. For cemented devices, the resulting larger cavity has less residual bone stock as the hole generated is usually 6 mm larger in annular dimension than the stem. There are also fewer chances for revision surgery if there is a need for replacement in a cemented joint.

Cementless installations are increasingly common as a smaller cavity can be created and there is no need for the cement in a compression set device. What is needed is a more precise control of the type of cavity produced. This requires more extensive use of alignment tools to insure a compression fit. There is obviously less necrosis potential from the cement in cementless installations, but the actual drilling procedures to create the cavity can also heat the surrounding bone stock.

There is a desire to compare the general performance of cemented versus noncemented joint constructions, and in many instances that is very difficult to do. Some comparison studies have considered which procedure is ultimately more expensive and from a performance perspective, which has led to less aseptic loosening, an indicator relating to osteolysis. In general there is no striking performance difference that would suggest one device performs better. One study compared cemented total hip arthroplasty (THA) implants assuming they were of equivalent design at 5 years of installation versus cementless at 3 years, as shown in Table 11.4. The limited number of cases of loosening was low and there was a subtle preference for cementless ones in terms of complete integration but the evaluation was done at two different time points [66]. A separate study found essentially no difference [67]. So in the end, what one gets is to some extent the patient's preference, the clinician's preference and experience level, and with some common negotiation, there is a selection of both a device and a process, assuming there is a need.

Table 11.4: Data from Pospula et al. [66] comparing cemented versus cementless devices. The cement less devices were assessed at 3 years and cemented devices at 5 years.

	Cemented # (%)	Cementless # (%)
Implant integration		
Cup and stem integrated	77 (88.5)	90 (95.7)
Possible cup and stem loosening	2 (2.3)	2 (2.1)
Definite isolated cup loosening	5 (5.7)	1 (1.1)
defininte isolated stem loosening	3 (3.5)	1 (1.1)

From data on about 180 implanted joints, there was a small preference for cementless devices that seemed better integrated at 3 years of follow up as opposed to 5 years post-op with cemented.

11.7 Point to the Future

Growth and evolution within orthopedic devices: If one considers the overall satisfaction linked with movement-based disorders, the highest potential for new developments seems tied to spinal augmentation. Pain tied to disk herniation, vertebral fractures, and the deteriorating quality of bone stock with age in the spine suggest that spinal load capacity needs further optimization. This is a lingering and pervasive problem and with the aging demographics in developed countries, streamlined processes to evaluate new and creative solutions to revitalize and stabilize existing spinal bone stock is well worth it.

In terms of joint replacements, there has already been a large effort to modularize components to create a system for more personalized care. Options that allow one to suggest individually sized cups and balls for hips based on the patient's needs and capacity, the ability to market gender specific components, and the potential to resolve long-term biomechanical alignment issues again through more modularity suggest a larger portfolio of devices and components to choose from as options and the ability to mix and match. At least in terms of typical joint replacements including hips and knees, evolutionary growth and system growth linked with alignment tools and robotic surgery seem to carry the day in terms of executing the wealth of currently performed procedures just a little bit better.

In terms of overall growth, TJR will expand in developing countries where these procedures are performed, and growth will occur in terms of the number of specialists who can perform joint replacements. In terms of growth areas relating to new joints or procedures, shoulder joint replacement is expanding in numbers and orthopedic device companies have directed new design efforts to replicate the joint in which the ball of the proximal humerus articulates against a socket embedded in the scapula. The design spectrum for shoulder replacement also includes swapping the articulating ball to the scapula and the socket to the humerus. Shoulder replacement in 2014 accounts for about 53K procedures in the United States, compared to almost 1M total hip and knee replacements annually [68]. The number of specialists in the United States is expected to grow, relative to more established joint replacement specialists in already established areas of joint replacement.

The bar for regulatory approval in shoulder joint replacement is low as the general materials strategies going into the design leverage materials being used in other joints already. Shapes, sizes, tapers, and profiles are all joint specific and shoulders should be no different. This shoulder operates in extension not in sliding compression, so the loading profile is quite a bit lower compared to knees and hips. The chance for dislocation is larger given the lack of compression during normal function. Attention to surviving ligament and soft tissue strength to maintain joint alignment are more crucial in shoulders than in knees and hips. There should be less wear overall even using the same articulating components in the shoulder and expected lifetimes for implants are expected to be longer than for knees and hips.

From an overall health care standpoint, it is interesting to consider the perceived value for hip and knee replacement over shoulder replacement. Ambulatory function is highly valued and has a huge impact on cardiovascular health and the cost to society for expanded capacity for wheelchair access is large. Patients with deteriorating shoulders are also in pain like those with lower back or knee pain but it is easier for them to get around. There may be a difference in how much the patient population is willing to subject themselves to in managing pain versus receiving a shoulder joint replacement.

In terms of joint replacement, dealing with the ravages of arthritis triggers is a competition between orthopedics, ergonomics, and immunology. If arthritis is a systemic condition, then replacing one joint may initially mitigate symptoms, but the source remains to cause joint deterioration elsewhere. The root cause for many types of joint inflammation disorders is linked with many different forms of autoimmune disorders including Lupus, Raynaud's syndrome, and more generally Rheumatoid Arthritis. Corticosteroids that lower the sensitivity of the immune system to trigger an autoimmune inflammatory response can work for acute periods, but they are concerns for long-term use. Separately, further amplification of inflammation can arise from overuse injuries and repetitive motion injuries that can lead one joint to be in much more need of medical attention than others. There is a general need to be aware that while larger use of joint replacement can be warranted, there might be other health interventions to reduce the demand and cost of treating the underlying conditions.

11.8 Thought Exercise: Short-Term Surgical Viability Versus Long-Term Survival

As a last thought exercise, it is worth considering more deeply this issue of implant lifetime. Currently, significant expense and qualification testing is performed to insure that constructed devices pass adequate sterility standards. Of the three most common sterilization methods, the temperatures achieved to perform steam autoclave sterilization are high enough to cause component distortion. Ethylene oxide gas sterilization is commonly available in the OR but there can be some residues from the gas exposure that are latently toxic which yields gamma irradiation as a dry sterilization method that can performed after complete packaging leading to a sterile package as well. The damage inflicted on the long-chain structure proteins and DNA linked with bacteria is high enough to render it and effective biocide. But there are consequences to the UHMWPE polymer chain length and structure particularly on machined surfaces. Lower molecular weight and potentially some additional secondary crystallization are noted, so the structure of the sterilized surface is less wear resistant than UHMPWE before sterilization. We observe that the initial wear rates of UHMWPE bearing surfaces in orthopedic devices are higher than in the bulk. That initial wear rate in the first year of usage is as high as five times that of a later year. If latent osteolysis potential is linked with producing enough particles to create an autoimmune response, maybe revisiting the process of how much to sterilize is worth considering.

For example, there have been comparisons of implant lifetime and the general consensus is that hips and knees last well past 20 years before a need for revision surgery presents in a large segment of implant recipients. It is complicated to get data on overall TJR performance when older patients are more commonly implanted. In recent history, there have been retrospective studies on younger patients (avg age of ~50) who have been implanted, and the data suggests that roughly 1 in 3 implants will last 30 years without revision surgery [69], as shown in Fig. 11.15. This is not to suggest that the group not being

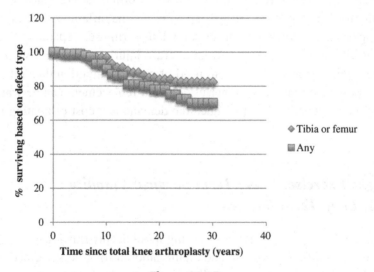

Figure 11.15
Example data on younger patients receiving knee implants. Data shows percentage free from revision surgery as a function of implantation time. The data suggests that roughly 2 in 3 have an expected implant survivorship of >30 years. *Data from W.J. Long, C.D. Bryce, C.S. Hollenbeak, R.W. Bener, W.N. Scott, Total knee replacement in young, active patients: long-term follow-up and functional outcome, J. Bone Jt. Surg. 96 (2014) e159(1−7).*

revised is pain free, but the results are promising. The general takeaway is that second generation devices created since the 1980s and 1990s, new surgical assist devices, and the knowledge gained from prior experience, new devices for similar joints have longer expected outcomes [69].

One reason why that outcome might not change is in part because materials development has been somewhat frozen given the large bar to increase the confidence in using any new material. These devices are sterilized to prevent infections introduced to the host during installation. During the last 30 years, manufacturing operations have become cleaner and larger use of gloves and handling equipment have reduced the potential for bacterial contamination on produced devices [70]. If 5 years of wear during the first year of device installation is produced, perhaps smaller irradiation doses could reduce that amount of wear and that one small change probably has a larger potential impact on implant lifetime than anything else one could propose. There is a trade-off between short-term concerns linked with immediate, postsurgical complications from installation and the long-term potential of an improved device lifetime. It is worth thinking about whether its worth sterilizing in a way that damages the implant components so clearly at the outset.

11.9 Other Schemes to Reduce the Wear on Sterilized Surfaces

With the idea that a sterilized UHMWPE surface is more likely to wear more upon installation, there have been efforts to use thermal treatments, the incorporation of antioxidants, and crosslinking schemes to reduce the cause the less wear resistant structures found on the bearing surface to be more resistant to wear. The rationale is that oxidized materials on the surface following sterilization are smaller in molecular weight and potentially more easily extracted from the bulk under wear conditions. The notion of the chemical crosslinking of the surface or heat treatment is to cause the higher energy oxidized chains to be interconnected [71] or engulfed in the bulk [72] of the structure presenting more of the virgin material back onto the surface. The annealing procedures are performed at temperatures either just below or just above the melting point ($\sim 140°C$ for UHMWPE) with the idea that the lower energy chains migrate to the surface and the oxidized chains dive into the bulk. Conceptually, this is a good idea, but how it is reconciled with the need for sterilization is somewhat unknown, as this subsequent posttreatment raises the question of whether the original radiation exposure was even needed.

A number of current studies have described the use of tocopherol derivatives based on vitamin E extracts in concentrations as high as 1% by weight as radical scavengers, although some of the early antioxidants considered are part of the Irganox series like Irganox 1010. Exposure to radiation to eliminate microbes that might be attached or incorporated within these resins has been done both with and without vitamin E [72]. The net effect of radiation damage shortening chains increases the level of the crystallinity on the surfaces. The presence of antioxidants appears to lower the amount of chain cleavage and levels of crystallinity are similar to that preradiation exposure. The takeaway is that through more advanced formulation including the use of potential antioxidants, more of the original wear resistant, long-chain architecture can remain on implant surfaces leading to lower effective wear rates during usage.

11.10 Conclusions

In this chapter, schemes to address trauma and chronic needs in orthopedics have been presented. Obviously traumatic injury large enough to trigger bone failure generally require a need to stabilize the failed bone region. There are other types of failures that relate to the ligaments and tendons that stabilize joints. Demonstrations of xenografting schemes are available, but it will be hard to replicate the functionality of current ligament autografts for performance. Presentations of solutions to stabilize vertebral compression fractures are also found in Chapter 11, Orthopaedic Biomaterials and Strategies.

Interventions to address more chronic osteodegenerative joint disorder and its corresponding pain include scheduled procedures to replace the articulating surfaces often by a series of integrated components required to create a bearing surface articulation usually matched to replicate lost joint function. A mature industry supporting hip and knee arthroplasty has developed and new opportunities exist for less commonly replaced joints including the shoulder, elbow, and ankle. The easy success and enormous impact achieved by liberating people from wheelchairs and allowing them to walk through hip and knee joint replacement has a tangible return on people's ability to navigate faster and more nimbly through daily activities. The impact from focusing on other joints from a development standpoint may not be as clear. But it is a ripe area of further experimental consideration and the human ankle, with its range of motion, its grueling performance standards for viability with such little bone stock is really an amazing feature of natural bioengineering.

11.11 Problems

1. A titanium/air composite is made using $E_{\text{titanium}} = 110$ GPa, that follows a "rule of mixtures" behavior, $E_{\text{composite}} = v_i E_i$, where v_i and E_i are the volume fractions and modulus of the ith, determine how much porosity is needed to match the stiffness of cortical bone.

2. Orthopedic UHMWPE erodes with a first year wear rate of 0.5 mm/year dropping linearly to a constant 0.1 mm/year at year 5 and beyond. The surface area of the acetabulum is a hemisphere 30 mm in diameter. Show a plot of the volumetric mass loss versus time eroded from UHMWPE over the first 10 years of life assuming even wear across the whole hemisphere. Calculate the cumulative particle emission process at 1 and 10 years assuming that the particles are 1 μm in diameter, what if they are smaller (0.3 μm in diameter).

3. Explain whether its more important to retain high strength or high modulus of elasticity in materials used in fracture fixation.

4. Obviously with an external fixator strategy, the transdermally installed pins run the risk of bacterial infection. Explain why a surgeon might recommend the use of an external fixator to address a fracture of a structural bone segment?

5. Explain why the use of injectable bone cements in kyphoplasty is considered safer than the same cement used as a grout in TJR.

6. If diagnostic imaging improves to the point of identifying degenerative joint disease earlier, explain what impact does this new knowledge has on future joint replacement surgeries. In other words, what therapeutic alternatives are there to TJR.

7. Tissue engineering efforts have been targeted augmenting schemes to upregulate cartilage growth and regeneration. Consider how one might be able to integrate biologically synthesized cartilage in vitro in degenerative joint disease and describe the technical challenges in yielding a stable and functional joint following some level of deterioration.

8. The construction of fracture fixation rods and plates with predrilled holes is commonplace. What impact does the presence of the unfilled holes have on plates loaded in bending?

9. Are larger or smaller holes better from a strength standpoint, all other things being equal.

10. The total joint recipient is commonly analyze diagnostically by X-ray annually to track bearing cup recession using polymer bearings. What kind of resolution is needed in X-ray to be able to assess wear if the hemisphere of the cup is 6 mm thick?

11. What kind of diagnostic assessment can be done in patients with metal on metal implants and what might one want to know after implantation?

12. Do some research and explain why synthetic total joints are so commonplace while so rare for ligament replacement in comparison to transplant?

13. An extracted ligament component has a very low modulus region if allowed to retract since it is isolated. Is there any benefit in replicating this unstressed toe-region response in a synthetic ligament?

References

[1] C.E.D.H. De Laet, B.A. Van Hout, H. Burger, A. Hofman, H.A.P. Pols, Bone density and risk of hip fractrue in men and women: cross sectional analysis, Br. Med. J. 315 (1997) 221.

[2] C.D. Newton, D.M. Nunamaker, Textbook of Small Animal Orthopaedics, Lippencott, Philadelphia, 1985.

[3] Helfet, D.L. Wrist Fractures, Hospital for Special Surgery 2014. Available from: <http://www.hss.edu/orthopedic-trauma-case46-wrist-fractures.asp>.

[4] A.E. Freeland, J.E. Torres, Extraarticular fractures of the phalanges, in: R.A. Berger, A.P.C. Weiss (Eds.), Hand Surgery, Lippencott, Williams and Wilkins, Philadelphia, 2004, pp. 123–138.

[5] J.B. Kamath, Harshvardhan, D.M. Nalk, A. Bansal, Current concepts in managing fractures of metacarpal and phalangess, Indian J. Plast. Surg. 44 (2011) 203–211.

[6] T.J. Bray, Techiques in Fracture Fixation, Gower Medical Publishing, New York, 1993.

[7] E. Arendt, R. Dick, Knee injuries among men and women in collegiate basketball and soccer, Am. J. Sports Med. 23 (1995) 694–701.

[8] Anterior Cruciate Ligament Repair. Available from: <http://www.nytimes.com/slideshow/2007/08/01/health/100230Anteriorcruciateligamentrepairseries_index.html>, 2007 (cited 06.04.15).

[9] ACL Graft Choices. Available from: <http://www.orthoassociates.com/SP11B35/>, 2015.

[10] I.H. Lieberman, S. Dudeney, M.K. Reinhardt, G. Bell, Initial outcome and efficacy of "kyphoplasty" in the treatment of painful osteoporotic vertebral compression fractures, Spine 26 (2001) 1631–1638.

[11] Rau, R. THe Human Mortality Database. Available from: <http://www.mortality.org>; 2015.

[12] J. Oeppen, J.W. Vaupel, Broken limits to life expectancy, Science 296 (2002) 1029–1031.

[13] Y. Robinson, C.E. Heyde, P. Forsth, C. Olerud, Kyphoplasty in osteoporotic vertebralncompression fractures—guidelines and technical considerations, J. Orthop. Surg. 6 (2011) 43.

[14] G. Lewis, L.H. Koole, C.S.J. van Hooy-Corstjens, Influence of powder-to-liquid monomer ratio on properties of an injectable iodine-containing acrylic bone cement for vertebroplasty and balloon kyphoplasty, J. Biomed. Mater. Res. Part B—Appl. Biomater. 91 (2009) 537–544.

[15] Z. Maric, R.J. Haynes, Total hip arthroplasty in juvenile rheumatoid arthritis, Clin. Orthop. Relat. Res. 290 (1993) 197–199.

[16] N.D. Clement, S.J. Breusch, L.C. Biant, Lower limb joint replacement in rheumatoid arthritis, J. Orthop. Surg. Res. 7 (2012) 27–34.

[17] A.F. Mourao, M. Amaral, J. Caetano-Lopes, D. Isenberg, An analysis of joint replacement in patients with systemic lupus erythematosus, Lupus. 18 (2009) 1298–1302.

[18] T.C. Cymet, V. Sinkov, Does long-distance running cause osteoarthritis? J. Am. Osteopath. Assoc. 106 (2006) 342–345.

[19] B. Fitzgerald, G.R. McLactchie, Degenerative joint disease in weight-lifters. Fact or fiction? Br. J. Sports Med. 14 (1980) 97–101.

[20] A.D. Woolf, B. Pfleger, Burden of major musculoskeletal conditions, Bull. World Health Organ. 81 (2003) 646–656.

[21] P.T. Williams, Effects of running and walking on osteoarthritis and hip replacement risk, Med. Sci. Sports Exerc. 45 (2013) 1292–1297.

[22] H. Koepp, W. Eger, C. Muehleman, A. Valdellon, J.A. Buckwalter, K.E. Kuettner, et al., Prevalence of articular degeration in the ankle and knee joints of human organ donors, J. Orthop. Sci. 4 (1999) 407–412.

[23] S.D. Bos, P.E. Slagboom, I. Meulenbelt, New insights into osteoarthritis: early developmental features of an ageing-related disease, Curr. Opin. Rheumatol. 20 (2008) 553–559.

[24] F. Hefti, Pediatric Orthopedics in Practice, second ed, Springer, Berlin, 2015.

[25] S. Boisgard, S. Descamps, B. Bouillet, Complex primary total hip arthroplasty, Orthop. Traumatol.: Surg. Res. 99 (2013) S34–S42.

[26] Behrang, A. Coxa Vaxa. Available from: <http://en.wikipedia.org/wiki/Coxa_vara#mediaviewer/File:FemurAngles.jpg>, 2011.

[27] Novick, N. Femoral Osteotomy: An Overview and an Interview with Robert L. Buly, MD. Available from: <https://www.hss.edu/conditions_femoral-osteotomy-overview.asp>, 2015.

[28] R.W. Crawford, D.W. Murray, Total hip replacement: indications for surgery and risk factors for failure, Ann. Rheum. Dis. 56 (1997) 455−457.

[29] F. Fassier, Z. Sardar, M. Aarabi, T. Odent, T. Haque, R. Hamdy, Results and complications of a surgical technique for correction of coxa vara in children with osteopenic bones, J. Pediatr. Orthop. 28 (2008) 799−805.

[30] M.E. Torchia, R.A. Klassen, A.J. Bianco, Total hip arthroplasty with cement in patients less than twenty years old. Long-term results, J. Bone Jt. Surg. Am. 78 (1996) 995−1003.

[31] J.C. Allard, G. Porter, R.W. Ryerson, Occult posttraumatic avascular necrosis of hip revealed by MRI, Magn. Reson. Imaging. 10 (1992) 155−159.

[32] J. Arlet, Nontraumatic avascular necrosis of the femoral head, Clin. Orthop. Relat. Res. 277 (1992) 12−21.

[33] W. Drescher, M. Alarifi, An update on femoral head necrosis, Minerva Ortop. E Traumatol. 64 (2013) 15−24.

[34] D. Weldon, The effects of corticosteroids on bone: osteonecrosis (avascular necrosis of the bone), Ann. Allergy Asthma Immunol. 103 (2009) 91−97.

[35] P.J. Favorito, W.M. Mihalko, K.A. Krackow, Total knee arthroplasty in the valgus knee, J. Am. Acad. Orthop. Surg. 10 (2002) 16−24.

[36] J. Charnley, Femoral Prosthesis, United States Patent 4,021,865, 1977.

[37] E.J. Harboush, Femoral Prosthesis for the Hip Joint, United States Patent 2,668,531, 1954.

[38] P. Frederick, R. Walter, D. Harwood, R. Kepley, Hip Replacement Incision Locator, United States Patent 7,901,411, 2011.

[39] I. Radinsky, M. Chasse, L.P. Amiot, D. Odermatt, Leg Alignment for Surgical Parameter Measurement in Hip Replacement Surgery, United States Patent 7,955,280, 2011.

[40] D. Odermatt, R. Bassik, C. Wu, D. Landeck, J. Wojick, Surgical Robotic Systems with Manual and Haptic and/or Active Control Modes, United States Patent 8,498,744, 2013.

[41] A.L. Lippincott, J.B. Medley, Low Wear Ball and Cup Joint Prosthesis, United States Patent 6,059,830, 2000.

[42] M.B. Sheldon, N.G. Dong, Acetabular Cup Assembly with Selected Bearing, United States Patent 6,475,243, 2002.

[43] H. Derar, M. Shahinpoor, Recent Patents and Designs on Hip Replacement Prostheses, Open Biomed. Eng. J. 9 (2015) 92−102.

[44] T.B. Pace, K.C. Keith, E. Alvarez, R.G. Snider, S.L. Tanner, J.D. Desjardins, Comparison of conventional polyethylene wear and signs of cup failure in two similar total hip designs, Adv. Orthop. 2013 (2013) Article ID: 710621, http://dx.doi.org/10.1155/2013/710621.

[45] K.F. Orishimo, A.M. Claus, C.J. Sychterz, C.A. Engh, Relationship between polyethylene wear and osteolysis in hips with a second-generation porous-coated cementless cup after seven years of follow-up, J. Bone Jt. Surgery 85A (2003) 1095−1099.

[46] T. Tateishi, T. Terui, H. Yunoki, Friction and wear properties for biomaterials for artificial joint, Bioceramics 2 (1990) 145−151.

[47] The US Food and Drug Administration, FDA. Information for Patients Who Have Metal-on-Metal Hip Implants. Available from: <http://www.fda.gov/MedicalDevices/ProductsandMedicalProcedures/ImplantsandProsthetics/MetalonMetalHipImplants/ucm241766.htm>, 2015.

[48] A.M. Crugnola, E.L. Radin, R.M. Rose, I.L. Paul, S.R. Simon, M.B. Berry, Ultrahigh molecular weight polyethylene as used in articular prostheses (A molecular weight distribution study), J. Appl. Polym. Sci. 20 (1976) 809−812.

[49] J.H. Dumbleton, M.T. Manley, A.A. Edidin, A literature review of the association between wear rate and osteolysis in total hip arthroplasty, J. Arthroplasty 17 (2002) 649−661.

[50] A.P.D. Elfick, S.L. Smith, A. Unsworth, Variation in the wear rate during the life of a total hip arthroplasty, J. Arthroplasty 15 (2000) 901−908.

[51] M. Jasty, D.D. Goetz, C.R. Bragdon, K.R. Lee, A.E. Hanson, J.R. Elder, et al., Wear of polyethylene acetabular components in total hip arthroplasty: an analysis of 128 components retrieved at autopsy or revision operations, J. Bone Jt. Surg., American 79 (1997) 349.

[52] C.J. Sychterz, K.H. Moon, Y.E.A. Hashimoto, K.M. Terefenko, C.A. Engh, T.W. Bauer, Wear of polyethlene cups in total hip arthroplasty, J. Bone Jt. Surg. Am. 78 (1996) 1193.

[53] Z. Lu, H. McKellop, Frictional heating of bearing materials tested in a hip joint wear simulator, Proc. Inst. Mech. Eng. 21 (1997) 101−108.

[54] G.G. Polkowski, J.J. Callaghan, M.A. Mont, J.C. Clohisy, Total arthroplasty in the very young patient, J. Am. Acad. Orthop. Surg. 20 (2012) 487−497.

[55] N. Bilsel, A. Gokce, H. Kesmezacar, E. Mumcuoglu, H. Ozdogan, Long-term results of total hip arthroplasty in patients with juvenile arthritis, Acta. Orthop. Traumatol. Turc. 42 (2008) 119−124.

[56] L.D. Dorr, M. Luckett, J.P. Conaty, Total hip arthroplasties in patients younger than 45 years: a nine- to ten-year follow-up study, Clin. Orthop. Relat. Res. 260 (1990) 215−219.

[57] L.D. Dorr, T.J. Kane III, J.P. Conaty, Long term results of cemented total hip arthroplasty in patients 45 years old or younger: a 16-year follow-up study, J. Arthroplasty 9 (1994) 453−456.

[58] H.P. Chandler, F.T. Reineck, R.L. Wixson, J.C. McCarthy, Total hip replacement in patients younger than thirty years old: a five-year follow-up study, J. Bone Jt. Surg. 63 (1981) 1426−1434.

[59] M.J. Chmell, R.D. Scott, W.H. Thomas, C.B. Sledge, Total hip arthroplasty with cement for juvenile rheumatoid arthritis: results at a minimum of ten years in patients less than thirty years old, J. Bone Jt. Surg. (Am.) 79 (1997) 44−52.

[60] D.H. Sochart, M.L. Porter, Long-term results of cemented Charnley low- friction arthroplasty in patients aged less than 30 years, J. Arthroplasty 13 (1998) 123−131.

[61] C. Ruddlesdin, B.M. Ansell, G.P. Arden, M. Swann, Total hip replacement in children with juvenile chronic arthritis, J. Bone Jt. Surg. 68 (1986) 218−222.

[62] J.D. Witt, M. Swann, B.M. Ansell, Total hip replacement for juvenile chronic arthritis, J. Bone J. Surg. 73 (1991) 770−773.

[63] I.D. Learmouth, A.W. Heywood, J. Kaye, D. Dall, Radiological loosening after cemented hip replacement for juvenile chronic arthritis, J. Bone Jt. Surg. 71 (1989) 209−212.

[64] P.F. Lachiewicz, B. McCaskill, A. Inglis, C.S. Ranawat, B.D. Rosenstein, Total hip arthroplasty in juvenile rheumatoid arthritis: Two- to eleven-year results, J. Bone Jt. Surg. (Am.) 68 (1986) 502−508.

[65] D.K. Halley, J. Charnley, Results of low friction arthroplasty in patients thirty years of age or younger, Clin. Orthop. Relat. Res. 112 (1975) 180−191.

[66] W. Pospula, T. Abu Noor, T. Roshady, A. Al Mukaimi, Cemented and Cementless Total Hip Replacement: Critical Analysis and Comparison of Clinical and Radiological Results of 182 Cases Operated in Al Razi Hospital, Kuwait, Med. Princ. Pract. 17 (2008) 239−243.

[67] C.M. Rorabeck, R.B. Bourne, A. Laupacis, D. Feeny, C. Wong, P. Tugwell, et al., A Double-Blind Study of 250 Cases Comparing Cemented With Cementless Total Hip Arthroplasty: Cost-Effectiveness and Its Impact on Health-Related Quality of Life, Clin. Orthop. Relat. Res. 298 (1994) 156−164.

[68] Wiater, J.M. Shoulder Joint Replacement. Available from: <http://orthoinfo.aaos.org/topic.cfm?topic = A00094>, 2011 (cited 2015).

[69] W.J. Long, C.D. Bryce, C.S. Hollenbeak, R.W. Bener, W.N. Scott, Total knee replacement in young, active patients: long-term follow-up and functional outcome, J. Bone Jt. Surg. 96 (2014) e159 (1−7).

[70] W. Whyte, H.H. Schicht, The Design of Cleanrooms for the Medical Device Industry, Cleanroom Design, John Wiley, New York, pp. 123−139, Chapter 5, ISBN: 9780471942047.

[71] O.K. Muratoglu, C.R. Bragdon, D.O. O'Connor, M. Jasty, W.H. Harris, A novel method of cross-linking ultra-high-molecular-weight polyethylene to improve wear, reduce oxidation, and retain mechanical properties—recipient of the 1999 HAP Paul Award, J. Arthroplasty 16 (2001) 149–160.

[72] E. Oral, B.W. Ghali, O.K. Muratoglu, The elimination of free radicals in irradiated UHMWPEs with andwithout vitamin E stabilization by annealing under pressure, J. Biomed. Mater. Res. Part B—Appl. Biomater. 97B (2011) 167–174.

CHAPTER 12

Neural Interventions

Learning Objectives

With so many other successes in other subdisciplines of medicine, including orthopedics and cardiology, the skeletal structure, and adequate cardiac perfusion can often be augmented or maintained to sustain average people well into their 80s and beyond. It is also evident that quality-of-life issues are just as related to cognitive function. Using an architectural analogy, it does not help much if the framing is solid and the water pipes are sound but nobody is home due to some profound functional neurological morbidity. This chapter presents the types of conditions that lead to clinical material needs in the neurovasculature, how those conditions are presented as symptoms, and the types of materials and deployment schemes that can lower the risk of ischemia and rupture. If untreated, the continued growth of aneurysms that can lead to significant functional morbidities and sudden death. As learning objectives, one should come away from reading this chapter with

- a larger understanding of both endovascular and exovascular procedures that are used to modulate cerebrovascular blood flow
- the types of materials involved in creating a functional response
- Potential risk/reward scenarios involved in neurological interventions
- Opportunities for the future

12.1 Introduction

Increasingly, there are needs to also modulate vascular circulation further downstream from the heart. We are learning more about typical and abnormal cerebrovascular architecture as well as vascular malformations identified in other areas through better diagnostic imaging modalities, particularly angiography and functional MRI as we can now link thoughts, sights, sounds, smells, actions, and reasoning to different parts of the brain mid-experience. Due to advances discussed in Chapter 3, Bones and Mineralized Tissues and Chapter 10, Nanomaterials and Phase Contrast Imaging Agents, patients who present both as ER-type trauma cases can be imaged and the severity or presence of a vascular bleed or vascular ischemia can be gauged. The types of conditions that can lead to a need for diagnostic imaging include severe headaches, imminent vision and speech problems, muscle weakness and partial paralysis, vertigo, dizziness, tinnitus, and moodiness, and irritability. When one is originally diagnosed identifying a vascular anomaly, the playbook includes confirming whether the presented symptoms correlate with any observed vascular malformation and assessments are also made about the relative urgency for intervention. Not to make interventional neuroradiologists out of anyone reading this book, but there is a lot to learn about the link between anatomy and physiology as our tools for diagnosis are developing real time. There are much more relevant clinical assessments at least relating to anatomy and readers are pointed to [1,2] for a much more detailed view of neuroanatomy.

From a vascular flow perspective, there are two main end points cerebrovascular clinicians focus on, including both ischemias (blockages) and vessel weakening (aneursysms) as potential locations for eventual rupture. In other words, clinicians are concerned with understanding the link between the symptoms observed and the presence of a blockage or other abnormality. Blockages are considered very urgent, requiring immediate intervention to restore normal cerebrovascular function and to later assess any functional morbidity. Ruptured aneurysms are also considered critical and other nonruptured aneurysms usually trigger an observation phase to assess the urgency for intervention. A stable aneurysm does not change shape or dimension, while a weakening one grows in size and thins the vascular wall even further.

Readers are probably aware of so-called clot-busting drugs (alteplase, for example) deployed for ischemic stroke patients who are routed to critical care facilities early on in the onset of their ischemia [3]. These drugs deconstruct the ischemia and if normal circulation is reestablished within hours of the blockage, functional morbidities can, in some instances, be minimized. It does not mean people fully recover but in many instances, the profound debilitating consequences can be averted. Key for this is rapid diagnosis to identify blockage during that critical time window.

Larger risks are associated with ruptures, often linked with aneurysm with physical examples of both fusiform and berry aneurysm defects shown in Figs. 12.1 and 12.2. The most common fusiform defect is that of the aorta but other bulging defects that do not lead to formation of a narrowing aneurysm neck are called fusiform defects. Berry or secular aneurysms, outcroppings from the vasculature that arise from a weakened blood vessel are the more common type experienced in the neurovasculature. It is thought that between 2% and 5% of the population is at risk for aneurysm formation, although a large percentage (as high as 80%) of these are unreported and it is the rupture that often commences with the initial diagnosis [4]. What is striking is that for cerebral aneurysms, they occur in people in the prime of their life, between 35 and 60 most commonly. Women, for whatever reason, encounter aneurysm over men by a 3/2 ratio [5]. For someone with a bleeding cerebral aneurysm rupture, the outcomes are much more stark and can lead to internal bleed-out and death in roughly 40% of cases and of those who survive, more than half will have some sort of neurological deficit as a result of the bleed [5].

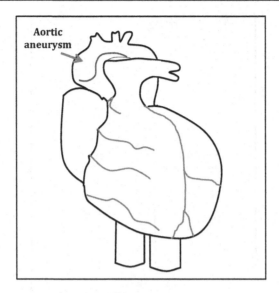

Figure 12.1
Fusiform aortic aneurysm seen as a bulge in the ascending aorta region in this representation.

There are many open questions about who is at risk for aneurysm formation. It seems reasonable to consider that those with hypertension and arthrosclerosis present higher arterial wall pressure and are stressing their vascular system more. Weakened vessels are more likely to distend in a hypertensive patient than one with normal blood pressure. There are a range of genetic connective tissue disorders such as Ehlers Danlos syndrome and Marfan's syndrome that seem to correlate with higher presentation for aortic aneurysm and other locations for aneurysms as well [6].

It is also worth noting that if one is diagnosed with an aneurysm, it does not mean that the aneurysm is destined to rupture. Neurologists discuss risk in the form of an accumulated living risk of about 1% chance for rupture per year one is living with the condition [7]. The larger the defect, the higher the perceived level of wall weakening and the higher the probability of rupture [8]. Some diagnosed aneursysms are congenital as one has been living with it all along. As one lives with the documented anomaly longer, there is a perceived reduction in the risk since if one reaches middle age with it failing, there is a growing sense that even though its an aneurysm, it might be stable and the risk/reward scenario linked with intervention isn't necessarily worth it.

A significant complication is that cerebrovascular brain access and heart access are quite different beasts. For a long time, the most common cerebrovascular intervention was by craniotomy, often an emergency procedure if presenting with an ischemia or a brain bleed in the ER. By then, things run their course and it is obviously an emergency case. Perhaps of more profound value are the instances in which these abnormalities have been diagnosed

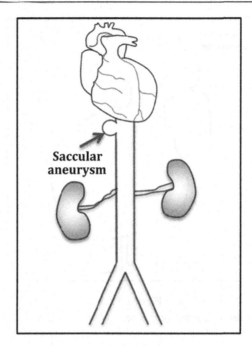

Figure 12.2
An example of a berry or saccular aneurysm—these usually form at the junctions of
y and t connections in the vasculature.

but have not led to either an ischemia or a rupture. In those instances, the neurosurgeons
have time on their side and can plan for more refined surgical interventions, faster recovery
times, and better outcomes.

12.2 Aneurysm and Cerebrovascular Modulation

Armed with good diagnostics to identify the vascular or cerebrovascular abnormality and
with some assurances that the defect is stable to imminent collapse or rupture,
neurosurgeons and radiologists can plan their strategy based on defect location, size, and
what is defined as eloquence, the attribute linked with how critical this location is to brain
function. Generally, the shorter the line of sight, the higher the likelihood that an
exovascular intervention will be easier to complete by a partial craniotomy in which the
cored bone segment can be reinstalled after intervention.

12.2.1 Clips

The exovascular approach to accommodate the presence of an aneurysm requires the
deployment of vascular clips that are placed at the neck of a berry aneurysm. Berry

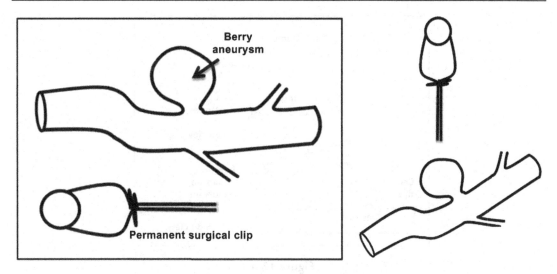

Figure 12.3
An example permanent surgical clip for isolating a berry aneurysm from the rest of the vasculature. Clipping the aneurysm reduces the pressure on the aneurysm wall and lowers the chance of a larger brain bleedout.

aneurysms resemble a balloon in which the distal orb of vascular wall expands into a sphere. In many instances, these berry aneurysms have a smaller junction with the vascular wall and comparisons are made about the radius of the balloon sphere or dome relative to the neck radius abutting the vessel wall. If there is a large disparity, the clip can isolate the weakened balloon region from the wall region and if the balloon ruptures, the clip is there to prevent a bleed out. An example is the Yasargil aneurysm clip system as shown below in Fig. 12.3 [9].

Examples of the clips deployed adjacent to models of aneurysms are shown in Fig. 12.4.

There are design details about the binding force for each clip, what it is made from, the tool that can be used to deploy it, etc. Metallic clips are produced from a range of alloys, including austenitic stainless steels, pure titanium and titanium alloys, and Co−Cr−Ni alloys. Undesirable alloys would include martensitic stainless steels that might be of the right composition but have a morphology that retains a high magnetic moment [10]. There have been prototype work to make hybrid polymer−metal clips from Co−Cr alloys and titanium as the spring component and the limbs of the clip from carbon fiber reinforced epoxy resin and polymethyl methacrylate [11]. Performance attributes of a competitive new type of clip would include constant clamping force, dimensional variance with clamping time, and reduced observable artifact during diagnostic imaging [11], A larger aneurysm might require more than one clip as part of the overall sealing strategy as shown in Figs. 12.5 and 12.6.

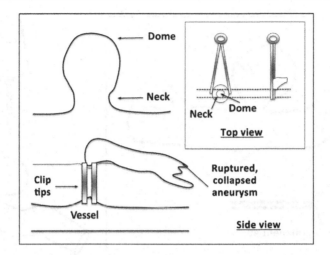

Figure 12.4
Schematic showing the berry aneurysm clipped and initially decaying. Plane and section views
showing the deployment of the clip from above and from the side also showing the decay
of the aneurysm isolated from the vasculature. If the residual aneurysm ruptures, the clip
prevents a bleed.

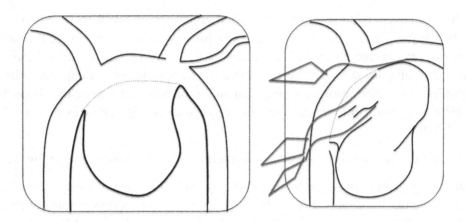

Figures 12.5 and 12.6
Treatment of an anterior communicating artery aneurysm by multiple clips. The aneurysm
is shown as a berry and the isolation from a group of 3 clips is shown From [12].

Better outcomes are found for clips when the vascular abnormality is closer to the skull
edge and easy surgical incisions can be made allowing access for deploying clips. Recovery
time is based on the ease of the surgical entry and functional morbidities are assessed along
with physical therapy as needed to enhance the recovery. But as with other surgeries, the
time for recovery can be on the order of weeks.

Some aneurysms that cannot be accommodated by clipping are called fusiform bulges with no real aneurysm neck. Fusiform aneurysms often have a smaller distinction between the radii of the defect and the vessel. The most common vessel forming fusiform aneurysms is the aorta, while berry aneurysms often form on the opposite side of a t joint with one artery feeding two adjacent ones. Deeper and more eloquent locations are also less promising as clippable sites as more gray matter is traversed in conducting the craniotomy to allow for installation. In recent years, more attention has been placed on so-called endovascular procedures.

Until the capacity to develop catheters that could be fed to the brain, there was not much that could be done to address patients with identified vascular malformations that were so deep or in such functionally relevant locations as to preclude any exovascular intervention. The collateral damage was often too great and so the involved neurologists attempted to manage symptoms that could include vertigo, tinnitus, and seizures, often through medications. Catheters are now sufficiently developed that allow for faster and more efficient transport to the brain by so-called flow-based catheters. In essence, by femoral catheterization, it is possible to direct functional catheters to areas of abnormal blood flow in the brain, where an aneurysm exists and fill it from the inside. There is a range of devices coupled with deployment catheters in which an embolic agent is added to trigger a clot within the balloon.

12.2.2 Coils

The most common choices for embolic agents are platinum-based coil rod stock that is fed through a catheter to fill the inside of the cavity formed by the aneurysm. The most common coils are what are defined as Gugliemi detachable coils, also made from platinum wire [13]. The platinum is produced in coiled rolls but the shape memory qualities of the metal allow it to bend and form an internal coil structure during deployment as shown conceptually in Fig. 12.7 [14]. It is defined as detachable and the material is susceptible to resistive heating at low currents allowing for its separation from the catheter. The interaction between the coil material and platelets triggers their activation and the goal is to fill sufficiently to clot within the interior portion of the aneurysm. Again, berry aneurysms are easier to fill with a discrete neck region than a fusiform aneurysm and once the clot is established, the vascular pressure displacing the aneurysm wall is decoupled by the presence of the clot. There are both continuous rod stock and discontinuous thin sections of extruded coil material that can present more surfaces to the platelets. Without direct line of sight as with craniotomy with the neurosurgeon capable of looking at the defect, there are needs for remote observational capacity that is accomplished by the continuous fluoroscopy that allows one to track both the catheter placement but the subsequent filling process.

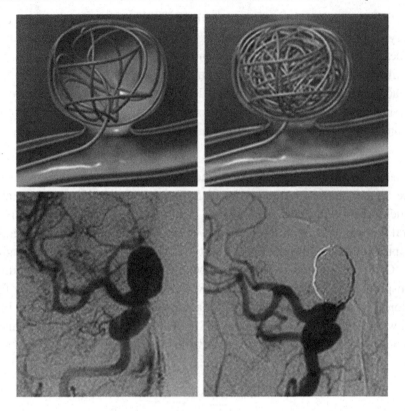

Figure 12.7
Schematic of partially and fully filled aneurysm and the bottom images are a representative berry aneurysm before and after coiling. The fast that the phase contrast fluid is not observed in the aneurysm after treatment confirms the decoupling of pressure on the aneurysm wall. *Reproduction courtesy of the Society of Neurointerventional Surgery, www.snisonline.org.*

More types of potential aneurysms can be accommodated using coils. If the neck of the berry aneurysm is large, it is possible to fill the interior of the berry with the coil materials and decouple the stress through a stent that helps to wall off the berry more effectively if the stent seals the internal vasculature from the berry [15] as shown conceptually in Fig. 12.8.

Coiling generally works very well. Complications with coils arise as reasonable volumetric filling of the aneurysm by the coil material is needed. The coil or wire needs to be engineered so that it does not perforate the already weakened vessel wall. Doing so essentially creates a physician-induced aneurysm rupture. There are other complications that can arise or the coil material is not homogeneously distributed sufficiently and thus the pressure remains on the wall. It is also possible that the coil material is not completely housed within the aneurysm. If some fraction of the coil material is misplaced and

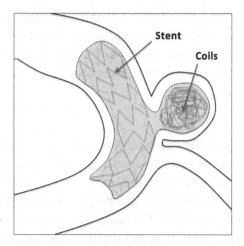

Figure 12.8
Schematic of a combined coiling and stenting procedure. Overall, the scheme is to eliminate pressure on the aneurysm wall.

protruding into the functional vasculature, there is a later inherent risk that clotting will occur downstream from where the aneurysm is located, as platelets, activated by their surface interaction, trigger a clotting cascade leading to a later ischemia.

From a materials development perspective, better coil materials than what is currently used will lead to a more robust and controlled coagulation response for successful aneurysm filling procedure. If the coil material was easier to dispense, had less chance to rupture the weakened vessel, and remained distributed within the aneurysm, these would positive attributes for any new embolic coil material.

What is amazing to consider is that the process of filling an aneurysm endovascularly is essentially an outpatient procedure. Yes, there are risks and complications from the installation of a functional catheter but this temporary installation requires effectively no surgery and recovery with monitoring is all that is needed to track the metabolism of the anesthesia. There is a wider volume of the brain that is capable of being treated endovascularly than with craniotomy, so recovery is much faster and the risks linked with functional morbidities to create line of site for clipping are superfluous. The capacity to develop endovascular interventions is a disruptive technology in neurosurgery and has real potential to reduce overall health care costs at least in aneurysm defects.

12.2.3 Embolic Fluids

If the placement of the hard coils runs the risk of rupturing the already weakened vessels, perhaps other softer, fluid-based deployment strategies can be employed that lead to fewer, rupture-based complications. The notion of fluids and dispersions that either passively or actively solidify into gels has been formulated have performed rather nicely. Here, the goal is not necessarily a clot-induced solidification but if the fluid can fill the defect and precipitate or gel, the same decoupling of fluid stress can be achieved.

12.2.3.1 Dispersion-based Embolics

The most successful dispersions have used biocompatible polymers dissolved in an appropriate biocompatible solvent that can dissipate in vivo. A common solvent is dimethyl sulfoxide, DMSO, a liquid that is both metabolizable and dispersible once injected. The notion is that solutions of soluble polymers like polyethylene vinyl alcohol copolymers or others for that matter, dissolved in DMSO or some other appropriate biocompatible solvent, can be directly injected into the aneurysm and that over time, the DMSO permeates other tissues away from the interstices of the berry aneurysm but solvent transmission does not allow for the separate permeation of the polymer which concentrates and ultimately precipitates in the aneurysm, as shown in Fig. 12.9 [16].

A sufficient amount of injected polymer can successfully isolate the aneurysm wall from the vasculature, thus reducing the potential for aneurysm rupture. Higher concentration polymer solutions are more viscous and difficult to dispense, so multiple injections of more dilute solutions has been common practice, The benefit of liquid filling aneurysm is that there is less potential of directly puncturing the aneurysm wall. The spurious transport of liquid media outside of the aneurysm and downstream is a recurring latent risk.

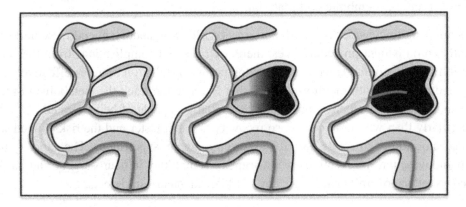

Figure 12.9
Schematic of injectable embolic therapy in which a dispersion precipitates into the aneurysm. A catheter is introduced into the embolism and the goal is the fill the aneurysm with fluid that will gel (in dark) and decouple the internal blood pressure from the walls of the aneurysm. The aneurysm is commonly filled in progressive stages going from left to right.

12.2.3.2 Reactive Liquid Embolics

The high viscosity of concentrated polymeric solutions suggests that perhaps there is a mix and set scheme that could yield low molecular weight reactants that are mixed or easily dispersed into the balloon cavity with the idea of a rapid polymerization or crosslinking reaction. There are already schemes for considering this using tissue sealants for anastomoses and other wound healing. The overall goal with this type of strategy would be a well-controlled, clinician-dictated procedure ideally in which the neurosurgeon can insure the resin is situated in the correct location prior to triggering the solidification reaction. Any other reactive resin would need a trigger like light, pH, or a temperature change for converting the resin, although the resin requires an invariance to the continuous fluoroscopy. Ideally, the catheter might also need to be adapted to include the potential the aspirate and redispense misdeployed resin.

The catheter design for a reactive embolic fluid dispensing is more complicated than simpler catheters that have fewer design requirements. Any requirements for mixing need to be addressed with the design, as does any other functional trigger such as a resistive heating element, light, acid, or base titration to somehow activate the resin, etc. The issue giving the clinician optimum control including the ability to dispense and redispense is probably best dealt with by a multilumen catheter and there are likely limits in the cerebrovasculature as to how large a multilumen catheter can traverse within its conveyance to the brain.

12.2.4 Filling of Other Defects

The capacity to fill or clip a vascular defect that is prone to rupture is appealing. Modulation of the vascular network is also warranted with other clinical conditions. For example, beyond aneurysms, there are so-called arteriovenous malformations (AVMs), congenital formations of vasculature that are comprised a range of arteries and veins that are interconnected together through a junction box called a nidus. The direct link between arteries and veins overpressurizes the veins in the nidus making them more susceptible to rupture causing a brain bleed but often not as life threatening as with normal aneurysms. There are also instances in treating primary malignant tumors in which the there is a perceived value in blocking the feeding pathways for the tumor, that often recruit their own blood supply to nourish it more effectively. In both instances, there is a larger desire to block the feeding arteries for the tumor or the nidus. In both instances reactive fluids, once injected, solidify either by interacting with clotting factors or through some other reaction mechanism. The most common reactive fluid for embolic therapy used today is N buty cyanoacrylate (NBCA), approved for usage in 2000 [17]. The resin is nominally filled with tantalum to allow for radiopaque tracing and reacts with proteins in solution to solidify forming a plug for feeding arteries of AVMs. Each embolization procedure is called a pellicle. Attributes of the materials included in dispersions include solubility in a solvent of limited toxicity, rapid transformational response, and forming either a gel or a harder structure. Ideally, the dispersion is easy to deploy by clinicians, has adequate shelf life and stability, and is invariant to how each clinician deploys them. Key control of both the injection pressure, temperature, and the virulence of the solidification reaction are all key as the goal is to actually seal off the blood vessel at some fixed distance downstream from the catheter, creating an embolism. An example of occluding a feeding artery to a vascular defect is shown in Fig. 12.10, where in this instance, polyvinyl alcohol dissolved in a solvent precipitates in the feeding artery occluding it for an AVM in this case [18].

Embolic fluids need to solidify in controlled and ideally robust ways once injected. Too virulent a crosslinking or solidification reaction and insufficient downrange distance covered by the embolic fluid and there is a chance that the catheter actually gets fixtured to the solidifying embolism. Too slow a kinetic conversion and it is possible to pass the embolic fluid past the ideal sealing location and after that, it is possible to overpressurize the nidus causing its rupture. Both would be considered complications and likely require an emergency craniotomy to stabilize the patient more directly. The key feature for any of these functionally transforming structures relates gauging the dynamic mechanical response with time once it is injected. A variety of both polymers and solvents can be considered as potential embolics and the overall toxicity is likely on a continuum of response.

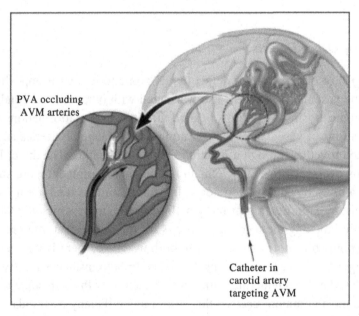

PVA occluding
AVM arteries

Catheter in
carotid artery
targeting AVM

Figure 12.10
Schematic for injectable therapy, where a fluid blocks a feeding artery to an AVM nidus.
Reproduced from the Aneurysm and AVM Foundation web site, www.taafonline.org.

Overall, there are reasons to modulate cerebrovascular flow which can be accomplished both endovascularly and exovascularly. There is significant individuality in diagnosis and postulated interventions. We have mentioned clips, coils, and embolic fluids which all have their capacity to address a latent risk about either hemorrhage or ischemia. There are other more active neural interventions both from a diagnostic front and in terms of therapy.

12.3 Neural Probes and Stimulators

Disease, debilitating neuromuscular atrophy as with Parkinson's disease and multiple sclerosis, trauma, and its associated pain have led to direct interest in how to modulate brain function through electrical stimulation to interfere with pain responses, upregulate productive neuromuscular signaling and the like [19]. There is significant interest in both receiving electrical signaling from normal and diseased brain function and interventional interest in creating new signaling pathways that can be synthetic. Probes are useful not only for therapy and pain management but also for diagnostics as in electrocorticography, where probes are placed directly on the cortex during signaling, yielding higher resolution than with electroencephalogram or EEG-type measurements. The history of these interventions dates back to the 1950s and continued progress has led to somewhat better outcomes in terms of probe construction, installation, and signaling performance.

From a hardware perspective, the signaling/receiving components are true haptic interfaces embedded or adjacent to brain tissues. Because these electrodes originally derived from typical conductor traces, they were produced from highly electrically conductive thin films from copper and gold. These traces were often attached to printed circuits and other schemes to create appropriate electrical signal transmission. An example of a typical probe is shown in Fig. 12.11 and described by Lai et al. [20]. The neural probe structures that have historically been embedded have possessed much larger mechanical mismatch compared with the surrounding tissue into which a probe is embedded. The typical modulus of even epoxy—fiberglass laminate material is on the order of 10s of Gigapascals (GPa) at body temperature while the neural tissue is on the megapascal to kilopascal (Pa-1MPa) range [21,22].

The general understanding is that the there is insertion damage to the surrounding cellular environment into which these probes are installed and there is a corresponding glial scar progression similar to that with pacemaker electrodes that grow to insulate the signaling sensitivity and resolution of these devices over time. The takeaway is that probes tend to function for a sustained period and then probe performance deteriorates due often to the local tissue environment that cannot be overcome by continued tuning.

Higher resolution and thinner devices that allow for larger electrode density per unit area are being developed. There are many both larger and smaller devices that are being developed, including those based on organic coatings on carbon fibers, including deposited

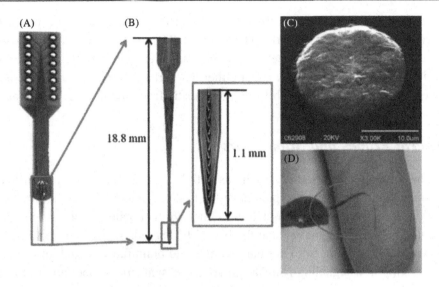

Figure 12.11

Schematic for a neural probe in which the probe is stiffer than the neural tissue into which it is deployed. *Reproduced with permission from* Lai et al, J. Neural. Eng. **9** *(3), 2012, 036001.*

films of ionomeric, polyethylene dioxythiophene-polystyrene sulfonate (PEDOT−PSS). This conductive organic thin film has been deposited more often given its robustness for deposition quality and the variety of substrates onto which it can be deposited. If deposited on carbon fibers, the fibers are themselves stiff even if the PEDOT thin film is somewhat more compliant.

The hypothesis that if the mechanical mismatch is so profound, then perhaps new materials composed of hybrid inorganic/organic structures should yield less modulus mismatch and the increased compliance might reduce glial cell lysis over time. Over the last 10 years, there have been a number of interesting strategies linked with increasing both the compliance and the overall biocompatibility of the components going into new probe design.

Rigid (A) and (B) flexible 3D electrode structures produced from a rigid silicon wafer and polyimide thin films accordingly from Takeuchi et al [23], shown conceptually in Fig. 12.12.

There have been schemes to produce 3D and 2D planar electrode arrays on next generation flexible circuits building on dielectrics such as silicones [24] and polyimides [23].

Haptic electrode interfaces have also been formed from conformal coatings on electrode surfaces such as parylene C [25]. Planar devices can be inserted on an end to construct deep brain stimulator electrodes, while 3D architectures are most promising in the area of organ

Recording
pad

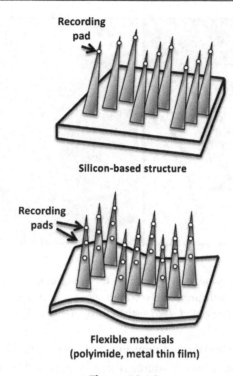

Silicon-based structure

Recording
pads

**Flexible materials
(polyimide, metal thin film)**

Figure 12.12
Schematic of conformal electrode surfaces allowing for planar sensation or signaling.

sensing/impulsing, where the capacity to sense or impulse larger discrete areas of brain, for example, without having to distort the organ for larger functional contact, an example of which are shown in the following in Fig. 12.13. Jeong et al have demonstrated examples of integrated sensor arrays attached over a curved substrate to represent whole organ electrical diagnostics [26], potentially a dramatic leap in diagnostic imaging performance with more discrete sensor attachments.

What is even more impressive using interconnection strategies linking discrete silicon impulse or sensor circuitry on flexible silicone substrates, coupled with the capacity to build and integrate components for higher fidelity. The potential to build these conformal electronic films could lead to dramatic breakthroughs in functional organ response, where more rigid structures have had either lower surface coverage or has mechanically manipulated the organ (brain, cortex, etc) in order to have a larger signal.

From a signaling perspective, the use of PEDOT−PSS substrates as relatively biocompatible and functional organic electronic assemblies has led to significant improvement in the use of integrated impulse probes in the treatment of Parkinson's disease, where the aberrant nerve signaling that leads to the profound motor skills problems

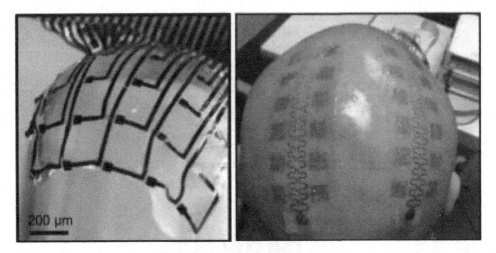

Figure 12.13

Examples of larger planar sensory configurations for compliant-shaped sensing. Much higher signal resolution is possible with printed electronic sensors and haptic interfaces are attached. *From Jeong et al. [26] Neuron **86**, 2015, 175–186.*

at are experienced including tremor and neuromuscular rigidity. The devices are relatively simple, driven by a battery as a power source, there is an impulse generator and leads that transmit the signal to the probe end. By interfering with the aberrant signal, there is profound reduction in the observance of the shaking tremors. Key to success by installing a deep brain stimulator is reducing the observable symptoms of Parkinson's while not compromising other facets of brain function [27].

12.4 Conclusion

There remain a number of challenges in producing neural probes on flexible substrates, such as relatively low resolution (dictated by contact printing methods), the inability to scale to the high number of channels necessary for comprehensive mapping of brain activity, and we know seemingly little about the overall biocompatibility of implantable components destined for the neurovasculature. What is impressive is that on the horizon, there appear to be both sensory systems and functional electrical signaling systems that have improved our understanding of brain function and perfusion in vivo and address symptoms linked with neuromuscular diseases such as Parkinsons's disease.

What is also key is that there is a large learning curve required to just understand the neural landscape. The number of potential tools and qualified materials solutions available to neurosurgeons is considered insufficient. Explaining this gap to designers and inventors isn't necessarily easy for clinicians to describe in digestible language as significant understanding of neuroanatomy, brain function, complications, and functional morbidities is required to participate. More comprehensive brain diagnostics will help to identify more of those in need of an intervention and as the number of potentially affected people rises, more attention will be directed to neuroscience and neurosurgery.

Here, we have mentioned modulating cerebrovascular flow, and sensing and inducing electrical signaling to characterize/augment brain function. Neural interventions are and will continue to be an important areas in clinical medicine for the foreseeable future, for as aspects of age-related cognitive deficit affect larger populations, the desire to change outcomes for older patients will be increasingly important.

12.5 Problems

This chapter does not lend itself to quantitative problems with so much embedded knowledge needed to solve it objectively. Consider for example, the simple process of injecting a plug of embolic fluid into the vasculature with the assumption that it solidified downstream at some distance. It would be desirable to know.

1. What is a typical velocity profile for blood in a blood vessel, with blood acting as a cellular fluid that shear-thins near the vessel walls. Depending on the size of the vessel relative to the cells, there are some differences but for larger vessels, a typical pipe flow profile is considered appropriate as a starting point.
2. What perturbations that exist if a patient has an AVM, where arteries are linked to veins without the aid of the pressure drop that occurs in the capillaries. Thus, venous flow in an AVM is usually much higher pressure than typical venous flow. That will affect the pressure drop term in the velocity profile. Recognize that hypertensive patients also have a separate internal pressure higher than average.
3. Embolic fluids injected require an active process of viscosity rise or gelation in blood or saline. Envision and describe what an appropriate data set might look like to characterize that type of response. There is a need to understand the volume fraction of the embolic fluid in the plug and what fraction is blood, if injected at a different temperature than body temperature, there can be temperature gradients that can also affect fluid viscosity. Consider how the gel time might be affected by concentration and temperature gradients if the blood is warmer within this moving plug.
4. Consider optimum outcomes from embolization. Describe what short-term and long-term attributes are linked with successful embolization and how is success graded (radiography, neurological tests, blood chemistry, etc).
5. Consider the same issues for a deep brain stimulator. Describe how one defines success and how is that graded.

Reduced tremors, less fatigue, better sleep patterns. One needs quantitative tools to assess these attributes, most often these are evaluated by a clinical 1−5 scale observation.

6. Describe how long do batteries last for a deep brain stimulator and how can the battery be effectively recharged?

7. A patient is treated with exovascular clipping procedures and cured for a period of 10 years. The patient had periodic follow up using an MRI unit with a field strength of 2.3 T. In the interim period following treatment, higher field strength MRI units capable of higher resolution are now available. Explain what potential complications arise, if any, for a clipped patient using a higher field strength?

8. What other pain-related clinical conditions might warrant impulse generators like deep brain stimulators. What is the optimum outcome from installation?

References

[1] P.P. Morris, Practical neuroangiography, LWW ISBN-13: 978-1451144154, 2013.

[2] A.G. Osborn, Cerebral angiography, LWW, ISBN-10: 0397584040, 1998.

[3] J. Wardlaw and the IST-3 collaborative group, Association between brain imaging signs, early and late outcomes, and response to intravenous alteplase after acute ischaemic stroke in the third International Stroke Trial (IST-3): Secondary analysis of a randomised controlled trial, Lancet 14 (2015) 485−496.

[4] Aneurysm Fact Sheet. 2015; Available from: http://www.ninds.nih.gov/disorders/cerebral_aneurysm/detail_cerebral_aneurysms.htm.

[5] Understanding: Brain Aneurysm Statistics and Facts. 2015; Available from: http://www.bafound.org/Statistics_and_Facts.

[6] M. Cury, F. Zeidan, A.C. Lobato, Aortic disease in the young: Genetic aneurysm syndromes, connective tissue disorders, and familial aortic aneurysms and dissections, Int J Vasc Med (2013), 267215

[7] G.J. Rinkel, M. Djibuti,, A. Algra, J. van Gijn, Prevalence and risk of rupture of intracranial aneurysms: A systematic review, Stroke 29 (1998) 251−256.

[8] D.O. Wiebers, J. P. Whisnant, J. Huston, 3rd, I. Meissner, R. D. Brown, Jr., D. G. Piepgras, G. S. Forbes, et al., Unruptured intracranial aneurysms: natural history, clinical outcome, and risks of surgical and endovascular treatment, Lancet 362 (2003) 103−110.

[9] YASARGIL Aneurysm Clip System. 2015; Available from: http://www.bbraun.com/cps/rde/xchg/bbraun-com/hs.xsl/products.html?prid=PRID00004559.

[10] Aneruyam Clips. 2015; Available from: http://www.mrisafety.com/SafetyInfov.asp?SafetyInfoID=229.

[11] A.C. Mamourian, N. Mahadevan, N. Reddy, S.P. Marra, J. Weaver, Prototypical metal/polymer hybrid cerebral aneurysm clip: in vitro testing for closing force, slippage, and computed tomography artifact, J. Neurosurg. 107 (2007) 1198−1204.

[12] Anterior communicating artery aneurysm clipping techniques. 2015; Available from: http://jtsciencevisuals.com/Content/Portfolio/f38cba12-3c58-48d0-838e-7a45fec765a3.fit-800x600.jpeg.

[13] Gugliemi detachable coils. 2/15/2015; Available from: https://en.wikipedia.org/wiki/Guglielmi_detachable_coil.

[14] Aneurysm treatment by coils. 2015; Available from: http://www.brainaneurysm.com/aneurysm-pictures.html.

[15] Endovascular aneurysm coiling. 2015; Available from: http://www.mayfieldclinic.com/PE-Coiling.htm-.VYreWevgC7M.

[16] Onyx liquid embolic system. 2015; Available from: http://www.joeniekrofoundation.com/treatment/onyx-liquid-embolic-system/.

[17] S. Vaidya, K.R. Tozer, J. Chen, An overview of embolic agents, Semin. Intervent. Radiol. 25 (2008) 204–215.

[18] Treatment of AVM. 2015; Available from: http://www.taafonline.org/am_treatment.html.

[19] P. Anikeeva, Biocompatible materials for optoelectronic neural probes, National Academy of Engineering. (2014). Frontiers of Engineering: Reports on Leading-Edge Engineering from the 2013 Symposium. Washington, DC: The National Academies Press. doi: 10.17226/18558.

[20] H.Y. Lai, L.D. Liao, C. T. Lin, J.H. Hsu, X. He, Y.Y. Chen, et al., Design, simulation and experimental validation of a novel flexible neural probe for deep brain stimulation and multichannel recording, J. Neural. Eng. 9 (3) (2012) 036001.

[21] M.A. Green, L.E. Bilston, R. Sinkus, In vivo brain viscoelastic properties measured by magnetic resonance elastography, NMR Biomed. 21 (2008) 755–764.

[22] G.H. Borschel, K.F. Kia, W.M. Kuzon, R.G. Dennis, Mechanical properties of acellular peripheral nerve, J. Surg. Res. 114 (2003) 133–139.

[23] S. Takeuchi, T. Suzuki, K. Mabuchi, H. Fujita, 3D flexible multichannel neural probe array, J. Micromech. Microeng. 14 (2004) 104–107.

[24] I.R. Minev, D.J. Chew, E. Delivopoulos, J.W. Fawcett, S.P. Lacour, High sensitivity recording of afferent nerve activity using ultra-compliant microchannel electrodes: An acute in vivo validation, J. Neural. Eng. 9 (2012), 026005

[25] B.J. Kim, J.T. Kuo, S.A. Hara, C.D. Lee,, Y. Lu, C.A. Guitterez, et al., 3D Parylene sheath neural probe for chronic recordings, J. Neural. Eng. 10 (2013), 045002

[26] J.W. Jeong, G. Shin, S.I. Park, K.J. Yu, L. Xu, J.A. Rogers, Soft materials in neuroengineering for hard problems in neuroscience, Neuron 86 (2015) 175–186.

[27] D. Prodanov, J. Delbeke, Mechanical and biological interactions of implants with the brain and their impact on implant design, Front. Neurosci. 10 (2016)Article 11

CHAPTER 13

Cardiovascular Interventions

Learning Objectives

The need to address cardiovascular flow arises from both issues in the cardiac muscle forcing oxygenated blood into the vasculature and separately in the vascular network as well. Within the realm of cardiovascular medicine, efforts have focused on facilitating blood flow through the heart and the rest of the circulatory system and included a variety of devices and interventions. On a peripheral vascular level, continued research is evaluating synthetic and hybrid schemes to replicate medium and small blood grafts as vessel replacements. Pharmaceutical interventions compete in addressing more systemic influences like arteriosclerosis.

In addressing individual concerns, there are instances of both errant and unproductive flow (vascular malformations), instances of inadequate flow (stenoses) and blockages (ischemias), and separately, there are instances where the vascular walls are weakened leading to aneurysm. Schemes to address inadequate flow within the network can include angioplasty and the installation of stents to reopen closing or partially blocked arteries. If the defects are not tied to the vasculature, there are more localized problems tied to cardiac output, valvular defects, and coronary artery disease. All those phase contrast agents discussed in Chapter 10, Nanomaterials and Phase Contrast Imaging Agents, are instrumental in gauging both cardiac and vascular health. Surprisingly, the general symptoms of high pulse rate, fatigue, and general weariness are indicators or symptoms of an overworking heart muscle, but the physical basis for what needs to be addressed can be much more nuanced. As a result, adequate diagnosis is critical.

The types of conditions leading to a need for intervention are the type discussed in Chapter 6, Environmental and Aging Effects on Tissues, and can be either sudden and acute, or progressive with advancing age. At its origin, effective perfusion can be compromised by insufficient coronary artery perfusion and blockages that advance oxygenated blood flow into the receiving organs and downstream vessels. Separately, aortic dissection or other aneurysms may or may not influence long-term health but are often fatal if they ultimately rupture. Torn or calcified leaflets leading to cardiac

Biomaterials. DOI: http://dx.doi.org/10.1016/B978-0-12-809478-5.00013-4

insufficiency and more nuanced arterial blockages called stenoses in arteries can form leading to the peripheral vascular perfusion problems. In this chapter, we will discuss design and use issues relating to stents, valvular repairs and replacements, and synthetic vascular grafting strategies. Like all grafting procedures, there is a competition between autografting and allografting of whole organs, so there is a need to value the types of interventions that are presented here, from needle and thread, to more invasive substitutions.

This chapter is organized around the three main themes of cardiovascular intervention. We will start at the pump and with all of the appropriate schemes for valvular repairs and replacements, and proceed downstream through vascular grafts most closely associated with coronary artery bypass surgery and aortic dissections, and follow that with needs to address stenoses further downstream. In each section, there will be a segment pointed to outcomes and to opportunities in the future to consider new types of materials and designs. Discussions about arterio-venous (A-V) shunts are presented in Chapter 14, Artificial Organs: Engineering and Strategies.

From reading this chapter, the reader should be able to

- Discern the distinction between autografting and xenografting as it relates to outcomes in coronary artery bypass graft (CABG) surgery.
- Understand the heroic interactions of the cardiologist in repairing torn leaflets, reshaping misshaped valves, and septal and interchamber defects that all lead to indications of regurgitation and cardiac insufficiency as an alternative to a synthetic replacement.
- Recognize the value of the heart/lung machine and new types of instrumentation such as left ventricular assist devices to allow for rest periods of the heart where surgical interventions are facilitated.
- Understand the linkage between reduced perfusion locally and the potential for both hypoxia and ischemic stroke to arise where blood flow is of a lower effective flow velocity.

13.1 Introduction

The pathway for cardiovascular intervention is essentially based on the development of heart bypass machines capable of redirecting flow to and from the heart while keeping the patient perfused. The development of machines to perform this function dates back well over 50 years, when the first known attempts to completely redirect blood flow through an external pump were conducted. The main blood-interfacing component is the tubing that is normally produced from plasticized polyvinyl chloride or silicone. The blood is extracted by cannula from the vena cava [1] normally feeding the heart and is driven by either peristaltic or centrifugal pumps, with the understanding that both of these pumps alter the hemodynamics of blood as it is propelled increasing the amount of hemolysis. There are a variety of membrane oxygenators that reoxygenate venous blood that is passed into an oxygenated reservoir. Oxygenated blood is reintroduced into a group of feeding arteries through one or a series of cannulae that are sutured into the arteries receiving from the heart [2]. Essentially, only one is needed and the preferred site in the ascending aorta, but if there is an aneurysm, arteriosclerosis, or other concerns about adding a cannula to the aorta, the femoral or iliac arteries have been shown to work as well, but with much higher complication rates [2]. Rerouted blood is usually cooled to reduce the level of hemolysis and induced platelet activation. Most blood contact is with these plastic tubes, and to a lesser extent, the cannulae that are place for reentrant blood. Schemes to prevent blood coagulation while on bypass are important. The anticoagulant heparin is commonly used not only dosed with the patient but heparin-bound vascular graft materials and oxygenation systems are also common, as are filters to isolate any coagulated blood.

To give an assessment of how much the heart bypass machine has impacted health care, statistics show that in developed countries, there are well over 100 coronary artery bypass surgeries performed per 100,000 people [3]. For the United States, that would put coronary artery bypass surgery at over 300,000 procedures/year alone, making it by far, one of the largest and successful elective surgeries in terms of the number of procedures. The numbers confirm the value of the intervention, with 4-year mortality rates from Coronary artery bypass graft (CABG) surgery of $\sim 7\%$, compared to 33% with candidates managed by only medical and pharmaceutical oversight [3].

With bypass units, the heart is temporarily and more readily available for valvular restorations, replacement, interchamber seal fixes, and CABG surgery. In this chapter relating to cardiovascular interventions, let's start with the heart. There are several reasons for intervention, and most conditions are triggered from some form of cardiac incompetence.

Heart valves can be compromised by either tearing of the flexible leaflets, or by the deposition of calcifications on the leaflets affecting both their sealing capacity and retarding their mobility. The aortic and mitral valves seem most susceptible to stenosis [4]. In terms of the comprehensive numbers of procedures, there were $\sim 330,000$ valve related procedures performed in the United States between 1998 and 2005 (~ 50K/year), with about 85% of them being replacement [5]. The trend or repair versus replacement is trending more toward repairs.

13.2 Valvular Repairs: Rationale for Intervention: Murmurs, Regurgitation, Congestive Heart Failure

13.2.1 Sutures to Address Leaflet Tears

While the protocols associated with what to repair versus what to replace continue to be refined, one can review how leaflet tears leading to regurgitation are being addressed though simple suturing. For suturing leaflets together, the preferred suture choice is a nondegradable one and the most common choice has been monofilament polypropylene. 4-0 Suture has been the recommended strengths and dimensions among many options [6]. Complications from suturing have included perforating the adjacent healthy leaflets induced by ends of the knots on the repaired one [7]. Perhaps other softer sutures such as multifilament braided structures including polyester [7] could be more effective if the strength of the alternative suture is not in question.

An example schematic on resolving a leaflet tear is shown in Fig. 13.1 [8]. Here the idea is to shape the torn leaflet segments to allow for a more seamless integration. A small tissue segment is excised near the tear as the margins are often ragged leading to resolution as the torn segments are reunited.

A separate consideration for the leaflets relates to the precipitation of calcium deposits on particularly the mitral and aortic valves, rendering them both harder, and often less capable to seal effectively. It is known that above pH 7.4, there is a larger driving force for calcium

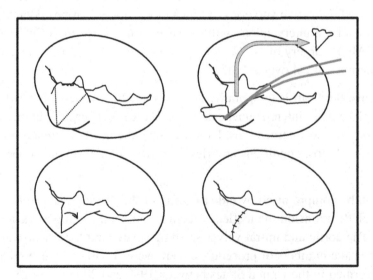

Figure 13.1
Schematic of leaflet repair using sutures, an increasingly common alternative to immediate replacement.

precipitation [9]. There are also drug therapies and diet that can influence serum calcium ion concentration which are also regulating factors [10]. Valvular stenosis is common, particularly in more aged populations. Clinicians can find some level of calcification on natural valve leaflet surfaces, and degenerative aortic stenosis is likely the most prevalent observable by clinicians. In more rare instances, clinicians can debride some amount of calcifications using ultrasonics to dislodge the precipitates from around the valve without tearing the residual tissue [11]. There is reference that suture placement for a valve replacement is easier, but debridement is not common. Obviously valvular stenosis is patient dependent and removing an individual series of precipitates doesn't necessarily reduce the root cause for precipitation, so more often, these valves are replaced.

13.2.2 Annulolasty Rings

Valvular dysfunction can also be amplified by misshaped valves, where the leaflets over time fail to overlap creating poorly sealing valves. With a misshaped valve, one can recreate a more cylindrical tube shape into which the valve seals by introducing an annuloplasty ring that can be sutured in and around the annulus of the valve. An example is shown in Fig. 13.2 [12].

Annuloplasty rings are made from a metallic C-shaped ring segment over which a Dacron PET braided mesh is woven. The current metal of choice is titanium, but others have been produced from surgical steels and even biodegradable structures have been proposed. The design goal for any ring is to be stiff enough that when stitched into the rest of the annulus, the stiffness of the ring will displace a more oval tube shape to represent that more of a cylinder. For the ring presented in Fig. 13.2, the interior segment is stiffer and the exterior regions are more flexible allowing the cardiologist or surgeon to load the oval region of the annulus along the major axis to stretch it.

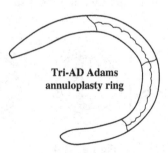

Figure 13.2

A schematic of the Tri-AD Adams annuloplasty ring. *Produced from Medtronic, Tri-AD Adams Tricuspic Annuloplasty Ring. Available from: <http://www.medtronic.com/for-healthcare-professionals/products-therapies/cardiovascular/heart-valves-surgical/tri-ad-adams/>, 2015.*

In some instances, the tears are profound and the use of both leaflet suturing and annuloplasty rings could be considered. An example of a more profound tear through a large region of a leaflet is shown in Fig. 13.3 [8]. The combination approach reinforces the leaflet segment where the crack extension is sharpest and can allow for a more comprehensive resolution of the tear following leaflet suturing. The takeaway message here is that the cardiac surgeon has tools to address valvular defects short of immediate valve replacement and diagnosis is a critical step in addressing cardiac anomalies triggered by regurgitation.

13.3 Prosthetic and Bioprosthetic Replacement Valves

It is clearly possible that upon diagnosis, the damage to the existing valve structure warrants a more comprehensive replacement. Examples of replacement valves are shown in Fig. 13.4 including the original Star-Edwards ball and cage type construction, which has been displaced by both bi-leaflet type constructions and the tilting disk arrangement.

The design environment is fairly harsh and these designs need to operate over and over again. In the materials realm, engineers talk about fatigue life, the ability of a device or a

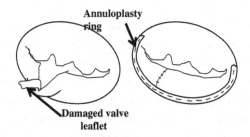

Figure 13.3
Schematic of repairing a torn valve through suturing of the leaflet and augmenting the valve support through the use of an annuloplasty ring that is sutured around the valve opening.

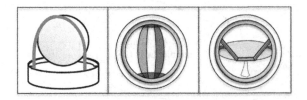

Figure 13.4
Various examples of heart valve replacements including left: a ball and cage design; middle: a bi-leaflet tilting disk assembly; and right: a single tilting disk assembly. Each design has a different hemodynamic flow pattern as blood is drawn through the valve region. Bioprosthetic devices are made by stitching a pericardial tissue segment over a valve template.

material to sustain many repetitive loadings, and the sum of those loading sequences represents a loading spectrum. The fatigue lifetimes of these components used as valves are crucial in that they must be constructed from robust materials capable of hundreds of thousands of performance cycles while at the same time not triggering the formation of clots and emboli that get sloughed off the device and delivered downstream where they subsequently trigger ischemic stroke (so-called thromboemboli). The majority of the xenograft materials in direct blood contact are machined from titanium bar stock, which is wear resistant making the valves less susceptible to erosion-induced valve leakage. Titanium is relatively averse to cellular attachment in blood, but different mechanical valves have different clotting potential. Titanium also rapidly oxidizes during manufacturing forming a stable TiO_2 layer that is hard, impervious, and relatively bioinert [13].

Another attribute of titanium is that physically deposited coatings can be grown on the surface of the metal leaflets in an attempt to further control both the rate of platelet activation and any cellular attachment. The variety of coatings produced from sputtering, pyrolysis, and chemical vapor deposition offer a wide potential for future patent protection linked with new device construction. It's been generally well accepted that variations on pyrolytic coatings of carbon [14] further reduce the potential that the new valve surface is the genesis of a later thromboembolism. Other types of diamond-like coatings have also been deposited [15]. This tailored surface approach might be in the long run better than requiring systemic treatment with anticoagulants to yield the same outcome.

The coatings tend to be well-adhered titanium surface and generally are not eroded over the life of the implant. The sheer variety of process conditions that can yield a functional coating leads to a larger number of continuing patent submissions for new ways to produce heart valves with improved surface qualities. Ratner et al. [14] go into extensive detail about the need to characterize surface structure and details relating to contact angle determinations to resolve the potential of droplet wetting on a solid surface are contained in Chapter 5, Property Assessments of Tissues. Other researchers have also probed surface structure [16].

Recognize that the hemodynamics of blood through these valves is quite different than with a viable natural valve, and there are issues about hemolysis from blood processed through these valves as opposed to the more flexible natural leaflets. Moreover, depending on how the valves open and close, it is possible that dead zones and eddy flows can be created which tend to also increase the chance of platelet activation and clotting, and thromboembolism.

13.4 Outcomes

In the end, after valvular intervention, the ultimate question is whether mortality rates are lowered by intervening. For someone with a failing valve, any intervention probably improves vascular circulation from the outset and they are likely healthier as a result. The larger question concerns whether one type of intervention, strategy, or prosthesis leads to a better outcome than some other. As a comparison, mortality statistics are used to justify the intervention. An example assessment is included below, which compares the mortality statistics of one group of patients receiving a specific Bjork Shiley spherical disk prosthesis versus a Hancock bioprosthetic valve. Assuming that the groups receiving each device are treated as equivalent, the comparison between device interventions can be done, as seen in Fig. 13.5 [17].

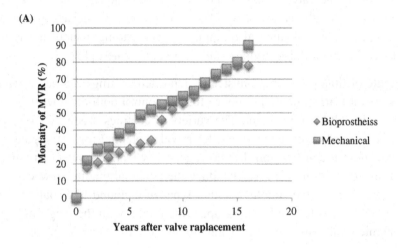

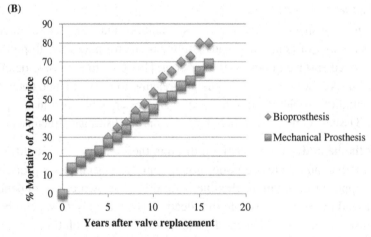

Figure 13.5

Mortality rates comparing the function of a bioprosthetic valve (blue diamonds, gray in print versions) versus a mechanical valve (red square, gray in print versions) for both the aortic valve (AVR) (A) and the mitral valve (MVR) (B) replacement. *Graph extracted and regraphed from K. Hammermeister, G.K. Sethi, W.G. Henderson, F.L. Grover, C. Oprian, S.H. Rahimtoola, Outcomes 15 years after valve replacement with a mechanical versus a bioprosthetic valve: final report of the Veterans Administration randomized trial, J. Am. Coll. Cardiol. 36 (2000) 1152–1158.*

There is a general acceptance that there is a continuing need for refining the patient pool tied to current cardiovascular health, age, BMI, other heath complications, as well as surgical refinements on how to execute each procedure, and whether they are best completed in harmony with other procedures (CABG, dual valve installations). When complications arise, there are key needs for further diagnostic determinations, retrieval studies, and pathology assessments.

13.5 Interchamber Defects

Intracardiac holes (septal defects) can form between the left and right sides of the heart chambers that can lead to profound inefficiencies that can also mimic congestive heart failure. It has been reported that atrial septal defects (ASDs) are identified in roughly 4 in 10,000 births making this a relatively commonly observed cardiac condition [18]. Ventricular septal defects (VSDs) are also observed. ASDs and VSDs are identified often early in life as congenital, others are less obvious or very small and are less revealing on a diagnostic EKG or maybe only under physiologic stress. There are interventions developed over the last 50 years that can help seal a range of these septal defects and the tools and materials for facilitating these repairs are improving [19]. It is possible to resolve these defects with sutures, assuming that they are relatively small, while increasingly, there are catheter-based friction fitting devices that can be deployed making the resolution more routine and less invasive.

To gather the locations around a septal defect together, it is necessary to apply tension to the septum to suture effectively or to add a patch to it accordingly [20]. Polypropylene (5-0) sutures seem a preferred suture for these defects; for more profound, larger holes, expanded polytetrafluoroethylene (ePTFE) patches are installed on one side of the septum and sutured in place to reduce how much tension is required to close the defect [21]. Comparisons between direct suturing and patch-based repairs have been made and the general recommendation is that for older populations who present later in life with septal defects that were not addressed early, patch-based procedures are preferred [22]. For ventricular septal defects, the surgical line of site is made by incisions into the ventricle. For other defects, likely other incisions are required followed by subsequent suturing at the end to repair the incision to allow the interior cardiac sealing. Suture-based septal defect repairs seem like very involved procedures, and it's remarkable how much cardiac surgery has progressed to the point that fixes on this level are even achievable.

More promising and less invasive schemes to address these defects require deployment by catheter to permeate the defect and to deploy seals on either side of the septal gap. Roughly 20 years ago, the Amplatzer dual disk assembly was built and configured from a Nickel/ titanium shape memory alloy meshes. The device transforms as it is deployed from a

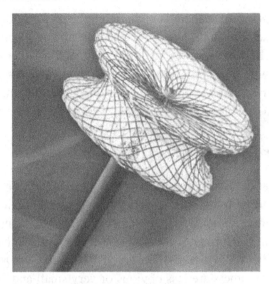

Figure 13.6
Transcatheter delivered into a septal defect after deploying the disk extensions. These types of disks are usually made from stent-like preforms adapted to the catheter. *Printed with permission from D.S. Moodie, Technology Insight: transcatheter closure of ventricular septal defects, Nat. Clinical Practice Cardio. Med. 2 (2005) 592–596.*

cylinder on the end of the catheter to a bulging lobed, dumbbell-like construction where the small diameter neck segment is situated directly in the septal defect, as seen in Fig. 13.6 [23,24]. The barbell disks overhang the gap defect. The bar segment attached to the barbells is fitted to situate within the gap itself, as shown in Fig. 13.7. Sealing has proven quite effective and it has revolutionized treatment of septal defects as a dramatically less invasive procedure with better outcomes and available for a much larger pool of potential recipients.

The size and hardness of the disks are such that their location of the installation site matters. Defects close to the valve regions can apply a moment to the valve dynamics leading to other challenges if the valve is somehow compromised by the installation of the septal occluder, and the mesh is much less compliant than the surrounding tissues. On top of the positional and hardness challenges, it also appears that a portfolio of disk sizes are required to deploy one and maybe this is an opportunity for composite solutions of meshes and conformal resins to provide for a more effective and softer haptic interface with the tissue.

13.6 Vascular Grafts

In moving from the heart downstream, the endothelium is a vast network beyond the physical dimensions of the heart. Estimates suggest that the endothelium has a mass of

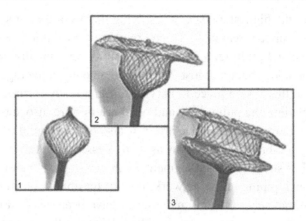

Figure 13.7
Scheme for how porous titanium preforms are ultimately deployed by balloon catheters to seal a septal defect. The interior section is of a smaller diameter to situate in the gap between chambers and the disks are designed after deployment to overhang the defect. *Permission asked for from Journal of Invasive Cardiology.*

$\sim$ 1 kg, and corresponds to at least 4000 m^2 when spread out [25]. By isolating the lengths of arteries, veins, and capillaries, it has been previously reported and carried forth that the length of the normal cardiovascular system is > 100 km [25,26], which is hard to imagine.

The largest concern with the endothelium corresponds to aging and its impact on vascular health, with the largest ties to arteriosclerosis. The reduced interior diameter of the lumen, caused by deposition of fatty plaques within the vessel wall of the endothelium, and increases the pressure drop for vascular transport making the heart pump harder to achieve the same level of perfusion.

Desirable design features for any replacement vascular graft include

1. The capacity to carry blood without leaking either within itself, or when, making graft/host connections known as anastomoses.
2. Softness and flexibility (E between 1 and 10 MPa).
3. Compliance, ideally matched to the pulsatile flow next to the adjacent arteries to which it is connected.
4. The capacity to retard platelet activation and clot formation, something linked to what is defined as patency, a continued openness of the vessel.

Regarding interventions, the choice remains between pharmaceuticals, transplants, and synthetic vascular grafting. More and more is known about peripheral vascular disease triggered by arteriosclerosis, and the pharmaceutical industry has invested a lot of money into identifying how to retard or dissolve precipitate plaques found with the endothelium.

Pharmaceuticals have the highest chance of resolving the disease on a systemic level. Everything else is a localized treatment. There are plenty of candidate vessels that need vascular augmentation and grafting. Vascular dimensions are typically defined as either larger or smaller. The aorta, being almost 25 mm in diameter on average, has no comparison in vivo so there is no place to harvest for an already formed autograft. The coronary arteries including the pulmonary and renal arteries are also substantial vessels. As flow is carried to the extremities, the iliac artery is also of substantial diameter. There are also a corresponding number of larger veins as well. Vessels generally less than 6 mm in diameter are defined as small diameter segments with capillaries generally much smaller than that. With so much piping in the network, it's not feasible to consider wholesale vascular replacement, but specific veins and arteries have been targeted in addressing overall health and replacements have been installed. With the thought of replacing individual segments of the piping network that have stenosed or are clogged, it becomes quite clear that we bias our interest on larger, more critical pipes and to a lesser extent, the capillaries.

The most common heterograft choices based on significant prior clinical experience have been grafts based on Dacron polyester, polypropylene, and ePTFE. For larger diameter grafts, these are all generally woven fabrics with pores larger than cell dimensions suggesting that there is some radial blood permeation along with the axial perfusion. As a result, these woven grafts are called porous or bleeding grafts, the porosity of which can be controlled by the type of knitting or weaving. The processes for making these woven constructs have been optimized over decades and are related to the orientation of the fibers, the weaving process to incorporate multifilaments into a repeating structure. Separately, there is a kinking process to form a corrugated structure that is more flexible than the multifilament weave. Once installed, the blood flows radially will help to seal the graft.

13.6.1 Dacron Grafts

Dacron polyester is also commonly impregnated with albumin, collagen, or gelatin to seal pores and prevent larger amounts of radial blood flow [27] and leaks relating to anastomoses. It is generally understood that smaller (<6 mm) vessels that have been replaced with prosthetic vessels have thrombosis rates that are greater than 40% within 6 months of installation [28]. The current state suggests that both pharma therapy and autografting and allografting are more likely to lead to successful outcomes. Opportunities exist in the realm of surface coatings to produce a more camouflaged surface. As the diameter of the vessel shrinks relative to the size of the cells contained in the blood, there is a higher probability that platelets will contract these surfaces and activate while encountering them. T and B cells linked with the immune system can also eventually target these foreign surfaces accordingly.

13.6.2 Expanded Polytetrafluoroethylene (ePTFE)

In comparing corrugated polyester-based pipe constructions, alternative grafts based on hydrophobic polytetrafluoroethylene that is stretched into a more compliant and porous, expanded form that was introduced as a lower extremity bypass graft in 1976 [29]. The process to produce expanded polytetrofluorethylene or ePTFE is essentially uniaxial or biaxial stretching of a melt extrudate from an emulsion polymerized resin, whether fiber, film, or tube, and coercing it into a porous, nonwoven networked fibril structure in which the distance between network nodes is on the order of 30 μm [30].

The introduction of porosity in ePTFE by processing increases its compliance and makes it easier to suture the graft. There is a direct correlation between the amount of stretching and the relative amount of the porosity in the emulsion polymerized structure. Typical porosity ranges from 75% with a draw ratio of 5 to as much as 90% for a draw ratio of 8.5 [31]

The critical evaluation for any vascular graft surface is its patency, the fraction of the lumen interior area that remains open over time. Thus, upon initial installation, one starts with 100% patency, and if the vessel promotes the growth of either bacterial colonization or triggers a clot formation, the patency is reduced with increased graft lifetime.

What is interesting to observe is that where these grafts are installed matters, comparing largest graft locations with other locations overall. Patency rates (the fraction that remain open and unoccluded) relating to Dacron polyester vascular grafts to address aortic dissection are approximately 93% at 5 years of service, life, and for ePTFE, between 91% and 95% depending on the study parameters [32]. But grafting from the femoral artery to the femoropopliteal artery in the leg led to 5-year patency rates of 43%, and for ePTFE, no better at 45% [33]. The outcomes are even worse for lower knee grafts. With two different polymer backbone chemistries including a polyester and a polyolefin, one that swells from hydrogen bonding and one that's hydrophobic, the outcomes are nearly the same as grafts in smaller arteries. Separate coating studies such as grafting the intimal surface with heparin seem to have some improved benefit [30], but even now, it appears that we are far from an optimum solution that won't require continued attention due to relatively rapid occlusion over time.

Promising products from mats of electrospun fibers and decellularized allograft tissue would seem to have potential, and many preclinical trials have been attempted along that front. Separately, there are efforts linked with the notion that biodegradable conduits that can initiate sufficient intimal recellularization could lead to temporary graft structures that are gradually replaced by the host [34]. For these, the typical choice of cell-grafted poly-α hydroxy acids (e.g., PLA-PGA) electrospun mats that gradually degrade over time is the preferred concept. Clearly whatever is being reduced needs to be metabolized into nontoxic products.

The takeaway here is that most of efforts toward a better vascular graft solution are research studies using synthetic materials that have been performed for much shorter periods when the patency difference is less, and potential complications are less observable. It would be most promising if these current studies showed continued patency over longer term, particularly for below the knee vascular graft locations and smaller graft dimensions. It is also possible that if interventions can be posed on a healthier population pool, outcomes might be better. But the successful identification of an appropriate vascular graft independent of graft location remains incomplete.

13.7 Stents

Milestones in the progression of adult arteriosclerosis include increasing loss in patency as plaques displace more and more functional cross-sectional area over which blood can perfuse. While coronary arteries can be repopulated through autografting procedures, that does not necessarily resolve the issue of peripheral artery blockages. It is thought that maintaining the intimal cross section in renal arteries, femoral and carotid arteries will increase the viability of the tissues fed by these arteries that suggests a strong payoff for even prophylactic stenting. It is thought that as many as 10M people in the United States (3%) are suffering from peripheral artery disease and if replacement vessels perform so poorly, the stop-gap measure is to maintain the integrity of the existing vasculature [35]. Stenting can be performed either as a stand-alone procedure, or as a finishing procedure following balloon angioplasty to augment the resistance to restenosis.

Many different devices that are in use and all of these are essentially deployed on balloon catheters. Examples of commercial stents and their base metal composition are shown in Table 13.1 [36]

The porosity, braid structure, compliance, and structural driving force to expand are all design attributes important in opting for one design over another. There is a history of use issue and clinicians more familiar with one of these are more likely to use it in the clinic. Examples of the devices used in a comparison study are shown in Fig. 13.8. Limitations include the diameter of the balloon catheter onto which these devices are installed.

The general outcomes from stenting procedures suggest that the stents keep the vessels open. As a result, it may well be that patients who receive carotid artery stents are less

Table 13.1: Self-expanding carotid artery stents used for model experiments

Stent	Manufacturer	Material	Design
Carotid Wallstent	Boston Scientific	Cobalt chromium alloy	Braided
Ezpander	Medicorp	Nitinol	Braided
Jostent Self-X	Abbott Vascular	Nitinol	Segmented
SMART-Stent	Cordis Cardiovascular	Nitinol	Segmented
Zilver_Stent	Cook Medical	Nitinol	Segmented

Tanaka, N., J.P. Martin, K. Tokunaga, T. Abe, Y. Uchiyama, N. Hayabuchi, J. Berkefeld, and D.A. Rufenacht, Conformity of Carotid Stents with Vascular Anatomy: Evaluation in Carotid Models. American Journal of Neuroradiology, 2004. 25: p. 604-607.

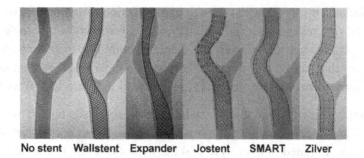

No stent   Wallstent   Expander   Jostent   SMART   Zilver

Figure 13.8

Conventional radiographic imaging to resolve the filling capacity and shape compliance of the different carotid artery stents. *Produced with Permission from N. Tanaka, J.P. Martin, K. Tokunaga, T. Abe, Y. Uchiyama, N. Hayabuchi, et al., Conformity of carotid stents with vascular anatomy: evaluation in carotid models, Am. J. Neuroradiol. 25 (2004) 604–607.*

likely to experience hypoxia as a result of an intervention. These devices are installed with less subtle enthusiasm because other procedures like surgery seem to have more favorable results at least in early trials for symptomatic carotid stenosis [37]. And prophylactically introducing stents into patients with low-grade hypoxia seems unrelated to a patient's health when they present with less extensive stenosis [38].

13.8 Drug Eluting Stents

Added functionality: If the main drawback in deploying bare metal stents is that the opened vessel can reclose or undergo restenosis, maybe the driving force for restenosis can be altered by introducing a drug released from the polymer coating on the stent to enhance the proliferative capacity of cells adjacent to the stent or to lower the clotting potential. The main polymer used as the vehicle is PLLA that slowly degrades within then vasculature allowing the release of any of a number of drugs as cell regulators including taxol and sirolimus [39]. Here there are questions about the molecular weight of the polyester, the drug loading content, the distribution of drug within the polymer coating, etc. The overall assessment is that the presence of a variety drug components in many different configurations released from the stent may improve the overall outcome over bare metal stents. As a result, the promise leveraged by hybrid drug and device combinations offers a broad intellectual property potential.

13.9 Added Constraints: Pediatric Cardiac Interventions

Permanent stents with a fixed extension distance once deployed serve a great purpose for adults with profound blockages. The larger dilemma arises when stenosis are encountered with pediatric patients. Maintaining the opening of a growing vessel is a separate added complication, highlighting the need to stabilize stenosed structures early in life, but creating deterioration mechanisms to allow the growth and evolution of the natural tissue as pediatric patients' progress in age. The options for a bioresorbable stent include ones designed to completely deteriorate away and there are both bare metal and bioresorbable polymer structures that can be considered as options. Comparisons between different viable alternatives for bioresorbable stent materials are included in Table 13.2 from Onuma [40].

Among deteriorating polymer structures, candidate bioresorbables have been produced from poly L-lactic acid, polycaprolactone, polytyrosine carbonate, and polyanhydride esters. These polymers are designed to hydrolyze and the hydrolysis rate is affected by the local pH, the polymer molecular weight, the degree of orientation, and latent crystallinity, if each can crystallize. The likely largest issue opting for a polymeric stent from a bare metal one is that the overall compliance of polymeric stents is much larger. The overall stiffness of polymeric stents as deployed will deteriorate with continued deterioration time, thus, efficiency as a stent is somewhat more fleeting, to the point that some companies producing these devices call them scaffolds and not stents at all, even though they are deployed as such. The polymeric stents can be also incorporated with drug and can be produced in a range of dimensions, all deployed by balloon catheter. Overall lifetimes for polymeric scaffold stents can range from weeks for polydiaxonone and PGA-PCL copolymers [41] to as long as 3 years for those based on PLLA [42], in the limited trials that have been performed so far.

To create the opening force, the typical strut dimensions for polymeric fibrils making up the expandable stent are larger (150 µm [43]) than that required for bare metal stents of higher modulus. The large fiber dimensions might be a limiting design factor in pediatrics due to the smaller blood vessel dimensions already. Typical molecular weight for the PLLA

Table 13.2: Mechanical properties and degradation time for different polymers and metals

	Modulus of Elasticity (GPa)	Tensile Strength (MPa)	Ductility (%)	Degration Lifetime
Poly L-Lactide	3.1–3.7	60–70	2–6	>24 months
Poly DL-lactide	3.1–3.7	45–65	2–6	6–12 months
Polyglycolide	6.5–7	90–110	1–2	6–12 months
50/50 Poly DL-lactide/ glycolide	3.4–3.8	40–80	1–4	1–2 months
82/18 Poly L-lactide/ glycolide	3.3–3.5	60–70	2–8	12–18 months
70/30 L-Lactide/e-caprolactone	0.02–0.04	18–22	>100	12–24 months
Cobalt chromium	215–235	1.45E + 03	40	Stable
Stainless steel 316L	193	690	40 +	Stable
Nitinol	45	700–1100	10–20	Stable
Magnesium alloy	40–45	220–330	2–20	1–3 months

Onuma, Y., J. Ormiston, and P.W. Serruys, Bioresorbable scaffold technologies. Circulaton Journal, 2011. 75: p. 509-520.

devices has been approximately 300 kDa, chain lengths more typical of bone implant devices than for biodegradable sutures. The deployment of these prototype stents requires heat to deploy. The stents can be formulated with drugs to elute out of the structure over time to prevent restenosis, and typical PLLA lifetimes. Clinical trials continue as the combined requirements of a small device and one that deteriorates with a controlled metabolism may not be achievable using hydrolytically sensitive polymers.

The alternatives are bare metal stents produced from bioresorbable metals. Most promising among them are magnesium and magnesium alloys [44]. Coalloyed with approximately 7% rare earth metals, these metals are much stronger than their polymeric counterparts allowing them to be miniaturized for smaller vessels while still remaining strong. Mg alloy stents are also soluble in saline allowing their effective metabolism over a period of several years where the need for a new one can be reassessed. In terms of functional metabolism, the presence of a degrading magnesium source in vivo might address a common dietary deficiency from the stent installation. The general assessment is that complete stent resorption only delivers approximately 5 mg of magnesium which is absorbed over the years of metabolism.

13.10 Pacemakers, Defibrillators, and Associated Hardware

Separate from the dysfunction in the cardiovascular system linked with regurgitation and blockages, there are cardiac problems that persist linked with an inability to signal the repetitive contraction of the heart muscle and new signaling strategies are needed. The impulse cascade of muscular contractions normally results in increased pressure in chambers filling the aorta which if linked with coordinated openings and closings of the valves leads to proper perfusion. If the involuntary neural signaling pathway that initiates pulses at the sinoatrial node of the heart is either irregular or somehow missing, there will be uncoordinated muscle contractions and arrythmias will result.

The major fixes for signal-based arrhythmias where appropriate signaling is ineffective are substitute electronic signaling pathways directed by both pacemakers and defibrillators. Pacemakers in their simplest forms include a battery, a clock chip, and a signal generator, leads to direct the generated pulsed signal to regions of the heart which will trigger a coordinated contraction cascade in the muscle, and a case or a housing to hermetically seal the electronics from the fluids contained in soft tissues which could compromise the electronics.

More sophisticated pacemakers would allow for surge pacemaking if under duress or load, or walking up stairs for example. The housing is typically made from titanium which is essentially bioinert although the leads which feed from the device are bathed in body fluids which could include both blood and interstitial fluids. The leads are essentially insulated wires and at the end, there is an electrode which forms the haptic interface where new signaling will result. There are a range of insulating resins which can be used to isolate the electronic signal including silicones, polyurethanes, and copolymer resins. The design requirements for the leads are much more demanding as the lead attachment has to flex with each successive heart contraction, and ideally, remain free of blood coagulants, ideally remain complaint and well adhered to the wire, and maintain its integrity as a lead material. The leads require hundreds of flexings per hour, thousands per month, and hundreds of flexing cycles over the lifetime of the device.

Implanted defibrillators are devices that are more sophisticated than simple pacemakers and contain more sensory functions to observe normal heart contractions, and are similar to pacemakers in that they also have a sealed set of electronics, leads, and paddle-based electrodes designed to defibrillate a heart undergoing random arrhythmias. The paddles are situated over segments of the heart muscle and when activated, strong signals are delivered to paddles internally, without requiring an external defibrillation strategy. For patients that suffer from periodic arrhythmias and atrial fibrillation, the installation of a monitoring device coupled with a defibrillator capable of shocking the fibrillating heart into a more coordinated rhythm is indeed value-added devices. Algorithms, software, and programming are needed to define under which conditions pacemakers function, and defibrillators are engaged and continued cardiac monitoring is needed to insure proper function of both of these devices. It is awesome to consider someone with a profound arrhythmia or fibrillation and through electronic bypass can be transformed from a congestive heart failure patient to a functioning member of society. Regardless of the type of electronic cardiac assist device is included, the biological response near the electrodes is often some growing level of scar tissue which can actually reduce the potency of the synthetic signal as more insulating connective tissue forms and lies between the signaling electrode and the semiconducting tissue.

13.11 Conclusions

In this chapter, schemes to address the repair of segments of the heart, primary arteries, and peripheral arterial segments have been presented. Cardiovascular surgeons are highly involved in coronary artery bypass surgeries and the alternative piping network maintained during bypass is crucial to successfully complete the repairs and to aid in the recovery of the patient. Separately, areas relating to vascular grafts, valves, and stenting were also presented. It is important to recognize that the cardiovascular surgeon's capacity to repair defects rather than replace the damaged regions is of increasing interest, and as a result, our interest in suture materials remain high. It is also clear that there is a competition in choosing between synthetic grafts and autografts and allografts for cardiovascular replacement tissues. Currently, the outcomes seem to suggest that autograft and allografts are preferred where possible in part due to the current inability to camouflage the surfaces to completely inhibit platelet activation and stenosis. There are areas where autografting of vascular structures is not possible though.

13.12 Pointing to the Future

The development of more catheter-based procedures and installations will displace other surgical interventions, primarily because of faster recovery times presented to the patient and lower potential from infection from open procedures. The push for new ways to treat common vascular diseases is one reason why there has been so much activity relating to the development of new stents not only for adults but for pediatric patients where there is a different vascular dimension and clearly a different design environment. It will be exciting to see how the challenge of vascular disease is addressed in the future.

On a more profound level, it is worth noting that tissue and cellular engineering will eventually have a larger role to play in the future in helping to repair regions of infarcted heart muscle damaged by ischemias and heart attack. There are ample research studies in both cell culture and in animal studies to consider roles of cell types, cell conditioning ex vivo, templating strategies of those cells on controlled morphology substrates with the idea that injectable or graft segment repairs could be performed in infarcted regions. The sheer volume of research will direct practitioners and budding tissue engineers to the most likely pathways that can effect real change in patients who have suffered from MI or other factors contributing to congestive heart failure. This work is important and needed.

13.13 Problems

1. Compare and contrast a bioprosthetic heart valve as opposed to a tilting disk assembly. Describe differences in terms of both hemodynamics and stagnant flow.
2. Why might repair over replacement of a heart valve be warranted?
3. You have a hypertensive patient undergoing bypass surgery, explain how might you accommodate the higher blood pressure in dealing with anastomoses?
4. You have a young patient who presented with congestive heart failure, explain what kinds of defects are likely and how might they be resolved
5. Why are the annuloplasty ring and other valve grafts often integrated with a fabric coating?
6. Explain ideal attributes for future small and medium diameter vascular grafts?
7. Explain the design environment of a stent and its stress state once deployed?
8. You have a drug eluting bioresorbable stent, describe how dosing or drug release by diffusion through the stent might be different than the bioresorption of the stent?

9. You are a cardiovascular researcher, choose and explain where you would want to invest your time and effort in solving a larger problem that exists based on what was presented here?

References

[1] Technical Aspects of Cardiopulmonary Bypass, 2015 (cited 2015). Available from: < https://www. openanesthesia.org/technical_aspects_of_cardiopulmonary_bypass/ > .

[2] E.A. Hessel, A.G. Hill, Circuitry and cannulation techniques, in: G. Gravlee, et al. (Eds.), Cardiopulmonary Bypass: Principles and Practice, 2nd edition, Lipincott, Williams, and Wilkins, Philadelphia, 2000.

[3] A.L. Hawkes, M. Nowak, B. Bidstrup, R. Speare, Outcomes of coronary artery bypass graft surgery, Vasc. Health Risk Manag. 2 (2006) 477−484.

[4] Facts and Figures: Cardiovascular Services. Available from: <http://www.johnmuirhealth.com/services/ cardiovascular-services/intervention/transcatheter-aortic-valve-replacement/facts-and-figures.html>, 2015.

[5] S.D. Barnett, N. Ad, Surgery for aortic and mitral valve disease in the United States: a trend of change in surgical practice between 1998 and 2005, J. Thorac. Cardiovasc. Surg. 137 (2009) 1422−1429.

[6] E.B. Savage, S.F. Bolling, Atlas of Mitral Valve Repair, Lippincott, Williams, and Wilkins, Philadelphia, 2006.

[7] B.K. Lam, A.M. Gillinov, D.M. Cosgrove, Failed mitral valve repair caused by polypropylene suture, Ann. Thorac. Surg. 76 (2003) 1716−1717.

[8] Aortic Valve Regurtitation (AVR). Available from: <http://www.indiahospitaltour.com/heart/pediatric-aortic-valve-replacement-repair-surgery-india.html>, 2015.

[9] J. Csapo, The influence of proteins on the solubility of calcium phosphate, J. Biol. Chem. 75 (1927) 509−515.

[10] H.M. Connolly, J.L. Crary, M.D. McGoon, D.D. Hensrud, B.S. Edwards, W.D. Edwards, et al., Valvular heart disease associated with fenfluramine−phentermine, New Engl. J. Med. 337 (1997) 581−588.

[11] F.J. Baumgartner, A. Pandya, B.O. Omari, A. Pandya, C. Turner, J.C. Milliken, et al., Ultrasonic debridement of mitral calcification, J. Cardiac Surg. 12 (1997) 240−242.

[12] Medtronic, Tri-AD Adams Tricuspic Annuloplasty Ring. Available from: <http://www.medtronic.com/ for-healthcare-professionals/products-therapies/cardiovascular/heart-valves-surgical/tri-ad-adams/>, 2015.

[13] N. Huang, P. Yang, Y.X. Leng, J.Y. Chen, H. Sun, J. Wang, et al., Hemocompatibility of titanium oxide films, Biomaterials 24 (2003) 2177−2187.

[14] B.D. Ratner, Biomaterials Science: An Introduction to Materials in Medicine, Elsevier/Academic Press, Amsterdam, 2013.

[15] R. Hauert, A review of modified DLC coatings for biological applications, Diam. Relat. Mater. 12 (2003) 583−589.

[16] M. Fedel, A. Motta, D. Maniglio, C. Migliaresi, Surface properties and blood compatibility of commercially available diamond-like carbon coatings for cardiovascular devices, J. Biomed. Mater. Res. 90 (2009) 338−349.

[17] K. Hammermeister, G.K. Sethi, W.G. Henderson, F.L. Grover, C. Oprian, S.H. Rahimtoola, Outcomes 15 years after valve replacement with a mechanical versus a bioprosthetic valve: final report of the Veterans Administration randomized trial, J. Am. Coll. Cardiol. 36 (2000) 1152−1158.

[18] M.S. Spence, S.A. Qureshi, Complications of transcatheter closure of atrial septal defects, Heart 91 (2005) 1512−1514.

[19] G. Webb, M.A. Gatzoulis, Atrial septal defects in the adult- recent progress and overview, Circulation 114 (2006) 1645−1653.

[20] R. Tanveer, A.U. Khan, T.A. Siddique, S. Siddique, A. Nasreen, Salman-ur Rehman, et al., Continuous versus interrupted technique of ventricular septal defect (VSD) closure in total correction for tetrology of Fallot pertaining to residual VSD, J. Pak. Med. Assoc. 60 (2010) 253−256.

[21] A. Haussler and R. Pretre, Surgical closure of a perimembranous ventricular septum defect with a running suture, Multimed. Man. Cardiothorac. Surg. 2008(523):mmcts.2006.002410. doi: 10.1510/mmcts.2006.002410.

[22] T. Kudo, M. Hashimoto, T. Uchino, T. Osada, N. Konagai, H. Hino, et al., Surgery of atrial septal defect in patients aged over 40 years: comparative study of direct suture and patch closure, Kyobu Geka, The Japanese Journal of Thoracic Surgery 44 (1991) 387–390.

[23] F. Praz, A. Wahl, M. Schmutz, J.P. Pfammatter, M. Pavlovic, S. Perruchoud, et al., Safety, feasibility, and long-term results of percutaneous closure of atrial septal defects using the amplatzer septal occluder without periprocedural echocardiography, J. Invas. Cardiol. 27 (2015) 157–162.

[24] D.S. Moodie, Technology Insight: transcatheter closure of ventricular septal defects, Nat. Clinical Practice Cardio. Med. 2 (2005) 592–596.

[25] W.C. Aird, Spatial and temporal dynamics of the endothelium, J. Thromb. Hemost. 3 (2005) 1392–1406.

[26] R.T. Jones, Blood flow, Annu. Rev. Fluid Mech. 1 (1969) 223–244.

[27] M. Prager, O. Polterauer, H.J. Bohmig, O. Wagner, A. Fugl, G. Kretschmer, et al., Collagen versus gelatin-coated Dacron versus stretch polytetrafluoroethylene in abdominal aortic bifurcation graft surgery: results of a seven-year prospective, randomized multicenter trial, Surgery 130 (2001) 408–414.

[28] J.T. Johanas, Characterization of silk-electrospun tubes for small diameter vascular tissue engineering, in: Mechanical Engineering, Tufts University, Boston, MA, 2008.

[29] H.E. Rodriguez, W.H. Pearce, J.S.T. Yao, The Ischemic Extremity: New Findings and Treatment, PMPH-USA, Shelton, 2010.

[30] L. Xue, H.P. Greisler, Biomaterials in the development and future of vascular grafts, J. Vasc. Surg. 37 (2003) 472–480.

[31] X. Hao, J. Zhang, Y. Guo, H. Zhang, Studies on porous and morphological structures of expanded PTFE membrane through biaxial stretching technique, Int. Nonwovens J. 14 (2005) 31–38.

[32] S.G. Friedman, R.S. Lazzaro, L.N. Spier, C. Moccio, A.J. Tortolani, A prospective randomized comparison of Dacron and polytetrafluoroethylene aortic bifurcation grafts, Surgery 117 (1995) 7–10.

[33] R.M. Green, W.M. Abbott, T. Matsumoto, J.R. Wheeler, N. Miller, F.J. Veith, et al., Prosthetic above-knee femoropopliteal bypass grafting: five-year results of a randomized trial, J. Vasc. Surg. 31 (2000) 417–425.

[34] H. Bergmeister, N. Seyidova, C. Shrieber, M. Strobl, C. Grasl, I. Walter, et al., Biodegradable, thermoplastic polyurethane grafts for small diameter vascular replacements, Acta Biomter. 11 (2015) 104–113.

[35] Peripheral Arterial Disease. Available from: <http://www.sirweb.org/patients/peripheral-arterial-disease/>, 2015.

[36] N. Tanaka, J.P. Martin, K. Tokunaga, T. Abe, Y. Uchiyama, N. Hayabuchi, et al., Conformity of carotid stents with vascular anatomy: evaluation in carotid models, Am. J. Neuroradiol. 25 (2004) 604–607.

[37] D. Yates, Stroke: Early trial results favor surgery over stenting for symptomatic carotid artery stenosis, Nat. Rev. Neurol. 6 (2010) 237.

[38] C.S. Powell, Carotid artery stenting, Tex. Heart Inst. J. 32 (2005) 620.

[39] A. Abizaid, J.R. Coste, New drug-eluting stents: an overview on biodegradable and polymer-free next-generation stent systems, Circulation: Cardiovasc. Interv. 3 (2010) 384–393.

[40] Y. Onuma, J. Ormiston, P.W. Serruys, Bioresorbable scaffold technologies, Circ. J. 75 (2011) 509–520.

[41] M. Zilberman, K.D. Nelson, R.C. Eberhart, Mechanical properties and in vitro degradation of bioresorbable fibers and expandable fiber-based stents, J. Biomed. Mater. Res. Part B, Appl. Biomater. 74B (2005) 792–799.

[42] J.A. Ormiston, P.W.S. Serruys, Bioabsorbable Coronary Stents, Circulation: Cardiovasc. Interv. 2 (2009) 255–260.

[43] P. Erne, M. Schier, T.J. Resnick, The road to bioabsorbable stents: reaching clinical reality? Cardiovasc. Interv. Radiol. 29 (2006) 11–16.

[44] A. Deynda, N. Deinet, N. Braun, M. Peuster, Rare earth metals used in biodegradable magnesium-based stents do not interfere with proliferation of smooth muscle cells but do induce the upregulation of inflammatory genes, J. Biomed. Mater. Res. 91A (2009) 360–369.

CHAPTER 14

Artificial Organs

Learning Objectives

There are several learning objectives in considering the wider use and application of artificial organs and the materials that constitute these. Diseases of vital organs are important to resolve; the word vital is not used lightly as organ failure can be a quick precursor to death. What has been learned from organ donation, tissue and blood typing, and the innate coupling between the virility of the immune system and its influence on viability of a transplanted organ has led to modern protocols making heart, lung, kidney, and liver transplants almost seem routine. The realm of artificial organs is deep with a dedicated journal of the same name and compendia of related research dedicated to asking "how" and "what if" with practically every organ.

The goal of this chapter is to think more strategically and present three different ways to consider how to view artificial organs as challenges to developing engineers to think broadly about the future where other opportunities exist to make a difference. The first considers kidney dialysis to replicate nature's filtration system. Current external dialysis, while touted as a successful intervention, consumes a lot of resources (clinical staff time, clinic infrastructure, and dialyzer time) and generates a lot of waste in the form of needles, tubing, and extracted biofluids handled as biohazards. The second considers metabolic organs like the pancreas that are instrumental in regulating both digestive and endocrine functions. A failure to regulate metabolism is not always observed as an acute symptom and this is one reason why diabetes is growing as a silent epidemic. The last organ discussed here, the bladder, is actually at the forefront of modern tissue and cellular engineering. The bladder is composed of two cell types making its replication conceptually easier than more complicated, metabolic organs. The bladder functions as a reservoir. Producing a tissue engineered bladder depends on the ability to coculture two different cell types together into functional prototypes that can be installed. There are many other organs that could be discussed and important research has been done to gauge the potential of many other organs targeted as replacements, but these three do a good job to establish the landscape.

In reading this chapter, three points are key. The first is in understanding that the mindset in replicating function is the overall goal. Any proposed artificial organ does not have to absolutely represent the shape and specific anatomical location. In fact, we might need to reconsider what is meant by implanted as well for "onboard" systems. Second, in many instances, artificial organs compete with transplants (particularly for heart, lung, and kidneys). With the playbook established on how to resolve donor/host issues through immune suppression and tissue typing, this pathway is preferred. But with long donor lists, stopgap measures to replace or augment function will continue to be needed. Third, it is worth noting the ancillary material and clinical impact required for successful use of artificial kidneys for example. Through this chapter, the reader can:

Recognize the need for artificial organs and their representation

Compare and contrast the success of a couple of examples of model artificial organs in terms of system complexity

Recognize that the design lifetime of different artificial organs are quite variable from days to years, and even those with a short design lifetime have some intrinsic value.

14.1 Kidney: Dialysis

There has been a revolution in how health care is dispensed, particularly as it relates to chronic organ failure. The kidney is critical to maintain health concentrations of metabolites as well as to regulate both fluid and salt content in vivo. The urine extracted per day includes a fluid volume of approximately $1-2$ L and contained within it are a range of different metabolites, inorganic salts, and other organic salts. Within the urine, typical extractions of the most common metabolites are included in Table 14.1 from Ref. [1].

Table 14.1: Types of metabolites and average excretion rates/day.

Component in Urine	Typical Daily Mass Range Excreted Grams
Urea	$20-35$ g
Uric acid	$0.3-2$ g
Creatinine	$1-1.5$ g
Creatine	$0.05-0.1$ g
Soluble cations	Na^+ ($100-150$ mmol), K^+ ($60-80$ mmol) NH_4^+ ($30-50$ mmol) Ca^{2+} ($4-11$ mmol) Mg^{2+} ($3-6$ mmol)
Soluble anions	Cl^- ($120-240$ mmol) SO_4^{2-} ($30-60$ mmol) HPO_4^{2-} $10-40$, depends on pH
Other organics	Ketones, amino acids, other trace metabolites

Going back 50 years, kidney failure was essentially a rapid death sentence contributing directly to 100,000s of deaths annually in the United States but tools to aid in external blood filtration were developing. Worldwide, the Dutch developed an external blood filtration machine late during World War II with small enough pores to retain the cellular components in blood [2]. The semiregular vascular access needed to tap the bloodstream for purification meant that clinicians were returning to the same veins that were increasingly scarred and difficult to access. A separate development of arteriovenous (A−V) shunts that allowed for veins to be more obvious increased the number of potential patients that could be treated [2,3]. With limited resources restricting who could receive the shunt and the access to the purifier, doctors were doing their own form of managed health care, and those without access generally succumbed quickly.

With landmark legislation passed in 1972 in the US giving, those with end-stage renal disease had more access to blood purification that was linked it to the Medicare program. Dialysis was to the eligibility of social security, and suddenly, a lot more affected people could be treated. There was a specific charge per purification session originally set by the legislation at $138 [2]. That meant that the cost of the clinician time, nursing staff, machine, and consumables was linked to a budget forecast of how much the sum of those components should be. The budget forecasting was woefully inadequate as it was anticipated that roughly 35,000 people would need the treatment and the budget to pay for this was ∼ $1 billion by the time the program was fully operational in the 10th year.

The net effect of expanded access was either a wild success or a financial disaster depending on how one looks at it. In 2014, ∼650,000 people in the United States are now diagnosed with end-stage kidney disease [4], that is a very large population, relative to what was anticipated in 1972. If people on dialysis remain viable longer, the number of direct deaths linked with end-stage kidney disease decreases, thus increasing the pool of affected patients that much faster. Chronic dialysis treatment has moved from hospitals to a variety of dialysis centers and clinics, and blood purification technology has advanced through companies such as Fresenius and DaVita. It has been estimated from DaVita, one of the larger companies performing dialysis in clinics that the cost of treatment annually in 2014 is ∼$83 K [5] leading to costs in the United States approaching $40 billion annually. Today, people subsist for years on dialysis (that is better than the alternative) and with the ranks of end stage renal failure (ESRF) patients rising from estimates of 20,000 new dialysis users per year, it is easy to understand how chronic end-stage kidney disease and its treatment is helping to blow up the federal entitlement budget. From a consumables perspective, the use of prosthetic renal systems is probably one of the largest areas of biomaterials usage on a volume basis. And the stark reality is that serving renal dialysis patients requires constant chronic care and living longer with a continuing need for dialysis care impacts the capacity to add new patients accordingly.

End-stage kidney disease is essentially a metabolic blood poisoning in which the kidneys can no longer effectively filter metabolites from blood. The origins of kidney failure can arise due to inflammation, due to clogging of the pores in the nephrons, the distributed functional filtration units of the kidney, housed in a subset of the kidney called the glomerular capsule, and other cytotoxic effects. In Chapter 6, Environmental Effects on Natural Tissues, we discussed that there is generally an innate decrease in filtration efficiency defined as glomerular filtration rate (GFR) with age. Generally, above age of 20, there is approximately a 10% decrease in GFR with each successive decade [6,7]. Some fraction of the pores in the filters clog. As a result, geriatric populations typically are already somewhat compromised in terms of kidney function. Of course, exposure to bacterial infections and other therapeutic or diagnostic drugs that are cytotoxic can create a separate acute damage within the nephron as well, as was mentioned in Chapter 10, Nanomaterials and Phase Contrast Imaging Agents. But the most common problems linked with kidney failure are hypertension and diabetes [5]. Within the clinic, diagnostic assessments of kidney performance are evaluated through urinalysis, including determinations of GFR, void volume, density salt content, pH, and specific analysis for individual metabolites including urea, uric acid, and creatinine. There are instances in kidney disease where void volume is reasonable but the density of the fluid extracted is lower indicating a higher threshold of nephronic size exclusion. In other words, only water and small metabolites can traverse the membrane. If metabolites are not excretable, they will accumulate in the bloodstream and lead to a form of blood poisoning very rapidly. The goal in internal medicine is to prevent acute renal problems from growing into chronic ones.

14.1.1 Dialysis Options

There are two main options relating to dialysis for people with compromised kidney function. For patients who can maintain good hygiene and can be taught how to perform fluid exchanges, there is a form of dialysis called peritoneal dialysis that allows for metabolite extraction in the peritoneal cavity. A much larger fraction of patients are directed to hemodialysis in which there is direct metabolite extraction from the blood.

14.1.2 Peritoneal Dialysis

The process of performing peritoneal dialysis requires an otherwise healthy, mentally alert, and physically capable patient to perform fluid exchanges. If the kidneys no longer allow ion and metabolite diffusion across an ensemble of functional nephrons, there are other large surface area membranes that can be substituted [8]. The peritoneal membrane is the next best hope, shown in Fig. 14.1. Peritoneal dialysis requires the installation of a transcutaneous silicone transfer tube with an injection port into the abdominal cavity now done through laparoscopic surgery [9]. After the port region heals and is capable of function, typically, up to 2 L of sterile dialysate fluid (mostly water, but some salts can be added to retain vascular salt content) is injected through the port and allowed to equilibrate for several hours [10].

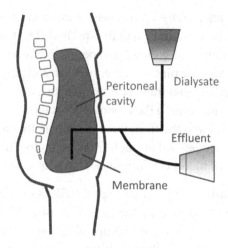

Figure 14.1
Peritoneal dialysis. Dialysate is loaded through a flexible injection port into the peritoneal cavity. By osmosis, metabolites are drawn through the peritoneal membrane into the dialysate fluid. Frequent dialysate fluid exchanges allow for a continuous metabolic extraction but significant time is required as is a large stockpile of supplies at home.

A 1D concentration gradient is established by metabolites in the blood and the fluid in the cavity across the thickness of the membrane which is linked to the mass flux. Normally, a higher concentration in the bloodstream than in the abdominal cavity is linked with a higher chemical potential and the metabolites will permeate across the membrane from the bloodstream into the cavity. By flushing the fluid in the cavity and then reinstalling fresh dialysate fluid, one can clear metabolites that accumulate during the equilibration phase while the dialysate collects them.

In a typical day, 4−5 fluid exchanges are needed to maintain healthy metabolite concentrations in the bloodstream, as such, each peritoneal dialysate patient has an arsenal of sterile liquids, needles, tubing, disinfectants, etc. to perform these functions at home and rigorous hygiene is required to ensure that the transcutaneous injection port does not get infected. The benefit of peritoneal dialysis is that a patient can live a normal life at home and can organize their life around when these fluid exchanges are performed. With only 3%−5% of dialysis patients undergoing peritoneal dialysis, it seems clear that it is not a particularly easy regimen to maintain.

14.1.3 Hemodialysis

Alternatively, hemodialysis is actually performed in the hospital or related clinic on a regularly scheduled basis. Similar to blood donation and other vascular access centers, hemodialysis patients are connected by venous needle incisions in their arms to a filtration unit with high surface area also containing a dialysate fluid. The functional filtration membrane typically has thousands of hollow, semipermeable tubes. The tubes are typically 200 μm in diameter with an annular pipe diameter of 5 μm and pore sizes <1 μm in diameter. Hemodialysis is also a 1D radial mass transfer process with axial flow of blood and radial flow of the metabolites perpendicular to the blood on a net basis [11]. Blood is conveyed by internal pressure from one arm into the filtration zone, where the metabolites and other soluble species within blood are pushed through from the hollow tubes into the surrounding dialysate fluid and the residual blood is reintroduced back into the receiving arm.

The patient's blood is typically circulated through the filtration zone a number of times during a single 4–5 h treatment period as shown in Fig. 14.2. The goal is to reduce metabolite levels gently, rather than a more abrupt filtration in a shorter period. The chemical composition of the dialysate fluid (salt for example) can be controlled, for example, to prevent extracting excessive salt content. Internally, the driving force for activating platelets to coagulate in the dialysis tubing is sufficiently large that the patients are put on anticoagulant therapy such as heparin to prevent ischemic stroke during treatment and immediately afterward. It is also possible through controlling the pressure of the dialysate fluid to control the amount of fluid extracted simultaneously.

The end result is a periodic, continuous (while they are hooked up) countercurrent extraction of metabolites, proteins, and fluid to replace kidney function. The quality of life both during

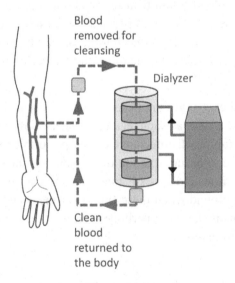

Figure 14.2

A schematic of hemodialysis showing arterial access, the pressurized flow to push the fluid through the filtration dialyzer, and returned through a venous port. Chronic dialysis patients often use cardiovascular shunts to make accessing the bloodstream more routine.

dialysis and away from the clinic is far from optimized. The typical schedule for dialysis patients is three times per week; so most patients are on a monday-wednesday-friday (MWF) schedule for uremic patients. Crisis levels of metabolites are usually not experienced until after at least four days, so scheduling these events every 2−3 days seems appropriate and works within the clinic scheduling. What it means is that each uremic patient needs access to similar filtration equipment on a semiregular basis, the hardware and the staff need to be in place for this to work. With the passing of blood through this fractionated filtration assembly in convective mass transfer, the blood spends a lot of time outside of the body of a warm individual and there is also convective heat transfer to the room that leads to cooler, filtered blood returning to the receiving arm. Often during dialysis, uremic patients are buried under several thermal blankets and after treatment are often quite fatigued as a result of each treatment. Travel is difficult to coordinate and needs to be planned with other dialysis centers to insure there is capacity for treatment. So while uremic patients can survive under current treatment protocols for years, their independence and quality of life are obviously compromised with their tethering to these purification clinics. This background is given, only to show that the current state of the art is not ideal and engineers need to be cognizant of opportunities for both new types of designs and materials that can lead to more efficient dialysis treatment, fewer side-effects, and facilitated logistics in increasing access.

The current list of cardiovascular components commonly used for dialysis include those related to the A−V shunt, the needles, tubing, clips, and other associated hardware to connect the shunt to the filtration system and the filter itself. An example A−V shunt access is shown in Fig. 14.3 [12]. All of these components of the exovasculature are blood contacting with the exception of the clips.

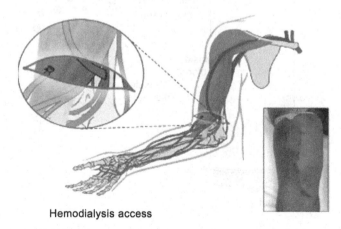

Hemodialysis access

Figure 14.3
Arterio-venous (A-V) shunt schematic showing how much easier blood access is after shunt insertion. *Published with permission from T Vachharajani, The atlas of hemodialysis access.*

The tubing, mostly made from silicone resins and previously plasticized polyvinyl chloride (PVC), needs to be flexible to accommodate where it is placed relative to the vascular access locations and ideally clear to allow for clinicians to observe continued flow. Ideally, clotting should be prevented in the tubing and schemes have been developed to create heparin-grafted internal surfaces of the tubing to reduce the driving force for clotting, but patients continue to be dosed separately. The filters are typically produced from synthetic polyethersulfones (PES) or from celluloacetates (CA). A baseline schematic of the membrane filter is shown in Fig. 14.4. These resins are produced in sufficiently high enough molecular weight to maintain their ductility and strength requirements when conveyed into the production of dialyzers.

From a long-term perspective, soft tubing such as silicone is the most commonly used and miles of disposable tubing are produced in high volume annually. There have been efforts to eliminate the use of plasticized flexible tubing, although those who are transfused are commonly exposed to trace amounts of plasticizer from plasticized vinyl blood bags.

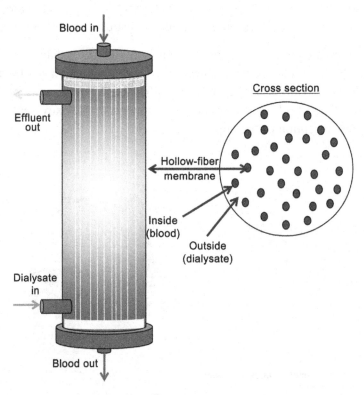

Figure 14.4
Schematic of a countercurrent flow showing axial of blood from one end to the other and the dialysate fluid operating by radial infusion and extraction.

There is a lot of process technology behind producing porous membranes of controlled pore size while still allowing the internal structures of the membrane to function without leaking. One scheme for producing porous membranes is to add a soluble dispersed phase into the molten polymer during extrusion which can be leached out later to create the pores. If the dispersed phase is a salt of controlled small particle size, the requirement for the process technology is to homogenize the salt distribution within the molten resin so that pores are of similar size after leaching and well distributed. By using a bimodal distribution of small particles in the molten resin, one might be able to regulate small molecule vs. larger molecule transport. Current design considerations are quite focused on regulating a larger number of potential metabolites beyond urea to include components like vitamin B12. Other engineering activity is focused on how to recycle and resterilize multiuse catheters which might have a small impact on the cost of performing treatment but probably do not have a large impact on making treatment either more efficient or more tolerable for dialysis patients.

The implanted A−V fistula or shunt is a critical piece of current hemodialysis paradigm allowing the hemodialysis clinic to have a more prominent vascular access location for these semiroutine trips for dialysis treatment. In many patients, a cardiac surgeon can directly connect a feeding artery to veins in the patient's arm. Without the pressure drop from capillary flow in the extremities, the vein responds to the arterial pressure by expanding several fold. Once healed, the larger vein protrudes in the arm and is a superhighway of vascular flow and even a blind nurse, or even worse, the author, could access this port from palpation only. For a subset of patients, this organic graft is not recommended and a synthetic vascular access region is created using either expanded polytetrafluoroethylene or polyester vascular grafts. The graft dimensions tend to be medium sized and with proper hygienic care, they can last for years. The same caveats for any cardiovascular implant are required as clotting and infection and general occlusion are key concerns for proper function of the fistula or shunt. It takes several months for the shunt to heal so the patient is tapped in other locations in the interim.

14.1.4 Continuous Metabolite Extraction

From a technological standpoint, the improved health of uremic patients is best addressed by considering that kidney function is a continuous, involuntary process, while dialysis is a temporary, external rerouting of the bloodstream; so, once the patient disconnects from the dialyzer, blood contaminant concentrations rise until the next dialysis treatment. Perhaps from an engineering perspective, more research could be placed on considering how to perform filtration *on board* using a bioartificial kidney (BAK) which leads to a whole new series of challenges but the payoff might be huge in terms of improved quality of life.

There are ongoing efforts linked with the construction of cartridge filters in series to isolate metabolites from the bloodstream linked with onboard filtration [13,14], an example of which is shown in Fig. 14.5. The first filter is essentially a size-exclusion filter and the second one allows for the permeation of metabolites through a layer of cultured epithelial cells to replicate the selectivity for metabolites through the renal tubules associated with normally functioning nephrons.

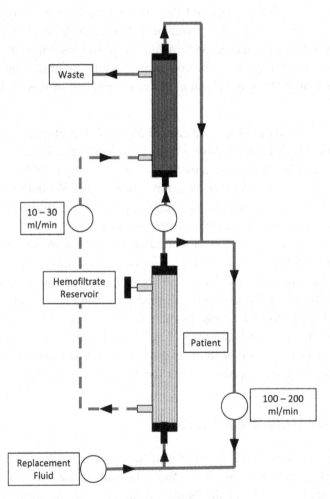

Figure 14.5

A schematic of a two-stage bioartificial kidney where blood flows from the bottom to the top of the picture with pumps represented by circles. The first stage is a simple hemodialysis filter to purify by size exclusion and then to redirect a fraction of the purified blood from the dialyzer into the bioreactor filtration cartridge downstream. The two-stage system has been suggested in several different schemes [14]

There are two main fluid streams, a purified cellular blood component and a second waste stream that is routed accordingly. The problems associated with artificial kidneys in development are related to the upregulation of inflammatory markers found in blood, including interleukin IL 1 and C-reactive protein, markers of biological stress [13]. Patients continue to be heparinized during treatment. The user is involved in programming extraction and flow rates and the device seems incapable of autonomous control during sleep hours. Any device will need a functional display to allow the user the ability to modify extraction conditions. The concerns about vascular inflammation give one pause. It might be possible to improve treatment by avoiding vascular access with the artificial kidney and relying on continuous or semicontinuous extraction by routing the dialysate fluid within the abdominal cavity. If there was a less ambitious scheme to leverage simpler filtration as opposed to using the renal cells as the filter, the ability to produce and maintain the system might be easier. But if the cells are required to extract the metabolites, then their need is clearly established.

To sum up, there is a growing clinical and financial crisis looming as new cases of end-stage kidney failure continue add to the clinical load, while transplanted organs continue to lag the need. The National Kidney Foundation reports that 3000 people per month are added to the donor list and annually, about half that total (17,000 in 2014) received a new kidney [5]. The dialysis treatment list gets longer each year with more people requiring dialysis with a cost of ~ $80 K/year (2014 dollars). There is still a cost for those getting transplants as the cost of antirejection drugs remains a recurring cost, but that is likely less than for the chronic care linked with dialysis. Lessons might be learned regarding other types of noncellular systems that have been produced. The most advanced type of device in this realm is the pancreas.

14.2 Artificial Pancreas

A similarly intractable and potentially even more expensive problem exists in dealing with diabetes, a disease that is growing at a much faster rate than even end-stage kidney disease. Diabetes is essentially a metabolic failure within the pancreas tied to resolving vascular blood sugar concentration [15]. Within the last 30 years, there has been an explosion in the consumption of larger amounts of sugar (up to 22 teaspoons of added sugar daily in the US diet as of 2009, adding up to 350 extra calories [16] in diets daily). The paradigm has been to reduce fat in diets, and adding sugar was a cheap and easy way to make fat-free foods more tolerable. As a result, general sugar consumption, in the United States at least, has risen sharply.

The pancreas is the organ most involved in distributed human alchemy, producing a range of different enzymes aiding in digestion (the exocrine system), and facilitating the regulation of serum blood sugar through exquisite control regulated by primarily the α and β-cell types found as islet cells of the pancreas [15]. These islet cell [15] secretions are released into the bloodstream and form part of the endocrine system. So-called α cells secrete a hormone called glucagon and β cells produce insulin. A third type of islet cell, the δ cell, regulates the activity of α and β cells. Overconsumption on a regular basis of sugar triggers the activation of α or β cells that can ultimately render them less or unresponsive over continued time, the origins of adult-onset diabetes.

It is worth noting that there are two types of diabetics, one group called type I or pediatric diabetes cases in which the β cells are not capable of regulating blood sugar and while there are degrees of dysfunction, it typically takes time and several blood tests to yield a confirming diagnosis. There is also a group of diabetics called type II or adult-onset diabetics, whose pancreases have atrophied, probably as a result of those high sugar diets. If through dietary intervention the dysfunctional cells can be repopulated quickly and perform normally, perhaps the long-term consequences of diabetes might be retarded. What seems alarming is that the term adult-onset probably needs refinement as type II diabetics are being diagnosed before age of 10 and the likely culprit is a diet saturated in excessive sugar. Diabetes is a silent epidemic requiring immediate intervention. If diabetes persists, diabetes will increase the number of people suffering from blindness, extremity damage and amputation, and often end-stage kidney disease which makes the earlier discussion about dialysis even more important. Parents and kids need to read labels and act accordingly.

The ramifications of metabolic regulatory failure are stark. The typical metabolic diagnostics are an endless series of blood prick tests coupled with readings of blood sugar content in sera. A $1 billion industry has developed consisting of pin prickers, diagnostic test strips, and readers of all kinds, colors, and shapes. The results of the readings lead to decisions and actions by the patient to inject insulin as a direct result of food that is consumed. Multiple pin pricks are needed per day for proper management until routines can be established and a patient can correlate their feelings and symptoms with needs to manage insulin content. Automation has come in the form of insulin pumps, conceptualized in Fig. 14.6 that have been developed to address the insulin deficiency [17].

These simple devices are designed to introduce either a sustained (small) regulatory dose or bolus over time and further programming can allow for periodic spikes to coincide with meal times (a surge bolus). The insulin pumps facilitate typical insulin loadings, but often continued blood chemistry assessments are still required to insure that the bolus distributions match the regulatory need. Insulin pumps do not factor in any imbalance between α and β cell secretions, which really require assessment in tandem. For type I diabetic children, it is the responsibility of parents to ultimately test and decide on behalf of their children whether and how much insulin their child receives, a thankless and often stressful task undertaken by the entire family. Bear in mind that it is this harmonic balance

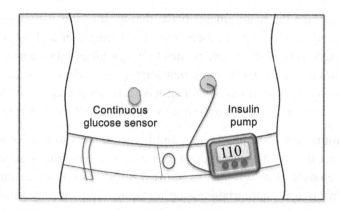

Figure 14.6
Schematic showing how an insulin pump gets a signal and released insulin as a result.

of insulin and glucagon that is required to maintain healthy sugar content in blood. Overinsulating can lead to diabetic comas and if it happens at night, often a sleeping coma can be induced in which a diabetic child does not wake up.

As an artificial pancreas, we could discuss here the idea of a series of immobilized islet cells, housed in some sort of implantable membrane through which we route blood through. There is this whole issue of what it takes to maintain this type of structure and there are likely countless research papers highlighting the potential. It is not the intent of the author to discount all of this activity that is laudable and worthwhile. But while substantial attention has been showered on cellular solutions that are years away, that turning point of a functional device never seems to get any closer to reality.

If the goal is refined to simply replicate the harmony of the metabolic secretions, that seems a much more achievable technological goal, even more so with the wealth of distributed computing power we regularly carry with us in our watches, our cell phones, our tablets, etc. Table 14.2 highlights the features and capacities of an idealized artificial pancreas

Table 14.2: Feature of an idealized artificial pancreas.

- On board
- Blood chemistry measurement frequently: 1/minute
- Ability to dose glucagon and insulin in controlled isolated portions
- No requirement on the user for measurement or regulation
- Dashboard and communicable readout Wi-Fi accessible
- Links with other vitals (BP, heart rate, pH, temp)
- Weekly volumetric capacity of glucagon and insulin
- Controlled insulin and glucagon levels within more narrow ranges than achieved by self-assessment

What is interesting about the requirements list is that most of this is already achievable, now just requiring integration, signal processing, developing user and control interfaces, and a functional algorithm. None of this relates to a Herculean transformation of new monolithic materials development or some new strategy for cellular engineering. Let's discuss the last few years of developments that have led to the creation of an onboard pancreatic assist device to regulate blood sugar without patient intervention.

One needs to monitor both constituents on a rapid enough basis to resolve spikes in either concentration during digestion, sleeping, and exercise. The decision to inject should be objective and there ought to be self-checks of the postinjection serum insulin and glucagon concentration to insure that appropriate dosing was done. The capacity to measure these constituents often is there but for an onboard system with a battery, there is a balance between too many measurements and a short battery lifetime.

The ability to design and develop a dual injection system does not seem to be much of a stretch from an insulin pump. There is a more involved signal-processing requirement to convert the measurements into an expert system that decides about an intervention (inject or not and how much) and needs to store and display functional data attributes. If the measurement, decisions, and injections can all be automated, then likely any user who can tolerate the placement of the injection ports can be considered a potential candidate, including those with dementia, children, infants, etc.

Finally, with so much new wearable technology available and apps being developed to harness the internal power of the components, what a great design challenge exists to resolve how a smart phone or equivalent device could function as a user interface and display. This was performed with the notion of replicating pancreas function synthetically [18] Here, design goals would include how to energize the pump systems and the measurement capacity, how to store and retrieve these data sets on the user's phone, how to allow remote access to probe functionality in the testing phase of these systems etc. For a device like an Apple iPhone, one only has the charging interface connector and the headphone jack as a DC power interface to work with and even the newest version has done away with the jack. To leverage a commercial device as a user interface is in the realm of systems engineering to solve how to harness the haptics. Such an undertaking was performed by staff at the Boston University (BU) School of Biomedical Engineering linked with Massachusetts General Hospital (MGH) who proved how to build and test an appropriate device with this control potential using earlier versions of iPhones. An example of the newest type of dual injection assist device is called the iLet device with an example output displayed on the unit along with subdisplays linked with individual hormones regulated by the device is shown in Fig. 14.7 (from [19]).

The proof is showing how well these devices work. In 2014 and 2015, demonstrations were conducted on the Boston peninsula with diabetics who were outfitted with a complete

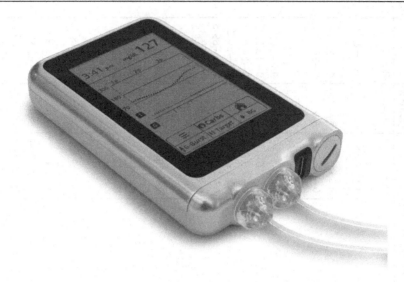

Figure 14.7
This is the iLet system that combines rapid and repeatable tracking of pancreatic markers like blood sugar and a dual pump system to replicate the function of the pancreas to express insulin and glucagon. *Courtesy of Beta Bionics Inc.*

onboard artificial endocrine hormone-replacing pancreas and allowed to vacation [19]. Hundreds of volunteers were asked to remain on the peninsula but roamed free otherwise. Their artificial pancreas systems were designed to both perform their regulatory function and allow the team to monitor the performance of the individual systems through Wi-Fi interfaces. The results have been outstanding, showing that the overall control of both glucagon and insulin concentration in the bloodstream were capable of being maintained with much tighter controls than with any of the same patients doing their own pricking, measurement, and deciding whether to inject or not. A summary of the data sets were published in [19] and some of that is shown in Table 14.3. The demonstrations have proven that blood component regulation through battery-operated, onboard electronic measurement and injection systems are possible. There are metabolic spikes but if large variances in dynamic hormone concentration correlate with lower endurance and larger malaise, the onboard strategy is ideal if these devices can be more widely approved for general use.

This story is just the beginning as further scale-up is required to more widely distribute and proof test these devices, resolve the limits of their performance, and also educate clinicians and insurance companies about their deployment. These are all milestones in the process of qualifying class III medical devices that have electronic biointerfaces through the US Food and Drug Administration. While these teams are developing new technology, there is just as much need to develop new pathways for device qualification, investigational devices, and tort liability, if new types of devices are going are linked to electronic user

Table 14.3: Output from Boston peninsula onboard pancreas clinical evaluation.

Variable	Adults N = 20				Adolescents N = 32			
	Bionic Prosthesis		Control		Bionic Prosthesis		Control	
	Mean	Range	Mean	Range	Mean	Range	Mean	Range
Day and night								
Plasma glucose on days 1–5								
Mean mg/dL	138	116–168			142	101–185	157	103–221
<60 mg/dL–% of time	2.3	0–8.9			2.6	0–11.5	3.5	0–17.2
<70 mg/dL–% of time	4.8	0–15			6.1	0–20	7.6	0–27.6
Carbohydrate interventions-#	2.2	0–10	3.4	0–10	3	0–15	6.6	0–20
Glucose level on continuous monitoring on days 2–5								
Mean mg/dL	133	114–152	159	105–225	142	117–179	158	95–222
<60 mg/dL–% of time	1.5	0–6	3.7	0–11.5	1.3	0–5.6	2.2	0–15.7
<70 mg/dL–% of time	4.1	0–12.4	7.3	0–16	3.1	0–9.6	4.9	0–24.4
70–120 mg/dL–% of time	47.7	29.4–65.5	30.8	4.1–67.4	42	31.3–63.1	30	9.6–56.2
70–180 mg/dL–% of time	79.5	69.3–98.2	58.8	35.1–82.7	75.9	61.4–94.1	64.5	29.5–89.5
>180 mg/dL–% of time	16.5	1.8–26.7	33.8	5.7–64.9	21	4.9–21.4	30.6	1.7–69.3
>250 mg/dL–% of time	4.9	0–12.7	12.3	0.1–32.7	5.9	0–21.4	10.8	0–35.6
Nighttime only								
Mean mg/dL	125	97–169			141	98–190	162	96–241
<60 mg/dL–% of time	1.7	0–22.2			1.3	0–10	2.2	0–30
<70 mg/dL–% of time	4	0–33.3			4.1	0–20	4.4	0–30
Carbohydrate interventions-#	0.3	0–2	0.6	0–3	0.8	0–5	1.6	0–7
Glucose level on continuous monitoring on nights 2–5								
Mean mg/dL	126	97–170	169	95–286	124	108–146	157	94–248
<60 mg/dL–% of time	0.4	0–1.6	3.3	0–15.4	1	0–4.9	1.7	0–17.7
<70 mg/dL–% of time	1.8	0–8.6	6.2	0–21.9	2.6	0–9.4	4	0–23.7
70–120 mg/dL–% of time	57.1	28.9–87	30.5	0–69.8	55.3	29.9–79.2	28.3	0–63.8
70–180 mg/dL–% of time	86.5	58.1–100	55.6	7–83.3	86.9	68.2–99.2	66.7	12.8–91.1
>180 mg/dL–% of time	11.8	0–39.8	38.2	1.6–93	10.5	0–26.8	29.3	0–87.2
>250 mg/dL–% of time	3.6	0–17.4	17.9	0–66.4	1.8	0–9.4	9.5	0–42.2

Data published in the New England Journal of Medicine, 2014; 371:313–325.

interfaces like smart phones and smart watches that are undergoing design changes at least on an annual basis.

There are several reasons why the technical challenges of building a group of developmental devices might be substantially easier to achieve than constructing a revolutionary business model for a biomaterials company leveraging smart phones as regulatory interfaces to dose any type of therapy. Probably of the highest concern are what happens to patients using devices that somehow lead to complications and what complications could arise. Doctors need appropriate training on installing devices correctly and patients/parents need user training to understand their responsibilities for maintaining the unit as well. Another challenge is qualification testing for an electronic drug distribution system with a functional biomaterial interface. One might expect that a simple insulin pump has a simplified electronic breadboard whose design is owned and built by the company supplying the device. All of the normal controls related to producing a device are spelled out in terms of regulatory legislation. But the process of leveraging off an established commercial device is brilliant but complicates who is liable if there is a system failure. This observation was the driving motivation for the team to produce their own display and drive system.

The sad truth is that in the event someone using one of these devices somehow has a complication, whether related to the device or not, it is possible that there is an embedded liability risk in a company building an artificial pancreas on an existing commercial device or platform they do not produce. It is worth noting that the status quo is hardly ideal or improving the long-term health for anyone and the health organizations, doctors, and patients ought to welcome new options even if there is a learning curve associated with how to deploy them. An example of such a dilemma is that each time Apple or another smart phone company comes out with a new connector interface, it might require companies deploying these devices as functional biointerfaces to redevelop their systems to achieve the same signal processing function with new hardware. Device upgrades usually come with longer battery lifetime and faster signaling processing so perhaps next generation user interfaces are linked with even more exquisite hormonal control.

It could be that as biomedical companies evolve from small enterprises to larger ones with more infrastructure, their capacity to more easily absorb development risk becomes more complicated. It is not a surprise to note that the developments linked with a smart phone-based artificial pancreas system arose out of a direct need of bioengineers with kids who were affected. Where would we be without the pioneers who are unsatisfied with the current state of the art? It is more challenging for an established biomaterials company with other products to accept this new type of liability risk in a new design paradigm.

The challenge is to have the same critical eye to envision how the other types of laboratory assessments can be automated and how the confluence of both new technology and materials could disrupt how we actually practice health care. Perhaps chemotherapy can be more controlled by linking infusion to true chemotherapy dose for an individual, perhaps antiseizure medication and pain medication can be more effectively controlled to prevent overdose and addition, perhaps we can think of ways to get patients more easily discharged from the hospital if their salt concentration or their hematocrit is too low by sending them home with an infuser. There seem to be an endless series of smart pump-type systems that could be considered with the demonstrations that have been presented here

14.3 Artificial Bladders

With the kidney dialysis and pancreas, it has been shown that synthetic and integrated synthetic solutions are possible, improving metabolic clearance and helping to use technology to maintain healthier levels of serum blood sugar. Protocols have been established as we have learned how to maintain people with compromised kidney and pancreas function. The goal for a prosthetic kidney is to convey a uremic patient to a successful transplant. With pancreas, this is not a viable option, nor is it with bladders.

Bladder cancer, like other cancers, can often be addressed by surgical resection to increase the chance for a longer life. Often large fractions of the bladder are taken and this can render the patient with much smaller capacity and if the nerves linked with sensation are consumed, it also renders the patient incontinent. The bladder acts as a reservoir of metabolites and fluids extracted in the kidney. The internal pressure rises as the extracted fluid volume increases and the stretching of the smooth muscle cells in the trigone region of the bladder creates an urge cue that it is time to find a bathroom. Depending on where the tumor is resected, the urge cue can remain even if the residual bladder reservoir is quite small. If the nerves in the trigone are severed, the urge sensation is also lost as a functional morbidity.

So the bladder is essentially an expandable bag with no metabolic function and its structure is otherwise unremarkable for filtration or other functional tissue requirement. If tissue engineering is going to be successfully deployed as a viable alternative to address disease in other more complicated metabolic organs, similar types of successful demonstrations will be needed similar to the pancreas. The anatomy of the bladder bag is essentially a thick, bilayered membrane. On the inside of the membrane are a series of epithelial cells which form tight junctions to prevent the bladder from leaking internally. Since these epithelial cells are found in the bladder, these are called urothelial cells. The structural rigidity and extensibility of the bladder derives from a colocation of smooth muscle cells which can extend as the bladder fills with continued kidney extraction and collection. From a tissue engineering perspective, the capacity to produce a bilayered structure relies on the ability to allow both cell types to flourish under coculturing conditions in the presence of the other.

Synthetic schemes have been developed to represent the lost bladder function using biodegradable polymer thin films from PLGA. The notion is that cells attach and proliferate on the polymer surfaces [20,21]. Generally, these schemes have not proven very successful. A cellular-based therapy would require the identification of a cell type that can proliferate accordingly, using stem cells derived from the patient to avoid potential immune rejection issues. Given the wide scope of places in which stem cells can be harvested, this challenge is easier achieved than first thought. Translating from the bench where issues of culture conditions and their effect on cell expression in producing prototypes that seem functional is crucial. The larger question is how well does something produced in the lab function in vivo. Animal trials have been ongoing since 2000 and human trials are now also being evaluated, all with very promising results.

In the first animal trials [20], approximately 90% of the bladders of healthy dogs were resected and viable cells from these tissues were isolated to yield stem cells spared as this location seemed to retain the nervous function to cue the urge response. Cells used to populate the artificial bladders were collected from biopsies prior to the surgery to allow for their coculture in vitro. As cells reached confluency on the surfaces of the 3D structure to represent the bladder (typically about 30 days), it was at that point that the cystectomies were conducted. Dogs were fractioned into three groups, those in which the trigone region was spared and the region was closed, and those in which a biodegradable membrane derived from a biodegradable (Polylactic acid/Glycolic Acid) copolymer (PLGA) representing the gross shape of the original bladder was installed were both considered controls. A third group had the bilayer cellular composite installed. Following recovery, the dogs were assessed periodically over a period of 11 months both for compliance in terms of a functional urge response and void volume.

The results were compelling. Even if the urge response was retained, there was insufficient capacity in the residual bladder to consider this viable and frequent needs for voiding were obvious, as observed in Fig. 14.8. With the biodegradable and cell-free bladder, only about half the original void capacity was retained and the results were quite variable with larger variance between animals and between observations. Upon recovery, almost 95% of the void volume capacity was retained in the dogs outfitted with the cellular graft over the 11 months of observation. Separate assessments of the gross anatomy after sacrifice were indistinguishable comparing cell composite tissue grafts [20]. Fig. 14.9 shows a prototype bladder being bathed in growth medium particular to specific cell types both inside and outside the polymeric membrane.

The playbook is established in that for patients that receive a bladder cancer diagnosis requiring resection, the goal would be to harvest a viable, cancer-free biopsy that contained appropriate cells that could be directed to yield both cell types in advance of the cystectomy. A company has been formed to produce these composites but the need

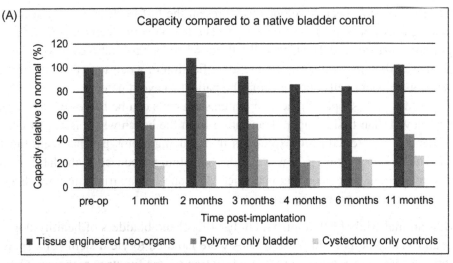

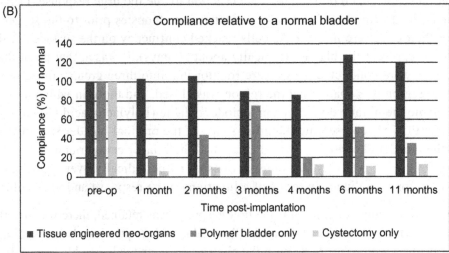

Figure 14.8

Clinical assessment of both capacity (A) and (B) compliance of beagles that underwent tissue-engineered bladder installation vs. controls. The capacity related to void volume and the compliance was tracked as a cue from the animal linked with an urge to void. *Data replicated from Oberpenning et al, Nature Biotechnology, 1999: 17:149−155.*

is currently unmet by the supply. After the cell-layered biodegradable composite reservoir is fully developed in co-culture to replace the resected bladder region, a cystectomy can be performed and the patient equipped with the graft bladder at the same time. Human trials have been ongoing since mid-2004 and perform cellular-based therapy in the form of tissue constructs to replace lost or diseased function seems increasingly on the horizon.

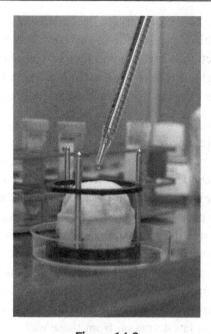

Figure 14.9
Tissue-engineered bladder construction with simultaneous coculturing of urothelial and smooth muscle cells on either side of a template bladder. *Courtesy of A. Atala and Beta Bionics.*

14.4 Pivoting to the future

In this chapter, three types of artificial organs have been presented including the kidney, the pancreas, and the bladder on a general continuum of performance. Alternative blood purification has been done for years, aided by improvements in machine technology linked with blood conveyance and metabolite extraction and those in A−V shunt technology to increase the viability of each uremic patient as a candidate for more routine dialysis. Treatment is satisfactory in maintaining patients indefinitely, but that sustenance comes with a cost. Design and development efforts to move from batch purification through blood recycling to a more continuous streaming purification might lead to a better ultimate outcome.

The development of onboard, dual-chemistry regulators to replicate pancreas function seems a very well thought out device design. The idea of using a well-characterized design interface like a smart phone and developing apps to harness its use as a display, a memory, and the autonomous decision maker is remarkable. And it is really encouraging to see the commitment to translating the original design concepts through the regulatory landscape and to consider how to scale up to larger populations of affected patients.

Finally, simple types of tissues like bilayer composites from epithelial and muscle cells cocultured to represent the bladder seem most achievable to pivot from the scope of more ambiguous tissue engineering to a more targeted need with an affected population (bladder cancer patients who require bladder resection to survive). The selection of the bladder with essentially no metabolic function is brilliant and lessons learned in coculturing one cell type in the presence of others might also pave the way to build cellular vascular grafts, other layered tissues, and even other organs if we could be so inclined to dream about.

As a last series of comments, it is worth noting that much of the original excitement relating to artificial organs stemmed from developments of the Jarvik 7 total artificial heart that was installed in a series of human patients that were terminal without a larger intervention in the early 1980s. These patients were counseled and ultimately offered to be implanted with an internal device to perform the perfusion of their damaged hearts and were equipped with a power pack to energize the device for larger mobility. A retired dentist named Barney Clark was the first volunteer implanted in 1982 living for nearly four months after installation. From those hopeful and highly publicized clinical trials on devices made from titanium and expandable chambers produced from a range of blood compatible polyurethanes, much was learned about managing patients and their blood chemistry, miniaturizing the power systems and diagnostic interfaces to perform the functions and increasing the experience. The latest version from those early trials is found at a company called SynCardia that has implanted more than 1000 recipients of a temporary total heart as a bridge to transplant and there are 4–5 other development companies producing variants, one recipient on the SynCardia web site is included in Figure 14.10.

SynCardia reports increased rates of installation of their devices under the auspices of an FDA trial [22]. Some patients with these devices continue to thrive more than three years after installation but the desire is to be implanted shorter rather than longer. The bridge period is regulated by the donor pool. The hope has to be that in the future, more viable donor organs are available as transplants to limit the time anyone has to bridge to a transplant. Whether on the bridge vs. transplant, the costs are in the $100 K to even beyond $1 million per procedure. The realm of transplants is expensive but an amazing confluence medicine, engineering, and innovation. Thanks, Barney for without you and the other volunteer recipients, this level of progress could not have been made.

14.5 Problems

1. Consider the term, mass flux, identified in the language of diffusion. This correlates to the amount of a constituent that passes across a certain surface per unit time. The units of flux are g/cm^2-s or $moles/cm^2$-s knowing the molar mass of the diffuser. Assume that diffusion only occurs across a dialysis tube containing 1000 fibers, each which is 250 microns in diameter and 20 cm long. Five hours of dialysis treatment yields 20 g of urea.

   a. Determine the mass flux of urea through this membrane (units of g/cm^2-s)

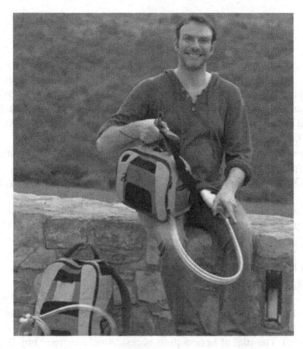

Figure 14.10
Frederic Thiollet who has lived with an implanted bridge device for over three years.
With permission from Syncardia.com.

   b.   The molar mass of urea is 60.06 g/mole. What is the molar flux of urea passing through the dialysis (units of mole/cm^2-s).

   c.   The molar mass of uric acid is 168.1 g/mole. Explain whether you would expect the mass flux of uric acid or urea is higher through the membrane

2.   Draw how urea concentration varies as a function of time over a week in the life of both a uremic patient undergoing two per week dialysis and one with a normal functioning kidney.

3.   The average measurement interval for an onboard pancreas system is 5 min. Explain the cost/benefit analysis of sampling glucagon and insulin chemistry more often.

4.   Congestive heart failure patients suffer from fluid accumulation in the lung. Diuretics like Lasix can flush both water and salt to the kidneys leading to higher lung capacity but overdosing (too much Lasix) can result in low blood salt concentration or a condition called hyponatremia and heart palpitations. Explain how might an onboard system like the artificial pancreas be developed to regulate salt content similarly?

5.   Explain the usage of other types of artificial organs like artificial livers used in drug assessment studies and their value in probing potential drug toxicities.

6.   Explain why tissue-engineered organs have lagged the more widespread use of transplants.

References

[1] Baig, Biochemical composition of normal urine, Nature Precedings, 2011, doi:10.1.1038/npre.2011.6595.1.

[2] R. Fields, In Dialysis, Life-Saving Care at Great Risk and Cost, ProPublica, Editor. 2010; Available from: https://www.propublica.org/article/in-dialysis-life-saving-care-at-great-risk-and-cost.

[3] Belding Hibbard Scribner. 2015; Available from: https://en.wikipedia.org/wiki/Belding_Hibbard_Scribner.

[4] United States Renal Data System, 2014 Annual Data Report: Epidemiology of Kidney Disease in the United States. 2014. National Institutes of Health.

[5] National Kidney Foundation: Kidney Disease Statistics. 2012. Available from: http://www.kidneyfund.org/about-us/assets/pdfs/akf-kidneydiseasestatistics-2012.pdf.

[6] E.M. Darmady, J. Offer, M.A. Woodhouse, The parameters of the ageing kidney, J. Pathol. 109 (1973) 195–207.

[7] R.J. Glassock, The aging kidney: More pieces to the puzzle, Mayo Clin. Proc. 86 (2011) 271–272.

[8] B.D. Ratner, Biomaterials science: An introduction to materials in medicine, Elsevier/Academic Press, Amsterdam, 2013.

[9] H.V. Harissis, C.S. Katsios, E.L. Koliousi, M.G. Ikonomou, K.C. Siamopoulos, M. Fatouros, et al., A new simplified one port laparoscopic technique of peritoneal dialysis catheter placement with intra-abdominal fixation, Am. J. Surg. 192 (2006) 125–129.

[10] J.B. Park, R.S. Lakes, BIomaterials, an introduction, Plenum Publishing, New York, 1992.

[11] J.F. Winchester, C. Jacobs, C. Kjeillstrand, K.M. Koch, Replacement of renal function by dialysis, Springer ISBN 978-0-585-36947-1, 1996.

[12] Vachharajani, T., 2010. The atlas of hemodialysis access. Available from: http://fistulafirst.esrdncc.org/wp-content/uploads/2015/12/Access-Atlas.pdf.

[13] H.D. Humes, D. Buffington, A.J. Westover, S. Roy, W.H. Fissell, The bioartificial kidney: Current status and future promise, Pediatr. Nephrol. 29 (2014) 343–351.

[14] Z.Y. Oo, K. Kandasamy, F. Tasnim, D. Zink, A novel design of bioartificial kidneys with improved cell performance and haemocompatibility, J. Cell. Mol. Med. 17 (2013) 497–507.

[15] The role of the pancreas in digestion and sugar metabolism. 2015; Available from: http://www.laparoscopic.md/digestion/pancreas.

[16] R.K. Johnson, L.J. Appel, M. Brands, B.V. Howard, M. Lefevre, R.H. Lustig, et al., Dietary sugars intake and cardiovascular health: a scientific statement from the American Heart Association, Circulation 120 (2009) 1011–1020.

[17] Insulin Pumps. 2015; Available from: http://www.diabetes.org/living-with-diabetes/treatment-and-care/medication/insulin/insulin-pumps.html.

[18] Kinder, L., 2014 'Bionic pancreas' passes test to help control diabetes, in The Telegraph, 16 Jun 2014, London, United Kingdom.

[19] S.J. Russell, F.H. El-Khatib, M. Sinha, K.L. Magyar, K. McKeon, L.G. Goergen, et al., Outpatient Glycemic Control with a Bionic Pancreas in Type 1 Diabetes, N. Engl. J. Med. 371 (2014) 313–325.

[20] F. Oberpenning, J. Meng, J.J. Yoo, A. Atala, De novo reconstitution of a functional mammalian urinary bladder by tissue engineering, Nat. Biotechnol. 17 (1999) 149–155.

[21] S. Sivaraman, J. Nagatomi, Polymer-based scaffolds for urinary bladder tissue engineering, in: S.W. Shalaby, K.J.L. Burg, W. Shalaby (Eds.), Polymers for vascular and urogenital applications, CRC Press, New York, 2012, pp. 175–199.

[22] SynCardia, FDA Approves the SynCardia Total Artificial Heart for Destination Therapy Study. 2015; Available from: http://www.syncardia.com/2015-press-releases/fda-approves-the-syncardia-total-artificial-heart-for-destination-therapy-study.html.

CHAPTER 15

Special Topics: Assays Applied to Both Health and Sports

Learning Objectives

From reading this chapter, one should come away knowing:

- How diagnostic assays can identify markers of aberrant health, and statistically different blood and urine chemistry.

- Recognize that there are legitimate health benefits for some banned substances for ailing individuals although doping of otherwise healthy individuals could raise both ethical and health concerns.

- Recognize this tense competition between those searching for a performance edge from an elixir and those tasked with maintaining the integrity of general sport.

- Gain a sense of the sophistication in elaborate schemes to skirt the rules.

- Recognize that much of what can be learned about how to upregulate cellular function could aid ailing individuals who are recovering from disease.

15.1 Introduction and Historical Basis

Elite athletes are found at the confluence of great genetics, amazing mental focus, healthy eating habits, and great training regimens. It is not a surprise to find that children of tall basketball players are also tall, and that children of athletes in one discipline are often accomplished in other sports as well. The allure to be the best in class has fame and great financial remuneration at the end of the rainbow in addition to the individual personal achievement. For whatever reason, society has tended to reward athletic performance. That observation has bred a certain extra desire on behalf of some to augment whatever natural talents they have, and this is nothing new, as reports of performance enhancing drug use dates back to the ancient Greeks [1]. In fact, the word doping derives from the Dutch word *doop*, meaning a viscous substance derived from opiates [2]. From restrictive diets, to health supplements to injections of therapeutics that affect both anatomical and physiological response, the goal of the umpires, referees, and officials of sports has been to

Biomaterials. DOI: http://dx.doi.org/10.1016/B978-0-12-809478-5.00015-8

insure that notion of a natural athlete still carries some meaning, sport is fair, and that everyone has an even chance. The International Olympic Committee (IOC) for example has created a list of banned, prohibited, or regulated substances [3] figuring that these things should not be found in normal amateur athletes who learn they are really good at swimming, running, rowing, or kicking a soccer ball. It's also bad for publicity if their next star athlete also has a raging addiction and can't control their impulses (Fig. 15.1).

More broadly, federal agencies have been tasked to insure that food is not tainted, with a similar sense that roadways, harbors and airplane taxiways are also safe for passenger travel. One can monitor vehicle emissions, air quality in mine shafts and more generally the workplace environment to ensure its safety for all involved, and that individual workers are practicing safe work practices which includes their own sobriety for example. What this has really meant is that those involved in monitoring these activities are capable of using analytical tools to probe the chemistry of human extracts to gauge their individual health, their exposure to toxins, and to establish a larger database of normal blood and urine chemistry. In other words, if we are what we eat, there should be residues resulting from the ingestion of both toxins and hormones, both legal and more questionable (Table 15.1).

The first focus is on urine chemistry and urinalysis, what we find unremarkable in normal urine, and a feature of other by-products that is also identified. It is also highlighted how urinalysis can monitor illegal drug use and how it has also been deployed to track the use of performance enhancing drugs (PEDs) and growth factors. It has only been through the

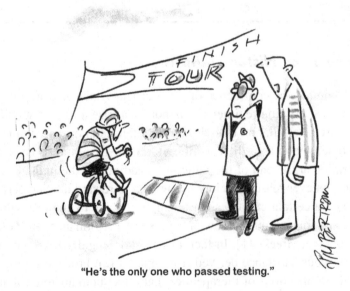

"He's the only one who passed testing."

Figure 15.1
The dilemma with drug testing in sports. *Reproduced with permission from www.cartoonstock.com.*

**Table 15.1: Classes of substances prohibited, or restricted
by the International Olympic Committee, including**

Prohibitions
  Stimulants
  Narcotics
  Anabolic agents
  Diuretics
  Peptide and glycoprotein hormones and analogues
Prohibited methods
  Blood doping
  Pharmacological, chemical, and physical manipulation
Classes of drugs subject to restrictions
  Alcohol
  Marijuana
  Local anesthetics
  Corticosteroide
  ß-Blockers

increasing accuracy and precision of analytical instrumentation that urinalysis can resolve unusual trace co-constituents found in excretions. *We are what we excrete in a way.*

It was already learned in chapters 6 and 14 that within normal urine, the typical levels of metabolites are excreted if isolated from urine. Most urinalysis is done on the liquid excreted and includes typically a determination of urine temperature (if fresh), pH (typically 4.5−8), a clarity determination, a density (typically $1.05−1.25$ g/cm^3), and measures of a range of organic and inorganic ionic constituents. There is usually a total protein assessment and since proteins are higher in density than water, the density of normal urine is typically slightly above 1 g/cm^3. Since a majority of urinalyses are used for primarily health monitoring assessments, the usual indicators being identified are things that should be normally found. Red blood cells found in urine could be an indicator of disease, trauma, or internal bleeding. Bacteria, yeasts, or white blood cells found in urine could indicate a urinary tract infection. The presence of aromatic urine or ketones is usually a metabolic indicator that could be indicative of diabetes. Low protein levels are an indicator of potential kidney failure when most of what is getting excreted is water. So the general health profile from a pee cup is quick and relatively inexpensive. There are further immunoassays that can be performed as part of employment verification and compliance programs and to screen for individuals with painkiller and other illegal drug additions, and controlled substances that are not normally present in typical urine.

Most early analyses of urine are done using gas chromatography linked with mass spectrometry. There is a residence time in the separation column and different molecules traverse through the column at different rates due to size, affinity to the column, etc. As improvements in machine quality and separations have evolved through the use of liquid chromatography linked with mass spectrometry (LC/MS), lower detection thresholds allow the determinations of trace contaminants at ever smaller concentrations. Hence there is more interest in evaluating athletes to insure that they are not harming themselves during training in their sport, and to insure some integrity to the game [4].

Within the last 20 years, much has been learned about how growth factors, steroids, and other hormone variants can influence cell and tissue behavior. Within muscle physiology, a regulating protein myostatin was identified that is involved in muscle breakdown and reduction [5]. An obvious target to maintain muscle mass might include regulating myostatin expression in muscle tissue. It is also known for example that injecting recombinant growth hormone, a protein with a molecular weight of about 22 KDa and a half-life of about 20 minutes once secreted or injected into blood [6], has a positive effect on muscle mass and function on adults deficient of growth hormone [7]. The short metabolic half-life suggests that it might be difficult to identify individuals injecting themselves long before a scheduled urine test.

If there is a balance between growth and regulating hormones, raising the growth factors relative to the regulating species will lead to higher muscle mass. Similarly, for bone, there is a well-defined pathway to upregulate new bone synthesis through the direct injection of components including bone morphogenic protein, BMP [8,9]. More generally, testosterone and other anabolic steroids that ultimately metabolize into testosterone have been shown to also improve muscle mass and strength in patients who are otherwise health compromised [10]. It is clear with all the science suggesting *body engineering* is quite achievable through injectable therapy, there are inputs and outputs to a hormonal intervention and the metabolites excreted are likely fingerprints of an earlier injection.

Two things are apparent. One is that these potent biological regulators need comprehensive assessments to identify latent risks related to their usage and these need to be explained to potential users. The other is regulating bodies in sports need to define appropriate limits for usage with the understanding that excretable metabolites are now within normal analytical detection limits. There might be justifiable reason for an athlete recovering from a bone fracture and who is not playing to receive BMP to speed their recovery. But there is a constant competition between analytical detection limits identifying new potential growth factors and creating proper regulatory rules at the same time within sports medicine, and general medicine as well.

With the capacity to accurately evaluate these established athletes, there is interest at both professional and amateur sports to validate those participating as free from hormonal engineering. Specific sports are regulated in terms of what is considered a health supplement, and what is considered food, and each sport seems particular about its rules, and how they are assessed.

15.2 What Can be Learned From Urinalysis?

15.2.1 Liquid Chromatography-Based Determinations

Liquid chromatography analyses of urine and spiked urine as controls, linked with the mass spectrometry signature have been identified for a number of potential doping agents, diuretics, narcotics, and pain modulators. An example of one anabolic steroid, calusterone, spiked in urine is shown in Fig. 15.2 [11]. The individual retention times and masses of innumerable compounds have been compiled and its an ever increasing list of potential hormonal regulators. As each hormone is characterized effectively and added to list of banned substances identified by the World Antidoping Agency, new ones that defy detection and are not on the list suddenly become more prominent in terms of distribution and usage.

It is not just the hormones and growth factors that are part of these cocktails that are used with performance enhancing drugs. In more sophisticated efforts to defy detection, the use of diuretics as fluid extractors to dilute excretions within urine are also on the rise, and the detection of these is also paramount to gauging the scope of performance enhancing drug usage.

To recap, there are a number of performance-enhancing drugs and related compounds that can be identified and quantitatively assessed in urine produced by athletes who use them. The preferred analytical techniques are focused on liquid chromatography linked with mass spectrometry and protocols are established on how samples are produced. Once collected, it

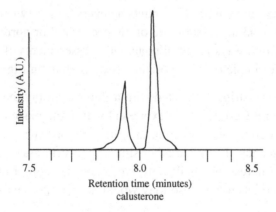

Figure 15.2

Data on the retention and observance of the anabolic substance calusterone spiked in urine. *Reproduced from Jeong, E.S., S.E. Kim, E.J. Cha, K.M. Lee, H.J. Kim, S.W. Lee et al., 2015. Simultaneous analysis of 210 prohibited substances in humanurine by ultrafast liquid chromatography/tandem massspectrometry in doping control. Rapid Commun Mass Spectrom, 29: 367–384. The spike at an earlier retention time of 7.9 minutes is linked with the steroid.*

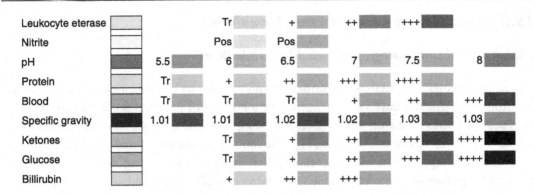

Figure 15.3

Colorimetric based analysis of urine where the concentration dependence of different constituents found in urine is noted. These assays are increasingly common for people who are independently monitoring metabolism. *Reproduced from the urinalysis tutorial [12]*

is incumbent on the analyser to maintain proper channels of safety, identification, and process protocols to insure that the correct athlete is identified and tested accordingly to accepted practices. Some 200 + compounds can now be screened, but that does not discourage the potential identification of new types of growth factors and other regulatory compounds that can help with increasing muscle and body mass, faster recovery time after overexertion, and increasing oxygenation potential.

15.2.2 Pee Strip Determinations

Most pee exposure assays are based on immunochemistry assays, where there is a fluorescent tag linked bound to the substrate of the pee strip. For normal urinalysis, there are pee-strip type colorimetric assays for semi-quantitative assessments of normal constituents tested within urine, an example of the colorizing assay is show in Fig. 15.3, from [12].

For pregnancy-based tests, strips are coated with a fluorescent tag that reacts with human chorionic gonadoprotein (hCG), which is expressed within the placenta during pregnancy. This is an example of a go/no go evaluation in which any presence of hCG for example is a likely indicator of pregnancy. There are other similar pee-strip assays for single constituents where the color of the fluorescence is linked to the concentration of ketones excreted in urine. These are also semiquantitative so they would not be likely used except for screening in evaluating athletes.

15.3 Blood Doping

There are more nuanced schemes to directly control blood chemistry to enhance performance that may be easier to obscure in subsequent urinalysis. Three potential schemes are available for those who are so inclined. The simplest way is simple acclimation at high altitude for extended periods prior to performance at a lower altitude. The amount of hemoglobin in mammalian blood and the corresponding measure of hematocrit are direct measures of oxygen carrying capacity and these vary with species, age, gender, pregnancy, and with resting altitude. An example of the potential payoff is shown in terms of middle distance (5 km) running times comparing the training vs performance location [13] for a group of runners who went through an altitude conditioning program, as shown in Fig. 15.4. In a group of 39 runners who were compared, 13 were unchanged in their time ($\delta t < \pm 15$ seconds), nine had slower times more than 25 seconds longer than their baseline sea level times after high altitude acclimation, and 17 had times that were more than 20 seconds shorter than their baseline times following the acclimation protocol (Fig. 15.4).

Typical human hematocrit levels for adult men range between 43% and 54% and adult women between 38% and 46%. During these high altitude acclimation periods, training creates a natural hypoxia that leads to larger expression of erythropoietin, a hormone to stimulate larger numbers of red blood cells to carry oxygen. There are a large series of studies that suggest over a period of weeks of training, a natural slight elevation as hematocrit levels (a ratio of the volume of red blood cells relative to the total volume in a sample of blood) can rise as high as 45%−61% in males, and between 46% and 50% in females [15]. Every extra capacity to carry oxygen allows endurance athletes to generally outperform others who have not had the same acclimation period. The general concept of altitude training arose from the siting of the Summer Olympics in Mexico City at a high

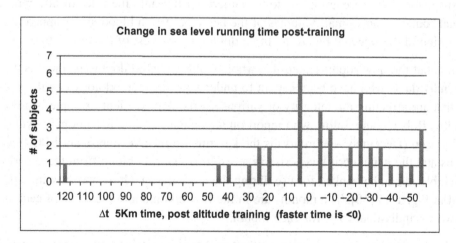

Figure 15.4

Examples of how altitude training affects performance of a group of trial runners who were retested at sea level following a high altitude acclimation. *From Chapman, R.F., Stray-Gundersen J, B.D. Levine, 1998. Individual variation in response to altitude training. J Appl Physiol, 85: 1448−1456.*

altitude (7300 ft, 2.25 km) in 1968 [16]. The performance in endurance events tended to lag prior records, but the anaerobic sprinting events saw no such drop-off. Also, most of the endurance medals were won by athletes from high elevation countries such as Kenya and Ethiopia [16]. The same type of acclimation can be achieved by athletes donning oxygen depleting air intake masks during training that limits their oxygen intake [17]. So training regimens and travel has been developed to allow athletes to naturally increase their blood oxygenation potential through these acclimation pilgrimages. The sad reality is that the longer someone is at lower altitude, the hematocrit level compensates for the richer air.

Less natural routes bypass those efforts to raise erythropoietin (EPO) levels which can be accomplished by directing injection of EPO at regulated times to recruit more and larger RBCs. In an open or detectable environment, those being injected with EPO to recruit new erythrocytes will excrete EPO and its metabolites at unnaturally high levels. The basis for using EPO actually is linked with chemotherapy patients with low hematocrit counts. Injection into these patients compensates for their extreme fatigue during recovery but they also express remnants of the EPO injection, not a problem if one is recovering from cancer.

One could extract the sera phase of blood and re-inject with normal blood to raise hematocrit but this would likely raise other cell types within blood and raise blood viscosity. Covert schemes to raise hematocrit by drug–induced EPO injections include performing most injections during the off-season to produce hematocrit-rich blood which can be stored and swapped into the individual during the performance season. The most direct way is simply to transfuse erythrocyte-rich blood and extract a similar volume. The goal, again under a covert operation is to raise hematocrit levels but not so much as to attract suspicion, and there are limits to hematocrit written into the rules of different individual sports. If only small volumes of the hematocrit-rich blood are swapped, the EPO concentration in the injected blood might be diluted by the rest of the circulating blood.

To learn about the how sophisticated this whole realm of blood doping is, there is a need to rely on individuals who have been caught to understand the methodology and the gaps in testing that are affecting the integrity of various sports. An excellent example is presented by Lundby, Robach, and Saltin, who report on an annual timeline for a doping cyclist [18]. The off-season (December–February) is the key time to receive significant EPO type injections and the hematocrit levels rise as a result. By storing blood from these periods, RBC-rich blood can be banked for use during the race season, (June and July in particular) as noted in Fig. 15.5 [18]. The months are in the first column and the dates of each month are shown for individual rows for each month.

For a calendar that has a single one-day event in April, a sustained cycling race over several weeks in July, there is the formation of an evolving pattern how to yield maximum performance while avoiding detection. While the data only speak on the issues directly relating to blood doping, there is no reason why other schemes to avoid detection of other

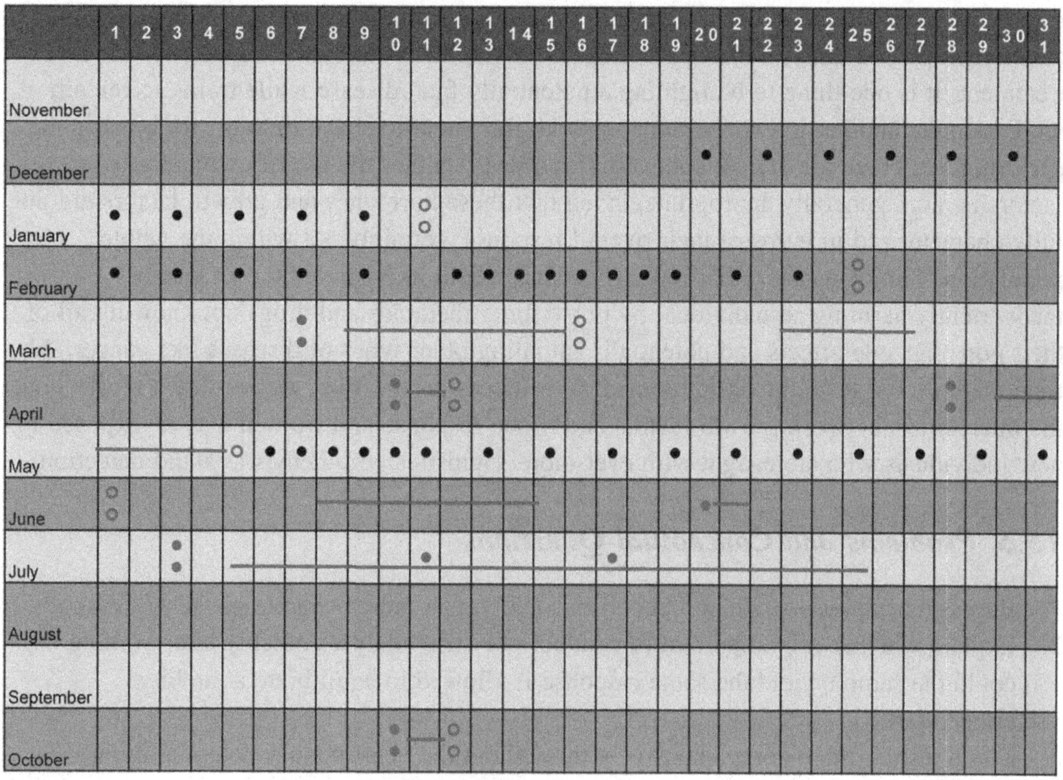

	1	2	3	4	5	6	7	8	9	10	11	12	13	14	15	16	17	18	19	20	21	22	23	24	25	26	27	28	29	30	31
November																															
December																				•		•		•		•		•		•	
January	•		•		•		•		•			○○																			
February	•		•		•		•				•	•	•	•	•	•	•	•	•		•			•	○○						
March							••	—	—	—	—	—	—	—	○○								—	—	—	—	—				
April									••	—	—	○○																••	—	—	—
May	—	—	—	—	○	•	•	•	•	•	•		•		•		•		•		•		•		•		•		•		•
June	○○									—	—	—	—	—	—	—					• —										
July			••	—	—	—	—	—	—	—	•	—	—	—	—	—	•	—	—	—	—	—	—								
August																															
September																															
October											••	—	○○																		

Figure 15.5

An example training/doping schedule for an elite cyclist training for bicycle races or events denoted as lines including the Tour de France race in July. The black dots correspond to EPO injections to raise blood hematocrit levels. The open red (grey in print version) circles correspond to blood draws and the filled red (grey in print version) circles are infusions. The goal is to raise hematocrit without causing a large spike in measured EPO. *Data re-tabulated from C. Lundby et al., 2012. The evolving science of detection of 'blood doping'. Br. J. Pharmacol. 165: 1306–1315.*

banned substances might be undertaken by athletes using a similar EPO injection calendar shown above.

There are other schemes used to mask an excessive concentration of EPO in urine, for example, by using diuretics to flush the kidneys thereby diluting the concentration of the components used in doping. It is for these reasons that diuretics are also considered *banned substances*.

15.4 Conclusion

Overall, there might be significant reason to consider the more widespread use of constituents that maintain youth and vigor for a longer period of life. There might well be reasons to incorporate growth factors into tissue-engineered constructs as well as to dose chemotherapy and dialysis patients with EPO, given their excessive fatigue following treatment. It is one thing to be fighting a potentially fatal disease while trying to remain vital, its quite another to expose someone with the intent to shave time off for a particular performance. There are ethical controversies about whether the use of external growth factors is more generally appropriate, given that these hormones and growth factors are not fully characterized in terms of their overall response, certainly not within the whole population. Clinicians are rather risk averse and would likely avoid the chance of inadvertently harming an individual by proscribing therapies and drugs not knowing all of their potential side effects and potentially initiating other types of diseases like cancer. As time marches on, from the basic biomedical sciences perspective, we will learn more about the interactions between growth factors and tissue response and we will also be exposed to new individuals who are caught with ever more sophisticated schemes to avoid detection.

15.5 Problems and Conceptual Questions

1. Between urinalysis and blood chemistry, which is a more accurate gauge of doping?
2. Explain whether it is important to conduct pee-strip analyses quickly after voiding or could the sample yield the same response if allowed to equilibrate at ambient temperature?
3. Could testing more comprehensively throughout the year identify potential doping events more often?
4. Explain whether more random testing will lead to higher identification of potential dopers?
5. If it is known that geriatrics lose muscle mass over time, how would myostatin regulation improve the muscle mass of these populations as compared to a younger population?

References

[1] Drug use in sports. 2013; Available from: http://sportsanddrugs.procon.org/view.timeline.php?timelineID = 000017.
[2] L.D. Bowers, Athletic drug testing, Clin. Sports Med. 17 (1998) 299–318.
[3] D. Catlin, T.H. Murray, Performance-enhancing drugs, fair competition, and olympic sport, JAMA 276 (1996) 231–237.
[4] C.K. Hatton, Beyond sports doping headlines: The science of laboratory tests for performance-enhancing drugs, Pediatr. Clin. North. Am. 54 (2007) 713–733 xi.
[5] G. Goldspink, B. Wessner, N. Bachl, Growth factors, muscle function and doping, Curr. Opin. Pharmacol. 8 (2008) 352–357.
[6] Human growth hormone (HGH) testing. 2015; Available from: https://www.wada-ama.org/en/questions-answers/human-growth-hormone-hgh-testing.
[7] R.C. Cuneo, F. Salomon, C.M. Wiles, R. Hesp, P.H. Sonksen, Growth hormone treatment in growth hormone-deficient adults. I. Effects on muscle mass and strength, J. Appl. Physiol. 70 (1991) 688–694.

[8]   W.A. Saltzman, Tissue engineering, Principles for the Design of Replacement Organs and Tissues, Oxford University Press, New York, 2004.

[9]   J.O. Hollinger (Ed.), An Introduction to Biomaterials. Biomedical Engineering Series, ed. M.R. Neuman, CRC Press, Boca Raton, Florida, 2012.

[10] O. Supasyndh, B. Satirapoj, P. Aramwit, D. Viroonudomphol, A. Chaiprasert, V. Thanachetwej, et al., Effect of oral anabolic steroid on muscle strength and muscle growth in hemodialysis patients. Clin. J. Am. Soc. Nephrol. 8 (2013) 271−279.

[11] E.S. Jeong, S.H. Kim, E.J. Cha, K.M. Lee, H.J. Kim, S.W. Lee, et al., Simultaneous analysis of 210 prohibited substances in human urine by ultrafast liquid chromatography/tandem mass spectrometry in doping control, Rapid Commun. Mass Spectrom. 29 (2015) 367−384.

[12] Urinalysis Tutorial. 2015; Available from: http://library.med.utah.edu/WebPath/TUTORIAL/URINE/URINE.html.

[13] J. Stray-Gundersen, B.D. Levine, Living high-training high and low" is equivalent to "living high-training low" for sea-level performance, Med. Sci. Sports. Exerc. 29 (1997) S136.

[14] R.F. Chapman, J. Stray-Gundersen, B.D. Levine, Individual variation in response to altitude training, J. Appl. Physiol. 85 (1998) 1448−1456.

[15] What is a normal hematocrit? 2014; Available from: http://www.emedicinehealth.com/hematocrit_blood_test/page3_em.htm - what_is_a_normal_hematocrit.

[16] D. Boning, N. Maassen, A. Pries, The hematocrit paradox − how does blood doping really work? Int. J. Sports Med. 32 (2011) 242−246.

[17] Sheppard, J.A. Elevation training mask and the effects: A case report. 2012; Available from: http://www.trainingmask.com/news/25/Elevation-Training-Mask-and-the-Effects%3A-A-Case-Report.html.

[18] C. Lundby, P. Robach, B. Saltin, The evolving science of detection of 'blood doping', Br. J. Pharmacol. 165 (2012) 1306−1315.

Postface

Going into the biomaterials discipline as an early learner, I was struck by how challenging it was to identify exactly why some devices and tools were fast tracked into clinical use, while thousands of good ideas languished as unutilized intellectual property. Even now, it is still a challenge to identify the cost of individual procedures even on a generalized basis. The lack of a value assessment makes it hard to choose where to invest one's time as a researcher or an engineer. This book has been written to provide a rationale for why at least point to a larger rationale for why medical advancement is at the confluence of both good technical ideas, linked with facilitating the need to intervene clinically.

Over my nearly 30-year career as an engineer and educator, I'm encouraged to see one can benefit the lives of others suffering from disease. From an academic perspective, emphasizing investigations on diseases among less served populations and orphan diseases might be even more applicable in executing the design process, without having such a competitive environment for intellectual property and patent protection.

Merit is generously handed out to the readers who have successfully completed this tome. In a way, this is one effort to address the interplay between three very large disciplines. They include the structure of living systems, the structure of synthetic substitutes, and the clinical connection that focuses on the overlap of the first two. I am afraid that the book is organized incompletely by design, to point to reader to the linkages between the design environment, competitive approaches to yield a successful outcome, and current schemes that consider the breadth of the materials genome applied in medicine.

In writing this book, any chapter here could be a deeper book on its own, and some chapters have multiple journals dedicated to advancing each subdiscipline. The goal has been to show the distinction and disparity between research efforts in these areas and often their disconnection to translational elements found in the clinics. Credit is also handed out generously to other authors who have advanced our understanding as it was those foundation textbooks on biomaterials that helped me to learn as well.

Challenges exist for any author embarking on such a broad sweep of materials in medicine. There are areas that could be expanded on but with limited time and as the only author, some topics could not be covered to the same detail. Of course the scope is targeted at the future, and perhaps as a result, there is less room for the complete historical perspective.

Histology has been largely deemphasized here as cell–biomaterial interactions are largely the realm of tissue pathology. It is true that most interventions that leave a implanted biomaterial will lead to cellular interaction and colonization on the surface. It is also true that biomaterial installations interact with the entire eukaryotic wound healing cascade, as well as with both probiotic and pathogenic prokaryotes. It is important to understand how cells interact with tissues and synthetic graft materials but decisions are often advisory and the timeline of cellular response depends on the level of vascularization in the region that is involved. It is left for the pathologists to gauge ultimately which combination of design and material are ultimately least harmful and most beneficial where they are deposited.

It is for the same reason that immunology and its corresponding response is also duly noted. Again the realm of pathology and immunology, we already know that even for tissue transplants, patients are often sufficiently immune-compromised as to prevent a host–donor immune response. A similar pathway exists for synthetic xenografts. Both histology and immunology are key considerations and milestones in biomaterial replacement, but ultimately the surface features, and their corresponding T-cell and B-cell interaction have less to do with the functional design principles.

Going forward students of biomaterials need to be both more quantitative in their skillsets and more discerning in the future. The metrics for success will include resolving how close synthetics, transplanted tissues and hybrid solutions come to replicating lost tissue, system, and organ function. There is no single solution that will win out; all can be viable. Biomaterial scientists and engineers might also note that comprehensive replacement in the long run might be less desirable if the capacity for early minor repairs resolves the original defect and its associated symptoms. That requires new thinking about how health care is delivered.

Alternative and earlier diagnoses in disease progression might lead to less need for larger interventions, comprehensive disease, and organ management. If early indicators for a particular disease can be correctly identified earlier in life and in the lifetime of the disease, perhaps interventions continue to tip the scales more in the form of tissue augmentation, regeneration, and repair, and less toward total replacement of tissues.

Nothing has been a bigger challenge for the author here than attempting to write the monograph, a collection of 15 enormous review papers that requires a breadth and depth to not embarrass one's self across disciplines. The book has been written aiming for the future in maintaining the currency for the book. The field changes in some areas overnight and in other areas, there has been little evolution once acceptable therapeutic protocols are established and insurance codes are created. Consider this dilemma as you read along. Finally, I would like to thank my editors, my colleagues, my students, and lastly my family who encouraged me along the way. Thank you for your time reading!

Index

Note: Page numbers followed by "*f*" and "*t*" refer to figures and tables, respectively.

Printed in the United States
By Bookmasters